Cardiology in Old Age

Cardiology in Old Age

Edited by

F. I. Caird
Southern General Hospital
Glasgow, Scotland

J. L. C. Dall
Victoria Infirmary
Glasgow, Scotland

and

R. D. Kennedy
Stobhill Hospital
Glasgow, Scotland

Plenum Press · **New York and London**

Library of Congress Cataloging in Publication Data

Main entry under title:

Cardiology in old age.

   Includes bibliographies and index.
   1. Cardiovascular system—Diseases. 2. Geriatrics. 3. Cardio-
vascular system—Aging. I. Caird, Francis Irvine. II. Dall, J. L. C.
III. Kennedy, Robert Davis. [DNLM: 1. Heart diseases— In old
age. WG200 C266]
RC667.C384   618.9′76′1   76-23094
ISBN-13: 978-1-4615-8779-8   e-ISBN-13: 978-1-4615-8777-4
DOI: 10.1007/978-1-4615-8777-4

©1976 Plenum Press, New York
Softcover reprint of hardcover 1st edition 1976
A Division of Plenum Publishing Corporation
227 West 17th Street, New York, N.Y. 10011

Foreword

As longevity increases, the scope of cardiac disorders extends more widely in the sixth decade and onward into the seventh and subsequent decades.

For example, as a result of effective cardiac surgery in childhood, congential heart disease is now found with increasing frequency in adults and not exceptionally in persons over 65 years of age. The frequency of aortic valve replacement for calcific congenital valve stenosis in subjects around 70 years of age illustrates the intrusion of congenital heart disease into the older age range. Thus, the publication of *Cardiology in Old Age* will be especially welcome at this time.

The Editors have assembled a formidable galaxy of experts to present the special problems of epidemiology, pathology, cardiovascular physiology and function, and of specific cardiac disorders in the elderly. The chapter on cardiac surgery is particularly appropriate to many current problems.

The whole subject must be of growing concern to all clinicians and health workers who have increasingly to deal with older patients who have cardiovascular disorders. Knowledge of the effects of aging on the cardiovascular system is therefore of great interest and the information given in this book undoubtedly will be of value to general physicians and cardiologists, who may be expected in the future to work more closely with geriatricians in the care of the elderly. Continuing research into the problems of aging is clearly also of great importance especially in the field of cardiovascular medicine.

It gives me great pleasure to wish this important book every success.

J. F. Goodwin

Professor of Clinical Cardiology
Royal Postgraduate Medical School
Hammersmith Hospital, London

Preface

The increasing life span of modern man and woman has brought with it many fascinating problems for workers in various disciplines. In medicine, this longevity has forced doctors to look afresh at health and illness in later years, and to review previously held opinions. This necessity to take a new look is particularly true for heart disease, the commonest cause of death and a major cause of ill health in old age. The importance of cardiac disorders in the elderly population is increasingly recognized by cardiologists and physicians with a special interest in geriatric medicine. Recent work has extended to elderly patients some sophisticated techniques of diagnosis and treatment not previously utilized for their benefit, and has clarified many problems. Major advances have taken place in the description of the numerous and varied pathological changes that may occur in the heart with aging, in the application to the older patient of cardiac pacing and cardiac surgery, and in the understanding of the rational basis of drug therapy in old age. In the elderly, new, noninvasive diagnostic methods are finding a place in the investigation of heart disease, and will without doubt assist in making diagnosis more precise, with resulting benefit to the patient. The aim of this monograph is to bring together current views on heart disease in later years, and to combine the scientific aspects of the subject with advice on the practical management of elderly patients.

One problem we have encountered results from the varied names of drugs used in the treatment of heart disease. We have attempted to resolve the difficulties created on both sides of the Atlantic by compiling a glossary combining the British and U.S. approved names, and the trade names, of all drugs mentioned in the text. This glossary will be found on pages 397–399.

We are most grateful to our contributors for the detailed attention they have give to the preparation of their contributions, to Mr. Roy Baker of Plenum Corporation for his help and encouragement, and to

Mrs. Elizabeth Young and Mrs. Catherine McPhee for their unflagging secretarial assistance.

Glasgow   F.I. Caird
                                                            J.L.C. Dall
                                                         R.D. Kennedy

Acknowledgments

Our thanks are due, for permission to publish illustrations, to the following publishers and editors of journals, and to the authors: *Acta Medica Scandinavica* for Figs. 4.2, 4.3, 4.5, and 4.6; Blackwell Scientific Publications for Figs. 2.10, 2.12, 2.19, 2.20, 2.25, 2.27, 2.28, 2.30 and 2.31, and 5.4; *British Medical Journal (British Heart Journal* and *Cardiovascular Research)* for Figs. 5.3 and 5.14; Churchill-Livingstone for Fig. 11.2; *Clinical Science and Molecular Medicine* for Fig. 5.1; Dr. G.W. Hayward for Fig. 12.4; *Journal of Chronic Diseases* for Fig. 5.5; *Journal of Electrocardiology* for Fig. 18.1; *Journal of Physiology* for Fig. 5.2; S. Karger A.G., Basel, for Tables 12.1 and 12.3; *The Lancet* for Figs. 5.7, 5.12, 5.13, and 12.3; and the *Quarterly Journal of Medicine* for Fig. 5.9.

                                                            F.I.C.
                                                         J.L.C.D.
                                                            R.D.K.

Contributors

F.I. CAIRD, D. M., F.R.C.P., Reader in Geriatric Medicine, University Department of Geriatric Medicine, Southern General Hospital, Glasgow, G51 4TF.

J.L.C. DALL, M.D.,F.R.C.P., Consultant Physician in Geriatric Medicine, Victoria Infirmary, Glasgow, G42 9TY.

M.J. DAVIES, M.D., M.R.C.Path., Reader in Cardiac Pathology, St. George's Hospital Medical School, University of London, Blackshaw Road, Tooting, London, SW17 0QT.

T. HANLEY, M.D., Consultant Physician in Geriatric Medicine, Harrogate District Hospital, Lancaster Park Road, Harrogate, HG2 7SX.

R. HARRIS, M.D., Clinical Associate Professor of Medicine, Albany Medical College; Chief, Subdepartment of Cardiovascular Medicine, St. Peter's Hospital, Albany, New York.

R.H. JOHNSON, M.A., M.D., D.M., D.Phil, M.R.C.P.(G), Senior Lecturer in Neurology, University of Glasgow; Consultant Neurologist, Institute of Neurological Sciences, Southern General Hospital, Glasgow, G51 4TF.

WILLIAM B. KANNEL, M.D., Medical Director, National Institutes of Health, National Heart and Lung Institute, Heart Disease Epidemiology Study, 123 Lincoln Street, Framingham, Massachusetts 01701.

R.D. KENNEDY, M.B., F.R.C.P., Consultant Physician in Geriatric Medicine, University Department of Geriatric Medicine, Stobhill Hospital, Glasgow, G21 3UW.

ROBERT LAWSON, F.R.C.S., Cardiopulmonary Surgery Fellow, University of Oregon Medical School, 3181 S.W. Sam Jackson Park Road, Portland, Oregon 97201.

M.S. PATHY, F.R.C.P.E., F.R.C.P., Consultant Physician in Geriatric Medicine, Department of Geriatric Medicine, University Hospital of Wales, Heath Park, Cardiff, CF 4XW.

ARIELA POMERANCE, M.D. M.R.C. Path., Consultant Histopathologist, Harefield and Mount Vernon Hospitals, Harefield, Uxbridge, Middlesex, UB9 6JH; Honorary Consultant in Cardiac Pathology, Northwick Park Hospital, Watford Road, Harrow, Middlesex. HA1, 3UJ.

T. SEMPLE, M.D., B.Sc., F.R.C.P., Consultant Physician, Victoria Infirmary, Glasgow, G42 9TY.

HAROLD SIDDONS, M.Ch., F.R.C.S., Consultant Surgeon, St. George's Hospital, Hyde Park Corner, London, SW1X 7EZ.

ALBERT STARR, M.D., Professor and Chief, Cardiopulmonary Surgery, Division of Cardiopulmonary Surgery, University of Oregon Medical School, 3181 S.W. Sam Jackson Park Road, Portland, Oregon 97201.

TORE STRANDELL, M.D., Assistant Professor, Karolinska Institutet; Head of Department of Clinical Physiology, St. Eriks Sjukhus, S-112 82 Stockholm, Sweden.

JOHN WEDGWOOD, M.D., F.R.C.P., Consultant Physician in Geriatric Medicine, Middlesex Hospital, London, W1N 8AA.

B.O. WILLIAMS, M.B., M.R.C.P., Senior Registrar in Geriatric Medicine, Victoria Infirmary, Glasgow, G42 9TY.

Contents

Epidemiology of Heart Disease in Old Age

F. I. CAIRD and R. D. KENNEDY

Introduction

Study of the epidemiology of heart disease in old age can contribute to the measurement of the size of the problem. The essential sources of information are studies of mortality, which are usually based on death certification, and of the prevalence of heart disease in groups of old people who have been examined specifically with regard to the cardiovascular system.

Mortality from Heart Disease in Old Age

Mortality statistics clearly show the importance and significance of heart disease as a cause of death in old age (Table 1.1; WHO 1974). In Scotland, death rates from heart disease rise almost exponentially with age, doubling with approximately every 9 years of age in men from middle age on, and every 7 in women (Table 1.2). Thus, the initially lower death rates for women approximate to those of men in extreme old age. Heart disease is the largest single cause of death over

F. I. CAIRD · University Department of Geriatric Medicine, Southern General Hospital, Glasgow, G51 4TF, Scotland.   R. D. KENNEDY · University Department of Geriatric Medicine, Stobhill Hospital, Glasgow, G21 3UW, Scotland.

TABLE 1.1. Causes of Death Worldwide[a]

	Age				
Rank	0–4	5–14	15–44	45–64	65+
1	Accidents	Accidents	Accidents	New growths	**Heart disease**
2	Congenital	New growths	New growths	**Heart disease**	Strokes
3	New growths	Congenital	**Heart disease**	Strokes	New growths
4	Pneumonia	Pneumonia	Suicide	Accidents	Pneumonia
5	Enteritis, diarrhea	**Heart disease**	Stroke	Chest infection	Chronic chest infections

[a] WHO (1974).

the age of 65 in both sexes (Table 1.3). The proportion is 36% in women, and varies little with age; it averages 37% in men, and falls slightly with age, from 39% at the age of 65–69 to 34% over the age of 85. In contrast, the proportion of deaths certified as due to neoplastic disease shows a striking decline with age in both sexes.

The predominant importance of ischemic heart disease is immediately apparent when the main diagnostic categories of heart disease are considered in relation to each other as causes of death in old age (Table 1.4; Registrar General for Scotland 1974). Ischemic heart disease accounts for 88% of cardiac deaths in men over 65, and 80% in women. In both sexes, the proportions fall with advancing age. Neither hypertensive nor rheumatic heart disease contributes more than 5% of cardiac deaths, but other forms of heart disease contribute

TABLE 1.2. Death Rates (per 100,000 per Year) from Heart Disease (I.C.D.[a] 390–429) in Scotland, 1973[b]

	Age						
Sex	25–34	35–44	45–54	55–64	65–74	75–84	85+
Men	12	97	411	1051	2235	4475	8489
Women	5	30	124	407	1095	2931	7269

[a] I.C.D., International Classification of Diseases.
[b] Registrar General for Scotland (1974).

TABLE 1.3. Deaths over Age 65 in Scotland, 1973[a]

			Percentage due to:							
			Heart disease (I.C.D.[b]: 390–429)		Neoplasms (I.C.D.: 140–239)		Cerebro-vascular disease (I.C.D.: 430–438)		Respiratory disease (I.C.D.: 460–519)	
	Total deaths									
Age	M	F	M	F	M	F	M	F	M	F
65–69	5,188	3,412	39	35	26	25	12	17	11	6
70–74	5,506	4,518	37	36	22	20	15	21	13	7
75–79	4,328	5,234	35	36	19	15	17	23	15	9
80–84	3,275	5,121	36	35	16	12	19	24	17	11
85+	2,609	5,822	34	36	10	8	20	25	17	11
TOTAL:	20,906	24,107	37	36	20	15	16	23	14	9

[a] Registrar General for Scotland (1974).
[b] I.C.D., International Classification of Diseases.

a greater proportion. Deaths in this miscellaneous category are mostly certified as due to "myocardial insufficiency," "congestive heart failure," or "left heart failure." They comprise 4–7% of cardiac deaths in the 65–69 age group, and 18–20% over the age of 85, the proportions being higher in women than in men at all ages. The increase with age is doubtless due to uncertainty in ascribing death from heart disease to customary categories, especially in extreme old age. Nevertheless, even over the age of 85, identifiable forms of heart disease are recorded for 80% of cardiac deaths. It is of interest that although death rates for ischemic heart disease in the elderly in Scotland have altered relatively little in the past 6 years, there has been a considerable fall in death rates from "other" heart disease (Table 1.5; Registrar General for Scotland 1969, 1974). This decrease may reflect lessening in the difficulties and uncertainties of diagnostic categorization, which is presumably contributed to, at least in part, by more adequate investigation of the elderly.

Heart disease is without a doubt the most important single cause of death in old age, and the most important form of heart disease is that due to coronary artery disease.

TABLE 1.4. Deaths over Age 65 due to Heart Disease in Scotland, 1973[a]

					Percentage due to:					
Age	Total deaths			Rheumatic (I.C.D.[b]: 393–398)		Hyper- tensive (I.C.D.: 400–404)		Ischemic (I.C.D.: 410–414)		Other (I.C.D.: 420–429)	
	M	F		M	F	M	F	M	F	M	F
65–69	2,028	1,219		1	5	2	4	93	84	4	7
70–74	2,060	1,626		1	3	3	5	90	83	6	10
75–79	1,529	1,896		1	2	3	5	88	82	9	11
80–84	1,173	1,820		1	1	4	5	83	79	12	15
85+	888	2,078		1	1	3	4	78	75	18	20
TOTAL:	7,678	8,639	AVG:	1	2	3	5	88	80	8	13

[a] Registrar General for Scotland (1974).
[b] I.C.D., International Classification of Diseases

TABLE 1.5. Death Rates (per 100,000 per Year) from Ischemic Heart Disease and "Other" Heart Disease over Age 65 in Scotland, 1968 and 1973[a]

| | | Age | | | | | |
| | | 65–74 | | 75–84 | | 85+ | |
		M	F	M	F	M	F
Ischemic	1968	1962	924	3704	2296	6829	6005
Heart	1973	2038	910	3824	2343	6628	5443
Disease							
Change (%)		+4.4	−1.5	+3.2	+2.0	−2.9	−9.3
"Other"	1968	162	129	594	507	1752	1909
heart	1973	115	95	457	382	1516	1494
disease							
Change (%)		−29.0	−26.3	−23.1	−26.6	−13.5	−21.6

[a] Registrar General for Scotland (1969, 1974).

Prevalence of Heart Disease in Old Age

Although differing methods and diagnostic criteria make rigorous comparison difficult, clinical examination of elderly populations has shown a high prevalence of heart disease (Droller and Pemberton 1953, Acheson and Acheson 1958, Kitchin et al. 1973, Martin and Millard 1973, Kennedy et al. 1974).

If ischemic heart disease is defined by the presence of angina pectoris or a history of past cardiac infarction, and/or abnormal Q/QS patterns in the ECG, its prevalence is about 20% in men and 12% in women over the age of 65 (Acheson and Acheson 1958, Kitchin et al. 1973, Kennedy et al. 1974). Kennedy and colleagues define hypertensive heart disease as a blood pressure of 180/110 mm Hg or more,

TABLE 1.6. Prevalence (Percentage) of Heart Disease in Elderly People Living at Home[a]

	Age			
	65–74		75+	
	M	F	M	F -
	(Number:	(Number:	(Number:	(Number
Category of heart disease	102)	167)	79)	153)
"Definite classifiable"				
Ischemic	20	12	20	12
Hypertensive	8	16	13	12
Valvular[b]	1	5	4	8
Pulmonary	2	0	4	0
Mixed[c]	2	2	14	12
TOTALS				
"Definite classifiable"	32	38	46	42
"Definite unclassifiable"[d]	8	4	10	8
TOTALS				
"Definite" heart disease	40	42	56	51
"Doubtful" heart disease[d]	8	9	6	8
No heart disease	52	50	38	41

[a] Kennedy et al. (1974).
[b] 10 cases of mitral, 12 of aortic, valve disease.
[c] Hypertensive and Ischemic.
[d] See text for definition.

together with an ECG showing "probable" left ventricular hypertrophy (i.e., high-voltage R waves and S-T-T changes; Kannel et al. 1970; Kennedy and Caird 1972). Its prevalence is 8–13% in men and 12–16% in women (Table 1.6). Over the age of 75, combined ischemic and hypertensive heart disease is also frequent.

The prevalence of rheumatic heart disease is of the order of 2–3% (Table 1.6; Droller and Pemberton 1953), a figure in keeping with estimates from studies of hospital patients (Bedford and Caird 1960). Aortic stenosis is found in about 4%, and again hospital and autopsy statistics are in agreement (Bedford and Caird 1960). Pulmonary heart disease is less common, and virtually confined to men (Table 1.6), despite a very high prevalence of chronic bronchitis in both sexes in the population studied (Caird and Akhtar 1972).

There remain two further groups of elderly people with heart disease, which may be termed "definite but unclassifiable" and "doubtful." "Definite unclassifiable" heart disease may be said to be present when there is clear evidence of cardiac abnormality, but a firm diagnosis cannot be given (e.g., left bundle branch block as an isolated finding). "Doubtful" heart disease may be defined as a possible abnormality of uncertain significance, such as radiological evidence of slight cardiac enlargement, or minor ECG abnormality (e.g., T-wave flattening). Kennedy et al. (1974) found "definite unclassifiable" heart disease in 4–8% of subjects aged 65–74, and in a higher proportion (8–10%) over the age of 75. "Doubtful" heart disease was present in a further 8–9% at ages 65–74 and in 6–8% over age 75.

These clinical studies thus show a very high prevalence of undoubted heart disease in relatively fit old people, approximating to 40% between the ages of 65 and 74, and 50% or more over age 75. Further evidence is provided by investigations of the ECG in the elderly. Studies of groups of elderly hospital patients or residents in institutions (Wosika et al. 1950, Fisch et al. 1957, Taran and Szilagyi 1958, Mihalick and Fisch 1974) are of less value in this context than studies of old people living at home (Ostrander et al. 1965, Kennedy and Caird 1972, Kitchin et al. 1973, Martin and Millard 1973, Cullen et al. 1974, Campbell et al. 1974). There are great advantages in the application of standardized methods of electrocardiographic reporting, such as the Minnesota Code (Blackburn et al. 1960, Rose and Blackburn 1968, Kennedy and Caird 1972).

The findings in the four studies set out in Table 1.7 derive from three continents, but are nevertheless in general agreement. Q/QS patterns are found in approximately 10% of elderly men and 5% of women; the correlation between these changes and the demonstration

TABLE 1.7. Percentage Prevalence of Electrocardiographic Abnormalities in Unselected Old People

Electrocardiographic abnormality	Men				Women			
	Age 70+[a] (Number: 127)	Age 62+[b] (Number: 214)	Age 70+[c] (Number: 213)	Age 65+[d] (Number: 872)	Age 70+[a] (Number: 162)	Age 62+[b] (Number: 268)	Age 70+[c] (Number: 190)	Age 65+[d] (Number: 1382)
Q/QS patterns	9.5	7.9	9.4	10.0	3.1	7.4	7.4	4.0
T-wave changes	36.2	23.3	24.0	19.2	32.0	29.8	15.7	12.6
Left ventricular hypertrophy	8.7	3.7	12.6[e]	6.7[e]	12.9	14.5	10.5[e]	10.3[e]
Right ventricular hypertrophy	—	—	—	1.4	—	—	—	0.3
1st degree heart block	10.2	3.7	5.2	1.5	7.4	3.0	4.7	0.6
LBBB[f]	0	1.4	1.4	1.6	3.1	0	3.7	1.2
RBBB[g]	4.7	2.3	3.3	2.7	1.9	2.2	2.1	1.2
Frequent ectopic beats (1 in 10)	11.8	—	4.2	4.0	3.1	—	2.6	2.5
Atrial fibrillation	3.1	2.3	5.2	2.1	4.3	2.6	3.2	2.4

[a] Ostrander et al. (1965).
[b] Kitchin et al. (1973).
[c] Cullen et al. (1974).
[d] Campbell et al. (1974).
[e] Includes Minnesota codes 3.1 and 3.3; others include only 3.1.
[f] LBBB, Left bundle branch block.
[g] RBBB, Right bundle branch block.

of past cardiac infarction at autopsy is reasonable (Kurihara et al. 1967, Horan et al. 1971). There is some variation in the reported frequency of T-wave changes, which are often of uncertain significance. Patterns indicative of left ventricular hypertrophy are found more commonly in women than in men, probably reflecting the higher mean blood pressure of elderly women (Hamilton et al. 1954, Master et al. 1958, Anderson and Cowan 1959). Criteria for right ventricular hypertrophy are difficult to define (see Chapter 10). Campbell et al. (1974) used the criteria of Goodwin and Abdin (1959) and found evidence of right ventricular hypertrophy in only 1.4% of men and 0.3% of women.

First-degree atrioventricular block is not uncommon (3% or so), but higher degrees of block, in contrast, are rarely encountered. The prevalence of second- and third-degree block together has been estimated as 0.03% at age 65–69, 0.04% at 70–74, and 0.11% over the age of 75 (Shaw and Eraut 1970). Ventricular conduction defects are common. Right bundle branch block has usually been found to be more common than left in old people at home (see also Edmands 1966); the contrary view (Björnberg 1960) is based on the study of old people in the hospital. Left anterior hemiblock with or without right bundle branch block is found in 4% of men and 1% of women (Campbell et al. 1974) and is probably the most frequent conduction defect (Kitchin et al. 1973).

The most common disorder of rhythm is frequent ectopic beats. Atrial fibrillation is found in 1.7% of subjects of both sexes aged 65–74, and in 4.8% over the age of 75 (Campbell et al. 1974).

These studies thus complement the clinical investigations in demonstrating a very high prevalence of heart disease. There is electrocardiographic evidence of cardiac abnormality in from 40 to 60% of apparently fit old people (Campbell et al. 1974).

Morbidity of Heart Disease in Old Age

There is relatively little information on the morbidity of heart disease in old age, although the incidence of cardiac failure is known to rise with age (Table 1.8; Klainer et al. 1965, McKee et al. 1971), and tends to be greater in men than in women (McKee et al. 1971). The same is true of congestive heart failure, as reflected in admissions to a geriatric unit (Bedford and Caird 1956); 14% of all such admissions had clinical signs of congestive heart failure, although this was not necessarily the principal reason for admission. Further evidence is provided by a study of disability in randomly selected old people

TABLE 1.8. Incidence of Cardiac Failure (per 1000 White Population per 6 Months) in Two U.S. Counties[a]

Age	Montgomery County, North Carolina, 1962		Caledonia County, Vermont, 1963	
	Population	Rate	Population	Rate
0–14	4287	0	7134	0
15–24	1987	0.5	2776	0
25–44	3489	1.1	5251	0.6
45–64	2794	12.2	4769	9.4
65–74	875	45.7	1686	43.9
75+	388	108.2	1142	95.4

[a] Klainer et al. (1965).

(Akhtar et al. 1973). Of 229 elderly people whose disability was such that they were unable to live at home without help, 20% had clinical evidence of heart disease that was considered to be a contributory cause of their disability, and affected their capacity for independent existence in the community.

References

Acheson, R.M., and Acheson, E.D. (1958) Br. J. Prev. Soc. Med. 12, 147.

Akhtar, A.J., Broe, G.A., Crombie, A., McLean, W.M.R., Andrews, G.R., and Caird, F.I. (1973) Age and Ageing 2, 190.

Anderson, W.F., and Cowan, N.R. (1959) Clin. Sci. 18, 103.

Bedford, P.D., and Caird, F.I. (1956) Q. J. Med. N.S.25, 407.

Bedford, P.D., and Caird, F.I. (1960) Valvular Disease of the Heart in Old Age, J & A Churchill, London.

Björnberg, O. (1960) Gerontol. Clin. 2, 133.

Blackburn, H., Keys, A., Simonson, E., Rautaharju, P., and Punsar, S. (1960) Circulation 21, 1160.

Caird, F.I., and Akhtar, A.J. (1972) Thorax 27, 764.

Campbell, A., Caird, F.I., and Jackson, T.F.M. (1974) Br. Heart J. 36, 1005.

Cullen, K.J., Murphy, B.P., and Cumpston, G.N: (1974) Aust. N.Z. J. Med. 4, 325.

Droller, H., and Pemberton, J. (1953) Br. Heart J. 15, 199.

Edmands, R.E. (1966) Circulation 34, 1081.

Fisch, C., Genovese, P.D., Dyke, R.W., Laramore, W., and Marvel, R. J. (1957) Geriatrics 12, 616.

Goodwin, J.F., and Abdin, Z.H. (1959). Br. Heart J. 21, 523.

Hamilton, M., Pickering, G.W., Fraser Roberts, J.A., and Sowry, G.S.C. (1954) Clin. Sci. 13, 11.

Horan, L. G., Flowers, N. C., and Johnson, J. C. (1971) *Circulation* **43**, 428.

Kannel, W. B., Gordon, T., Castelli, W. P., and Margolis, J. R., (1970) *Ann. Intern. Med.* **72**:813.

Kennedy, R. D., Andrews, G. R., and Caird, F. I. (1974) Unpublished.

Kennedy, R. D., and Caird, F. I. (1972) *Gerontol. Clin.* **14**, 5.

Kitchin, A. H., Lowther, C. P., and Milne, J. S. (1973) *Br. Heart J.* **35**, 946.

Klainer, L. M., Gibson, T. C., and White, K. L. (1965) *J. Chronic Dis.* **18**, 797.

Kurihara, H., Kuramoto, K., Terasawa, F., Matsushita, S., Seki, M., and Ikeda, M. (1967) *Jpn. Heart J.* **8**, 514.

Martin, A., and Millard, P. H. (1973) *Age and Ageing* **2**, 211.

Master, A. M., Lasser, R. P., and Jaffe, H. L. (1958) *Ann. Intern. Med.* **48**, 284.

McKee, P. A., Castelli, W. P., McNamara, P. M., and Kannel, W. B. (1971) *New Engl. J. Med.* **285**, 1441.

Mihalick, M. J., and Fisch, C. (1974) *Am. Heart J.* **87**, 117.

Ostrander, L. D., Brandt, R. L., Kjelsberg, M. O., and Epstein, F. H. (1965) *Circulation* **31**, 888.

Registrar General for Scotland (1969, 1974) *Annual Reports, Part 1: Mortality*, H.M.S.O., Edinburgh.

Rose, G. A., and Blackburn, H. (1968) *Cardiovascular Survey Methods*, WHO, Geneva.

Shaw, D. B., and Eraut, D. (1970) *Br. Med. J.* **1**, 144.

Taran, L. M., and Szilagyi, H. (1958) *Geriatrics* **13**, 352.

World Health Organization (1974), *World Health Statistics Report* **27**(9), 563.

Wosika, P. H., Feldman, E., Chesrow, E. J., and Myers, G. B. (1950) *Geriatrics* **5**, 13.

2

Pathology of the Myocardium and Valves

ARIELA POMERANCE

Introduction

The abnormalities found in the elderly heart include virtually every condition occurring in younger adults, in addition to those peculiar to the geriatric population. A full account of all these pathological processes is clearly beyond the scope of this chapter; readers requiring further information on any of the many abnormalities common to all age groups are referred to standard textbooks on cardiac pathology. Hudson (1965, 1970) summarizes the literature up to 1969; more recent advances, up to 1975, are included in Pomerance and Davies (1975). This chapter will concentrate only on conditions found exclusively or predominantly in people over 65 years of age, and on certain aspects of others that are characteristically associated with the elderly; it will briefly mention some uncommon conditions that occur, but tend not to be considered in this age group.

Many cardiac abnormalities, when considered in isolation, appear to be of clinical significance only when very well marked. The functional effects in most cases of aortic valve or mitral ring calcification, amyloidosis, or mucoid degeneration of the mitral valve, for example, seem insufficient to produce cardiac failure. Multiplicity of abnormalities is a feature of cardiac pathology in the elderly, however,

ARIELA POMERANCE · Pathology Department, Harefield Hospital, Harefield, Uxbridge, Middlesex, UB9 6JH, England.

as it is of the pathology of this age group generally, and the majority of cases of cardiac failure have more than one abnormality in the heart (Pomerance 1965, Linzbach and Akuamoa-Boateng 1973). It seems likely that even the lesser degrees of these changes do affect cardiac function to some extent, and if the changes are multiple, their cumulative effect then becomes sufficient to precipitate failure.

The Normal Heart in Old Age and Normal Aging Changes

Most of the findings generally regarded as typical of the elderly heart are not expressions of normal senescence, but of pathological processes that show increasing incidence with age. The normal standard for any age group should be set by the least degree of abnormality found. All pathologists with extensive autopsy experience are well aware that age cannot be reliably assessed from inspection of the heart. Many nonagenarians and even centenarians have coronary arteries almost free from atheroma, normal-sized hearts and valves, and endocardium showing no more thickening than cases half a century younger.

Despite the known decline in cardiac efficiency in old age, few changes attributable to biological aging alone can be seen; this absence probably reflects the limitations of current techniques. Quantitative changes in myofiber enzymes with aging have been demonstrated experimentally (Limas 1971), but the only constant myofiber change noted in man is an increase in lipofuscin (Strehler et al. 1959). This substance appears as yellow-brown granules at the poles of myofiber nuclei in routinely stained sections and is autofluorescent under UV light. It is not found in childhood, but is universal in the elderly and is unrelated to sex, race, other cardiac pathology, or myocardial function. This accumulation of lipofuscin is responsible for the brown color noted in atrophic hearts (brown atrophy). The frequent findings of small atrophic hearts in the elderly, however, is merely related to the high incidence of death from diseases associated with generalized wasting and is not an expression of senescence. In the absence of hypertension or ischemic or valve disease, heart weight remains proportional to body weight.

In the atria, there is an increase in interstitial elastic, collagen, and fat, and a decrease in muscle (McMillan and Lev 1962, Davies and Pomerance 1972). Occasionally, the increase in fat may mimic a tumor and be associated with arrhythmias (Page 1970).

Aging changes in the cardiac skeleton consist of increasing

density and sclerosis of the collagen. Fine foci of calcification are common (Sell and Scully 1965).

The endocardium of the atria and the atrial surface of the atrioventricular valves thickens progressively with age (McMillan and Lev 1959). Histology shows increased collagen and elastic fibers. These changes seem to be an irritational hyperplasia in response to blood flow.

In the valves, the effects of repeated contact and flexion are seen as nodular thickenings on the closure lines of the atrioventricular valves and palpable ridges along the attachments of the aortic cusps (McMillan and Lev 1964, Pomerance 1967). Hemodynamic factors are also responsible for the appearance of lipid in the collagenous layer (fibrosa) of both aortic and mitral cusps. This is seen macroscopically in the anterior mitral cusp as yellow plaques on the aortic surface (see Fig. 2.27); the size of these plaques increases with age.

Congenital Abnormalities

Congenital abnormalities other than bicuspid aortic valves are naturally uncommon in the elderly; they consist mainly of minor anatomical variations, such as quadricuspid semilunar valves, intra-cavitary cords, and small atrial septal defects. These are usually of no functional importance. Although unexpected survival with malforma-tions such as Fallot's tetralogy, patent ductus, or coarctation of the aorta are occasionally reported (Fontana and Edwards 1962, Perloff and Lingren 1974a,b; see also Fig. 2.12 in this chapter), the only major abnormalities seen with any frequency in the elderly are atrial septal defects. The oldest case seen personally died at the age of 87 with the defect occupying two-thirds of the septum secundum.

Myocardial Pathology

Cardiac Hypertrophy

The causes of ventricular hypertrophy in the elderly are the same as in other adults. Most cases of left ventricular hypertrophy are due to systemic hypertension, ischemic heart disease, or aortic stenosis. Lesser degrees of hypertrophy may occur with chronic anemia, thyro-toxicosis, myxodema, and most of the conditions listed as secondary cardiomyopathies (see pp. 23–24). Right ventricular hypertrophy is comparatively uncommon, and almost invariably associated with chronic obstructive airway disease.

Ischemic Heart Disease

Although this disease can no longer be regarded as almost synonymous with geriatric heart disease, it is undoubtedly the most important single cardiac abnormality in this age group in functional terms. In this hospital, as in a similar investigation a decade earlier, ischemic myocardial pathology was found in about half the geriatric patients dying in cardiac failure (Pomerance 1965, Pomerance and Hodkinson 1976), and was the only cardiac lesion present in 22%. As would be expected, the proportion is higher in cases of sudden death not in the hospital. Of a personally reviewed series of 380 sudden deaths in people over 65 years, 62% were due to coronary artery disease. An interesting observation, but perhaps not a surprising one, has been the lower incidence in extreme old age; in the tenth and

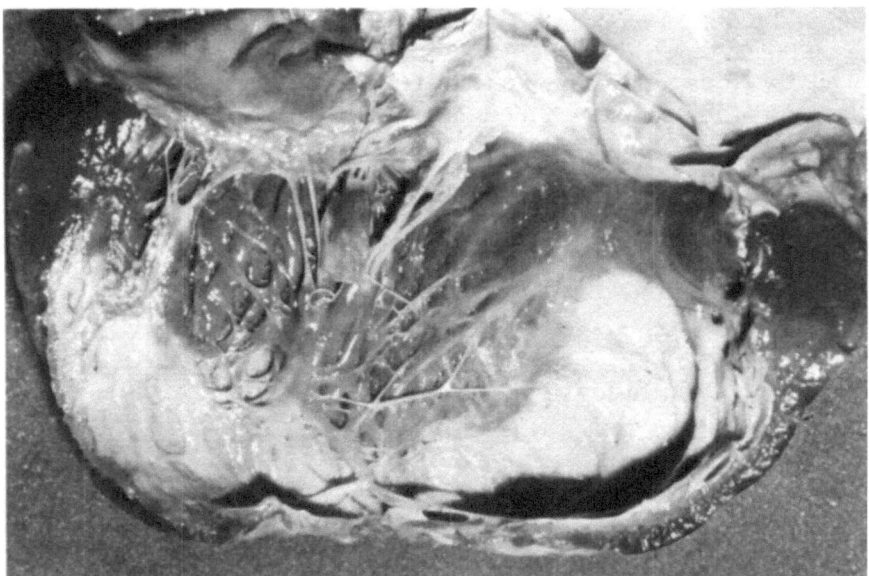

Figure 2.1. Large fibrous aneurysm of the left ventricle. From a 90-year-old blacksmith, fit and active until his sudden death. No suggestion of myocardial infarction in his past history.

eleventh decade, ischemic heart disease was found in only one-third of subjects in the combined hospital and coroner's autopsies.

Apart from the case of sudden death in which severe coronary artery narrowing is found without visible myocardial changes, the clinically significant lesions are usually relatively large areas of recent necrosis or fibrous scarring. The small foci of myocardial fibrosis common in elderly hearts are found with equal frequency in patients with and without cardiac failure. These lesions, the incidence of which increases with age, correlate poorly with coronary atherosclerosis (Schwartz and Mitchell 1962). They are probably the end result of the small foci of myocardial inflammation commonly noted in a variety of causes of death.

The aspects of ischemic myocardial pathology that are particularly characteristic of the elderly reflect the well-recognized atypical or absent symptoms in this age group. Autopsies are likely to reveal a high incidence of clinically unsuspected ischemic pathology unless ECGs are routinely performed. The figure in most series has been about 20% (Gjol 1972).

Large fibrous aneurysms, as illustrated in Fig. 2.1, are seen mainly in elderly subjects; often, there is no history indicating past infarction, although these lesions are clearly a consequence of extensive transmural necrosis. The aneurysm walls consist of fibrous tissue, often heavily calcified; the cavities may be filled with laminated thrombus, which, however, rarely seems to give rise to emboli.

External cardiac rupture (Fig. 2.2) is an uncommon complication of myocardial infarction except in the elderly. Its incidence has been calculated as increasing by 3.6% per decade (Sievers 1966). The reason for this increase is obscure. Aging alone does not cause thinning, muscle loss, or fatty infiltration of the left ventricle and, although it has been suggested that age-related alterations in cement lines and intercalated discs might increase the liability of myofibers to fragmentation (London and London 1965), there is at present no actual evidence for this relationship.

At autopsy, the most striking feature of rupture is the tense purple pericardial sac, distended by blood clot. The rupture site appears as a ragged tear, most often on the anterior wall of the left ventricle. Sectioning shows a ragged transmural hemorrhagic track, the appearances suggesting that the process is one of gradual dissection, rather than of a "blowout." Although rupture is always through or at the edge of an area of infarction, this area may be surprisingly small, as may the size of the occluded coronary artery. Rarely, the rate and extent of hemorrhage are restricted by fibrous intrapericardial

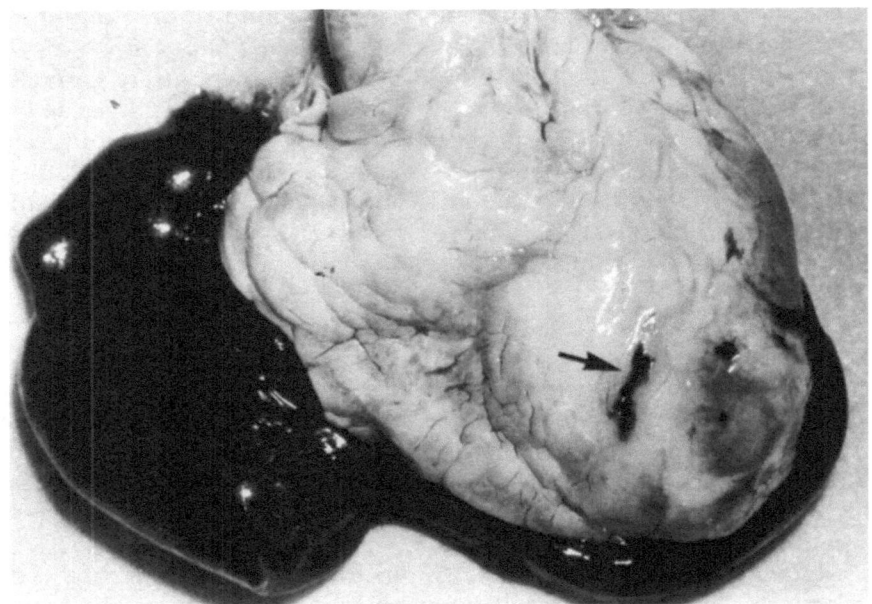

Fig. 2.2. Ruptured heart. There is an irregular tear in the anterior wall of the left ventricle (arrow). The heart is surrounded by clotted blood that filled the pericardial sac. From a previously well 82-year-old woman who died suddenly.

adhesion, and a false aneurysm forms. Successful repair is then possible (Van Tassell and Edwards 1972).

In most recent reviews, external cardiac rupture has been found in from 7 to 9% of fatal cases of myocardial infarction. The incidence was highest in medicolegal autopsies and in elderly psychotics. It was much commoner in women, and the most constant predisposing factors were postinfarction hypertension or physical activity and absence of previous ischemic episodes. Personal experience agrees with these findings. It appears that past ischemia has a protective effect in this context, because of the resulting increase in fibrous tissue.

Transseptal and papillary muscle rupture also occur in the elderly, but these complications, unlike external cardiac rupture, are no more frequent than in younger patients.

Cardiac Amyloidosis

As in younger patients, cardiac involvement may occasionally be found due to secondary or myeloma-associated amyloidosis, and rarely in the "typical" disseminated primary form with massive cardiomegaly. Amyloid is very common in the elderly, however, in the form of senile cardiac amyloidosis. This form of apparently primary amyloidosis is, for all practical purposes, confined to the heart, and its distinctive age and pathological distribution have justified its separate consideration. First recorded by Soyka (1876), amyloid has shown a subsequently reported frequency ranging from 2 to 83%. This enormous variation is clearly due to differences in sampling and staining techniques. Currently available methods for identifying amyloid are inversely related in respect of sensitivity and specificity. In our experience, using a new technique that has proved both specific and highly sensitive (Pomerance et al. 1976), amyloid was seen in 42% of over 300 geriatric autopsies. The deposits were minor and limited to the atria in 20%, however, and heavy ventricular involvement was present in only 5%. The early deposits were not associated with arryhthmias or digitalis sensitivity, and were clearly of no clinical significance. Patients with marked ventricular involvement had usually been in cardiac failure, but other cardiac pathology had often also been present, as in other recent studies (Serentha et al. 1973, Wright and Calkins 1975). Heart block and sino-atrial arrhythmias may be found with heavy ventricular infiltration, but seem to occur in only a minority of such cases.

In our material, senile cardiac amyloidosis as a whole was more common in women (51% compared with 33% in men), but when only well-marked ventricular involvement was considered, the frequency in men was over twice that in women. This finding suggests that although women are more prone to develop amyloid in the heart, they may be more resistant to its progression to clinically significant severity.

Grossly, the heart is usually of normal size. Microscopy shows deposits of material with the staining reactions and ultrastructure currently accepted as characteristic of amyloid, i.e., metachromasia with methyl or crystal violet, green birefringence with Congo red and polarized light, fluorescence with thioflavine T, positive reaction for tryptophan, and green color with sulphonated alcein blue. The earliest deposits are seen in the atrial capillaries and as fine interstitial strands between atrial myofibers. More advanced cases show broad bands

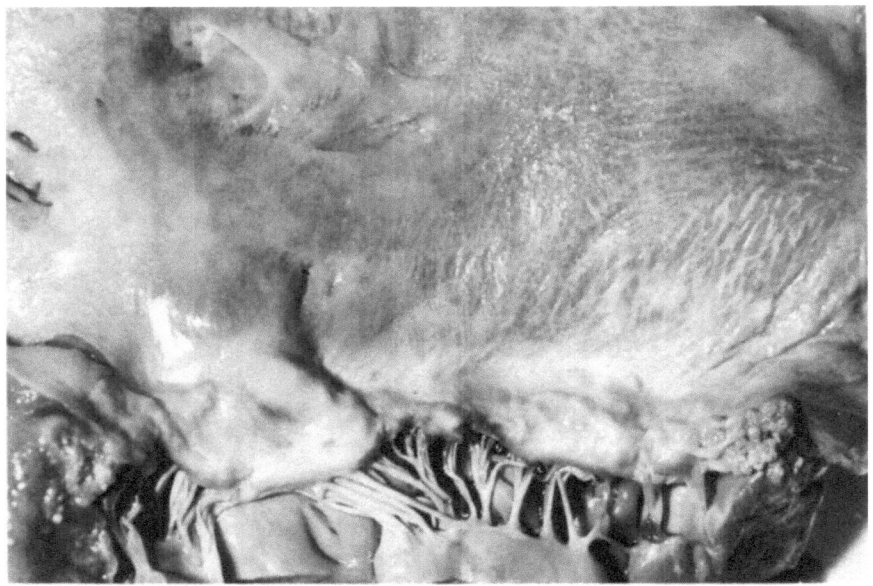

Fig. 2.3. Senile cardiac amyloidosis showing numerous small, closely set grayish nodules of amyloid in the left atrium. Mitral ring calcification is also present. From a 72-year-old woman who died in congestive cardiac failure.

surrounding and often compressing myofibers and nodular masses of amyloid in atrial endocardium, which can be seen macroscopically as minute translucent foci (Figs. 2.3 and 2.4). In the ventricles, early deposits appear as delicate networks around small, widely separated groups of myofibers. These deposits increase progressively in number, size, and thickness, finally resulting in compression atrophy of the myofibers (Fig. 2.5). Endocardial involvement is not a feature. In a minority of cases medium-caliber and small vessels are involved; rarely, this pattern may predominate. The myofiber atrophy accompanying increasing amyloid deposition accounts for the lack of cardiac hypertrophy. Usually the only naked-eye indications of even severe cardiac amyloidosis are the minute atrial nodules, and these may easily be overlooked.

Minor extracardiac involvement is found in about a third of cases with severe cardiac involvement, but this most often affects the lungs only, and amyloid is rarely visible in the usual biopsy sites. Clinical diagnosis is unsatisfactory at present since the total amount of amyloid is too small to influence the Congo Red test, electrocardiographic changes, in our experience, are varied and inconsistent (Raftery, personal communication), and the only biochemical abnormality found has been an elevated serum alkaline phosphatase (Hodkinson and Pomerance 1974).

The pathogenesis of senile cardiac amyloidosis remains obscure. The condition also occurs in certain strains of other species (Thung 1957, Schwartz 1970), and all studies agree that it is found only in the elderly and that its incidence increases with age. The sex differences and known existence of familial forms of amyloidosis suggest that genetic factors may be concerned. It is now generally accepted that amyloidosis is related to immunological dysfunction (Franklin and Zucker-Franklin 1972, Glenner et al. 1973), and senile amyloid may therefore be an expression of the immunological alterations occuring with senescence (Walford 1969). No correlation with serum protein or immunoglobulin levels has been demonstrable, however, in our material (Williams and Maughan, personal communication). At present, the disease is regarded as a form of primary amyloid, and there was no association with chronic infection or malignancy in our 120

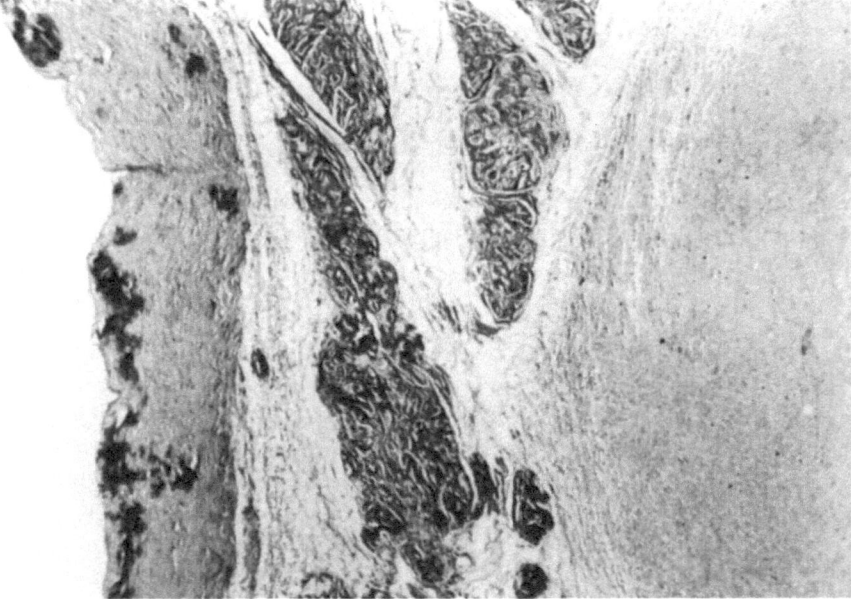

Fig. 2.4. Section shows dark-staining areas of amyloid in atrial endocardium and surrounding myofibers in the atrial septum. (S.A.B., × 80, approx.).

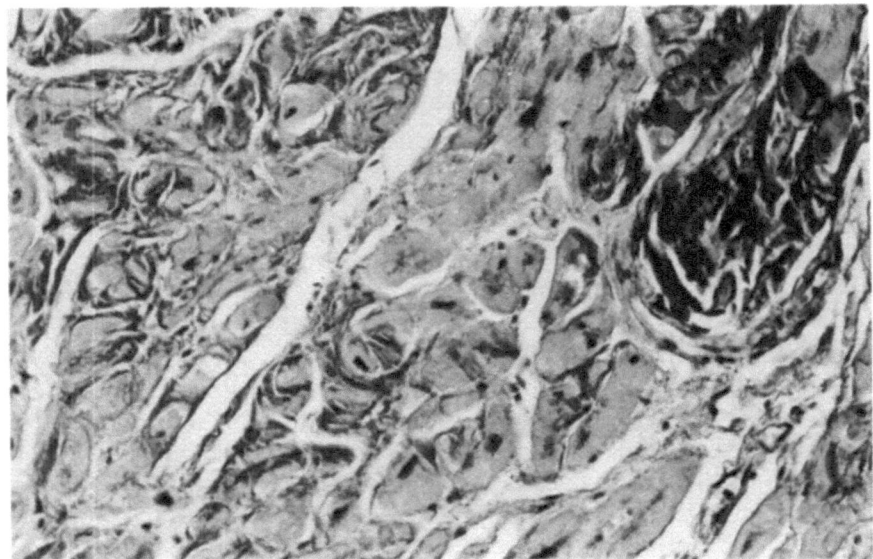

Fig. 2.5. Ventricular myocardium showing bands of dark-staining amyloid deposition surrounding myofibers. A group of fibers (upper right) have completely atrophied and been replaced by amyloid (S.A.B., ×180)

cases. Rosenthal and Franklin (1975), however, have recently reported an age-associated increase in a serum factor related to secondary and some familial forms of amyloidosis. It is clear that further studies of senile amyloidosis, using these sensitive techniques, are needed.

Cardiomyopathies

Both hypertrophic and congestive primary cardiomyopathies occur in the elderly.

Hypertrophic Obstructive Cardiomyopathy (HOCM, idiopathic hypertrophic subaortic stenosis, asymmetric septal hypertrophy) is not a common disease at any age, and is more familiar to pathologists than clinicians, since many cases seen at autopsy were clinically silent. Once regarded as a disease of young adults, it is now well recognized as not rare in the elderly; between 7 and 32% of patients in several recent large clinical series were over 60 years of age (Whiting et al. 1971, Pomerance and Davies 1975). The pathology differs in several respects from that typically found in younger patients. The hearts tend to be heavier, and hypertrophy of the free wall of the left ventricle is usually present, obscuring the classic asymmetrical septal hypertrophy. The typically short, thick, abnormally branched and orientated myofibers can still be found histologically, however, if sufficient blocks are examined. A striking and diagnostic macroscopic feature is a subaortic septal fibrous band (Fig. 2.6), which was present in 11 of the 15 cases over 60 years studied personally. Characteristically, the lower part of this band is a mirror image of the aortic aspect of the anterior mitral cusp, and it has clearly formed as a result of the systolic contact between cusp and septum that occurs in this condition. Once formed, the band remains, even if the ventricle dilates and the obstructive element is lost. It is therefore a useful indicator of the correct diagnosis in an age group where the possibility of hypertrophic cardiomyopathy might otherwise be overlooked.

Congestive Cardiomyopathy is a diagnosis rarely made in the elderly, since it demands exclusion of atheromatous myocardial dis-

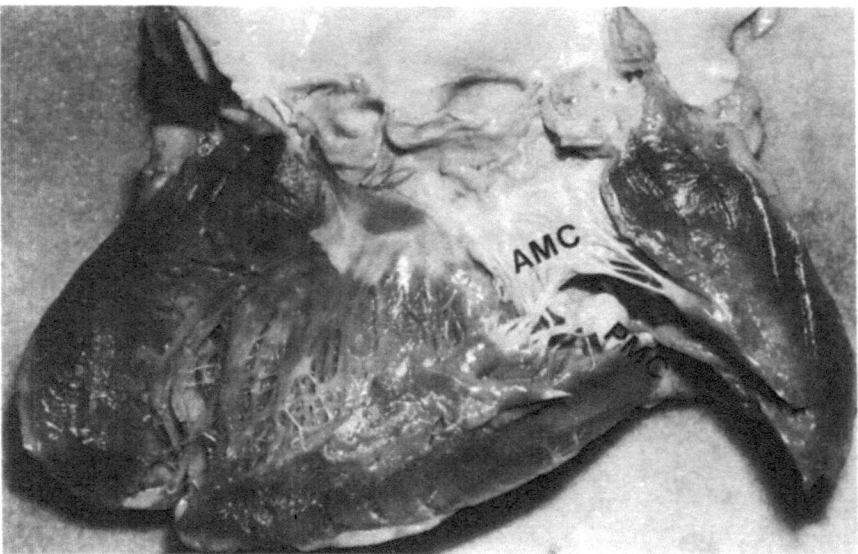

Fig. 2.6. Hypertrophic cardiomyopathy (HOCM) in an 84-year-old woman who died of gastrointestinal hemorrhage associated with acute on chronic bronchitis. The heart shows hypertrophy, most obviously of the anteroseptal wall; the cavity is relatively small, and there is a well-defined fibrous band high on the outflow tract of the left ventricle, corresponding to the lower edge of the anterior mitral cusp (AMC). A mild degree of ballooning deformity of the posterior mitral cusp (PMC) can also be seen.

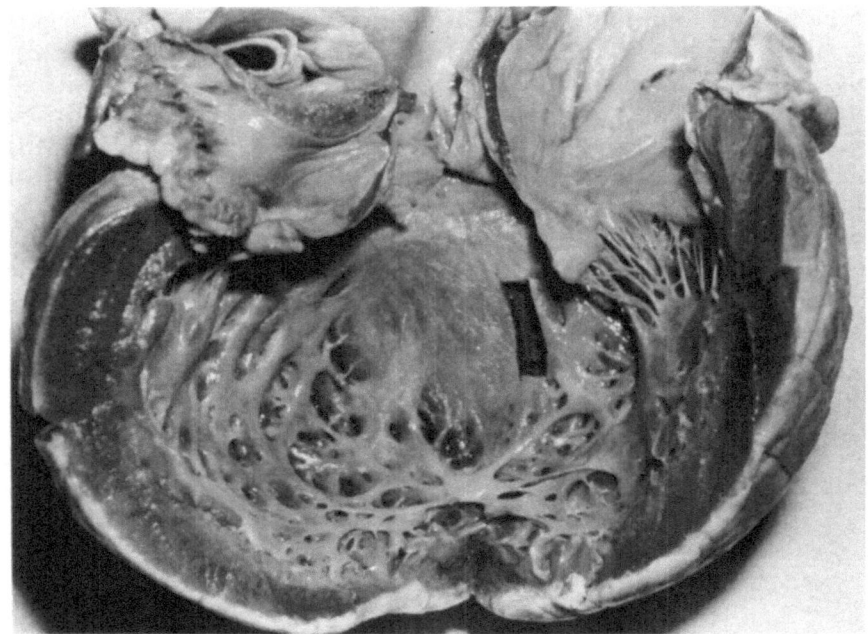

Fig. 2.7. Congestive cardiomyopathy in an 82-year-old woman with a history of angina and congestive cardiac failure. The heart is globular, with dilated left ventricular cavity and small white foci of endocardial fibrosis. The coronary arteries were widely patent, showing mild atheroma only.

ease. Such cases are occasionally seen (Fig. 2.7), however, and Roberts and Ferrans (1975) describe an example in a woman aged 96. In contrast to the appearances in hypertrophic cardiomyopathy, the heart in congestive cardiomyopathy is strikingly globular, with a large, dilated left ventricular cavity. Small areas of endocardial fibrosis may be seen in both ventricles, together with small thrombi adherent to the interstices of the cavities. The coronary arteries are notably free from atheromatous narrowing. Histological features are nonspecific, as might be anticipated in a condition that is probably the common end-stage of various etiologies.

Secondary Cardiomyopathies

As in other age groups, the heart may be involved in many systemic diseases, of which only the genetically determined neuromuscular and metabolic diseases need not be considered in the elderly.

Myocarditis (Fig. 2.8) may occur in a large number of virus and rickettsial infections (Gore and Saphir 1947, Kline et al. 1962), of which Coxsackie B is probably the most frequently encountered in Western Europe and the North American continent (*Br. Med. J.* 1971). Small foci of myocardial inflammatory cells, which do not justify diagnosis as myocarditis, are also not uncommonly seen in patients dying with a wide range of noninfective diseases. Myocarditis with giant cells as a conspicuous feature occurs in sarcoidosis and tuberculosis, as well as in the idiopathic form. Unsuspected tuberculosis remains a comparatively common condition in the elderly. Myocardial granulomas similar to the subcutaneous lesions may occur in patients with severe rheumatoid disease. Syphylitic gummas have become one of the least common types of cardiac pathology, but the occasional cases encountered are mainly in elderly patients. These last two lesions often form in the upper interventricular septum, causing heart block.

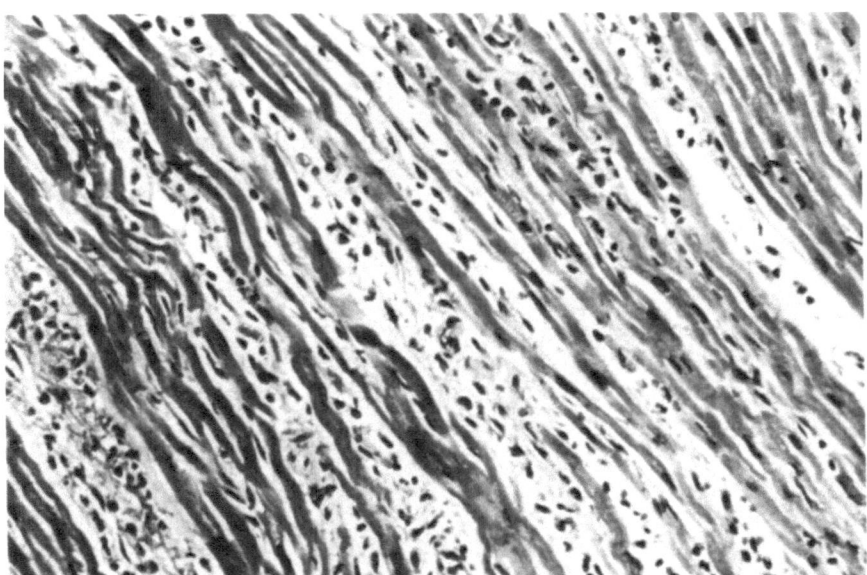

Fig. 2.8. Focal acute myocarditis. Numerous polymorphs and chronic inflammatory cells present between the myofibers. From an 81-year-old man with ulcerative colitis and suppurative pyelonephritis. (Hematoxylin and eosin ×80)

Metabolic Diseases affecting the heart are, in general, rare in the elderly. A notable exception is diabetes mellitus, which is a well-recognized risk factor in atheroclerosis (Robertson and Strong 1968), and so is associated with an increased incidence of ischemic heart disease. Primary hemochromatosis is an occasional cause of cardiac failure, and patients are often in the geriatric age group (Di Giorgio 1973). Pathologically, the heart is strikingly brown, and histology shows large amounts of brown pigment in myofibers, interstitial connective tissue, and conducting tissue; this pigment stains blue-green with acid ferricyanide. Changes that are pathologically indistinguishable from those of primary hemochromatosis may develop in patients with long-standing anemia following multiple transfusions. Oxalosis from chronic renal failure may also affect the heart, provoking myocardial fibrosis (Salyer and Hutchins 1974).

Nonspecific Myocardial Changes are seen in many diseases associated with cardiac failure. These changes usually appear insignificant in relation to the degree of cardiac dysfunction. The diseases commonly encountered in the elderly include thyrotoxicosis, myxedema, anemia, and chronic alcoholism. In all these conditions, small foci of myofiber degeneration and vacuolation may be present. In addition, interstitial fibrosis is often present in alcoholic heart disease (Schenk and Cohen 1970), fatty degeneration of myofibers is common in anemia, and myxedematous hearts may show an unusually well-marked degree of basophilic mucoid degeneration of myofibers (Haust et al. 1962); a mild degree of this change is very common in the elderly and has no diagnostic connotation (Rosai and Lascano 1970).

Cardiac Tumors

Most tumors found in the heart are metastatic. Careful examination in patients dying with disseminated malignant disease has shown cardiac metastases in a surprisingly high proportion of cases (see Davies 1975). Pancreatic, mammary, renal, and pulmonary tumors are the most frequent primary sites in the elderly.

Primary cardiac tumors are rare, although no less so than in younger ages. The most common are atrial myxomas. Hudson (1965) illustrates a case of a woman age 95. Myxomas usually form rounded masses attached to the margins of the foramen ovale (Fig. 2.9); with large tumors, the appropriate atrioventricular valve cusps are usually thickened. Myxomas are distinguished from large thrombi by their firm attachment, often by a distinct pedicle, and by the absence of rheumatic deformities or true stenosis of the mitral valve macroscopi-

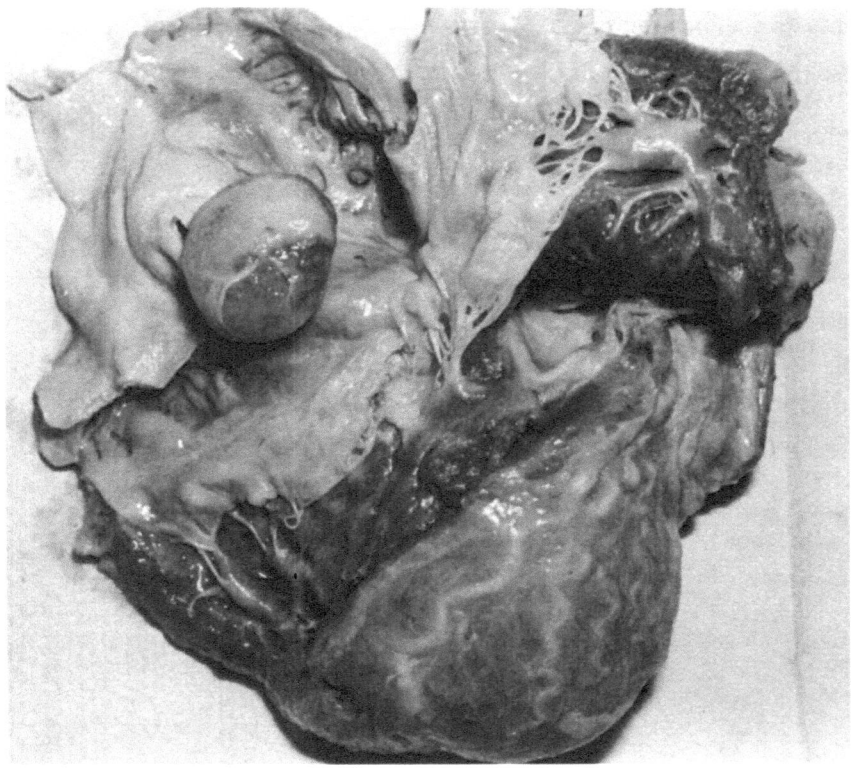

Fig. 2.9. Myxoma of right atrium. A pedunculated tumour showing superficial ulceration is arising from the atrial septum. The heart is atrophic, with gelatinous epicardial
fat and tortuous coronary arteries, and the myocardium was noticeably brown. From a
67-year-old man with progressive generalized debility.

cally, and by the presence of the characteristic lepidic cells in the
myxomatous stroma on microscopy.

Valve Pathology

Degenerative calcification is the most common single pathological
abnormality found in the elderly heart. From personal experience,
about a third of patients over 70 years of age have at least some degree
of macroscopically identifiable calcification of either aortic or mitral
valves. Mostly, this calcification is minor and of clinical significance

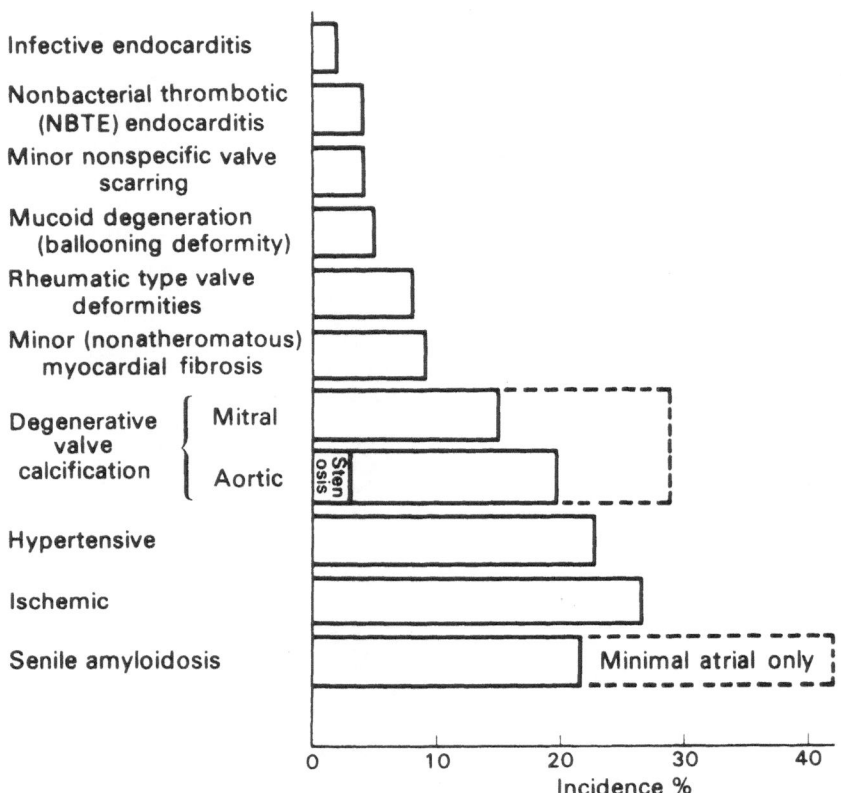

Fig. 2.10. Incidence of common types of cardiac pathology in 305 patients over 65 years of age (Northwick Park Hospital, 1972–1975).

only in generating murmurs; however, all forms of degenerative valve pathology predispose to thrombotic, and therefore to infective, endocarditis.

Aortic Sclerosis

This somewhat imprecise term has been applied to all forms of valvular thickening, from the palpable basal ridge that is almost universal by middle age to extensive calcification that is not quite sufficient to immobilize the cusps. Microscopy (Fig. 2.11) shows amorphous areas of calcification in the cusp fibrosa, usually most extensive in the basal part and not involving the free edge. This

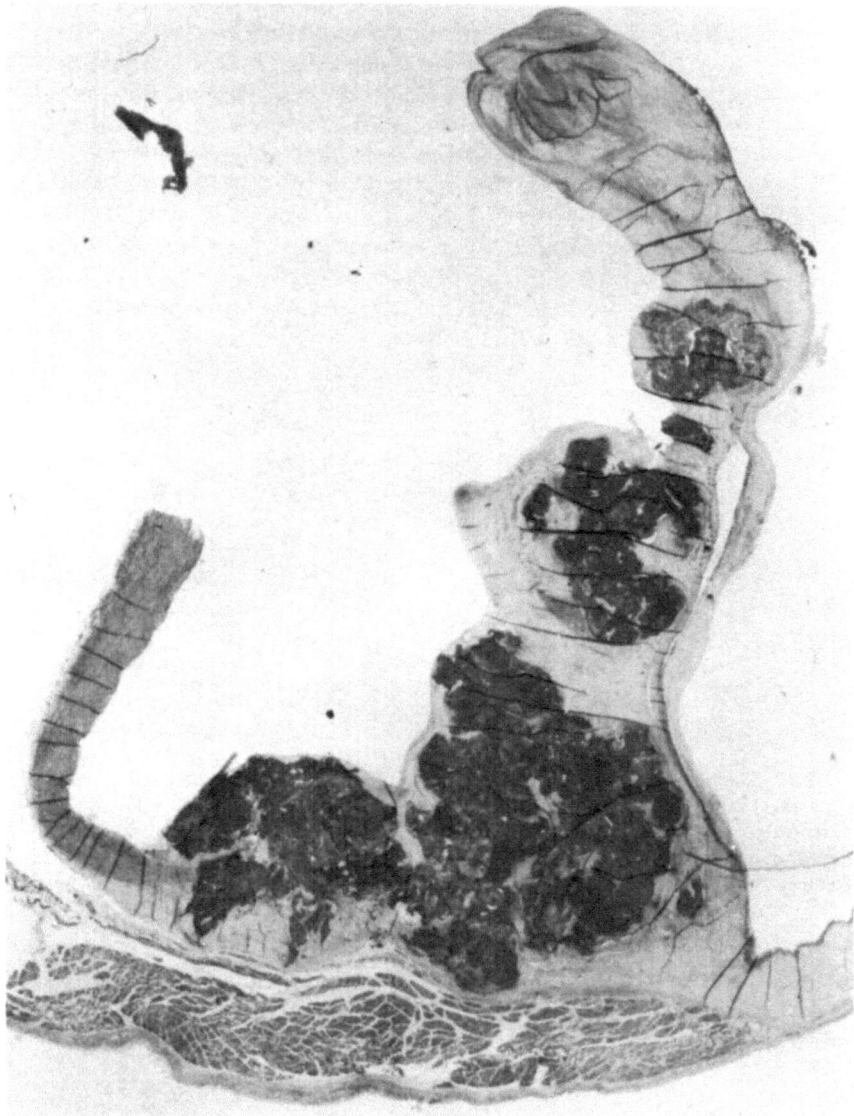

Fig. 2.11. Degenerative aortic calcification. Section through aortic cusp and base of aorta, showing nodular masses of calcification in the fibrous plate of the cusp and ulcerating into the aortic sinus.

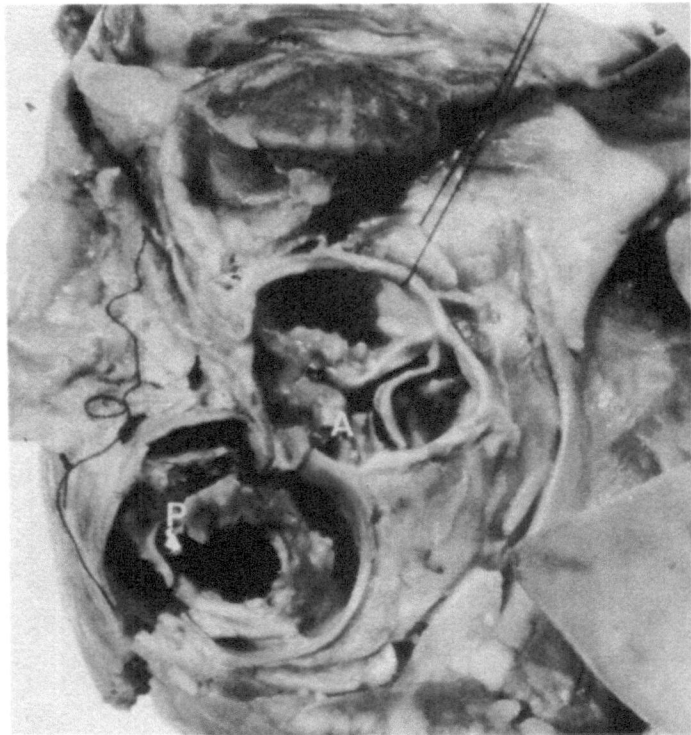

Fig. 2.12. Degenerative aortic stenosis (A). Three separate, equal-sized aortic valve cusps are present, with nodular calcification of cusps and in aortic sinuses. A mild degree of congenital pulmonary valve (P) stenosis is also present. From an 82-year-old man, known to have had heart disease since childhood. (Specimen by courtesy of Dr. R. Balcoln.)

calcification appears to be a form of dystrophic calcification, and to be related to the repeated flexion and mechanical stress of normal valve action.

Aortic Stenosis

This condition is found in about 4–6% of elderly patients (see Bedford and Caird 1960, Pomerance 1965, Pomerance and Hodkinson 1976). Mönckeberg (1904) is generally credited with the first attempt to determine its etiology. Over the next half century, a voluminous literature accumulated, in which the merits of degenerative and inflammatory etiologies were debated (see Roberts 1970), but the possible importance of the congenitally bicuspid valve was unaccountably ignored. The erroneous conclusions reached by most of the early investigators clearly arose from failure to separate isolated aortic stenosis from that associated with mitral valve disease, and from acceptance as evidence of past rheumatic carditis of lesions now recognized as nonspecific. We now know that isolated aortic stenosis may be due to degenerative calcification alone, to degenerative calcification superimposed on a congenitally bicuspid valve, or to past valvulitis, rheumatic or nonrheumatic. In individual cases, the etiology can usually be easily determined by simple inspection of the unopened valves from above, since each pathology results in a distinctive orifice shape. Stenosis due purely to degenerative calcification occurs in an otherwise normal three-cusped valve. No commissural adhesions are present, nor is cusp retraction; the orifice is

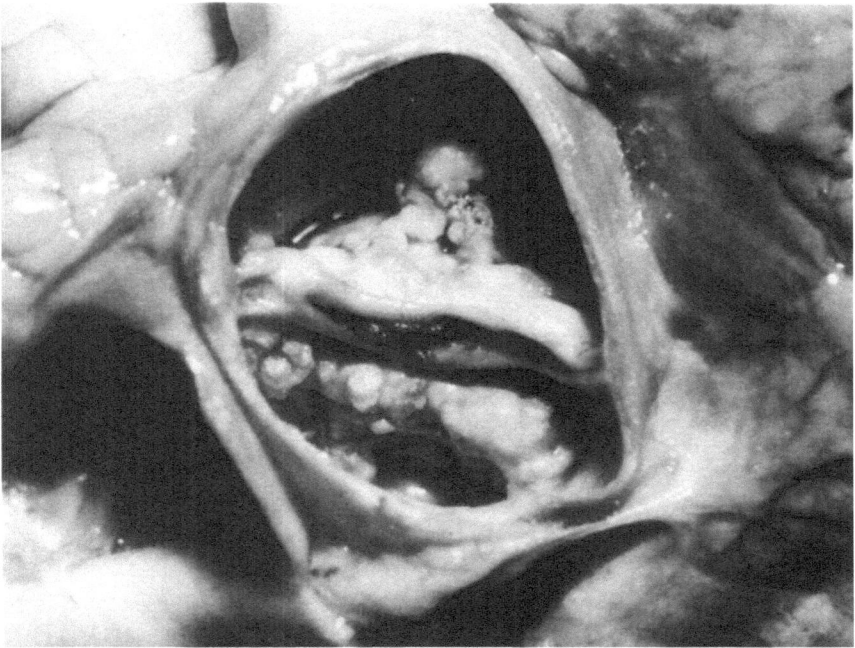

Fig. 2.13. Aortic stenosis due to degenerative calcification in a congenitally bicuspid valve. A calcified raphe divides the congenitally fused cusps (top), and the single cusp is also heavily calcified. The slitlike lumen is further obstructed by thrombotic endocarditis (NBTE).

therefore triradiate (see Fig. 2.12). This form of aortic stenosis differs only quantitatively from the calcification in aortic sclerosis, and is found only in the oldest patients. It is, however, by far the most common type in patients over 75 years of age (Pomerance 1972).

When stenosis is the result of degenerative calcification in a congenitally bicuspid valve, two almost equal-sized cusps are present (the larger having a fibrous ridge or raphe on its aortic aspect), and the orifice therefore forms a transverse or slightly crescentic slit (Fig. 2.13). The calcification is also of the same degenerative type as in the purely "senile" aortic stenosis, but has developed prematurely because of the abnormal mechanical stresses occurring in this deformity. Congenitally bicuspid valves are not inherently stenotic, and calcification is

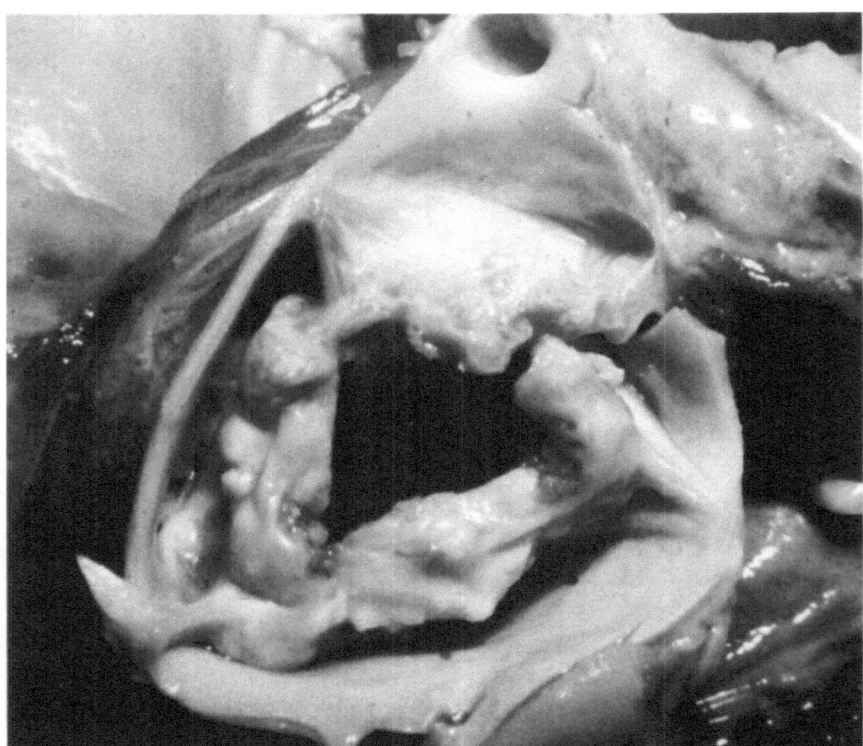

Fig. 2.14. Postinflammatory aortic stenosis. All three commissures of the originally equal-sized cusps are fused, and there is calcification of the commissures and cusp edges.

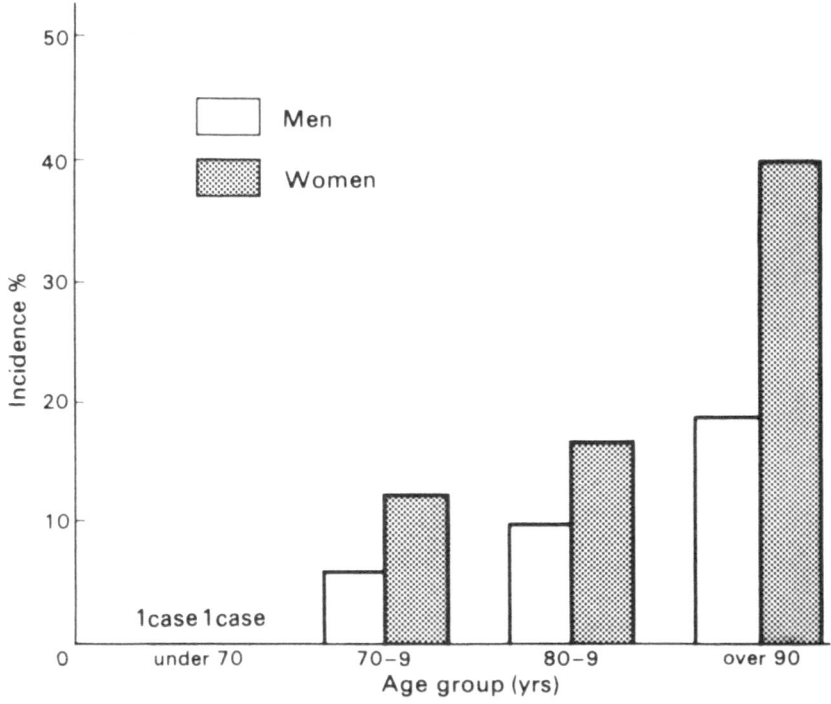

Fig. 2.15. Incidence of mitral ring calcification in relation to age (45 cases).

not invariable; uncomplicated examples are seen even in the elderly. The congenital nature of the fusion can be confirmed histologically in elastic van Gieson-stained sections. Normal valve architecture is absent from the ridge, in contrast to the picture in acquired valve fusion, where the remains of normal collagen and elastic layers are demonstrable even in heavy calcification (see Pomerance 1975 for illustrations).

In postinflammatory aortic stenosis, commissural fusion and cusp contraction have occurred in a three-cusped valve, and the orifice is therefore a central triangle or circle (Fig. 2.14). If fusion has not occurred equally at all commissures, the result is eccentric buttonhole or angled orifice, the apex of which remains approximately central. This form of stenosis is the least common type found in the elderly. The original inflammatory process may have been rheumatic, but nonrheumatic infections are more likely in the majority of cases. Isolated aortic stenosis is a well-recognized sequel of brucella and

rickettsial endocarditis (Peery 1958, Kristinsson and Bentall 1967) and
it is likely that, as in rheumatic-type mitral deformities, other cardi-
otropic infections may be implicated.

Mitral Ring Calcification

Degenerative mitral calcification occurs in the valve ring; the
cusps are involved only when calcified masses distort or ulcerate
through them.

Recognition of mitral ring calcification is generally attributed to
Dewitsky (1910). A historical review is included in the paper by Korn
et al. (1962). It is a common finding in the elderly, reported in up to
10% of autopsies on patients over 50 years of age (Pomerance 1970),
increasing sharply in frequency with increasing age (Fig. 2.15), and
much more frequent in women. Sex ratios have ranged from 2:1 to
3.5:1; all the 14 cases of clinically significant mitral ring calcification
reported by Korn et al. (1962) were women.

The degree of calcification varies from small, localized nodules or

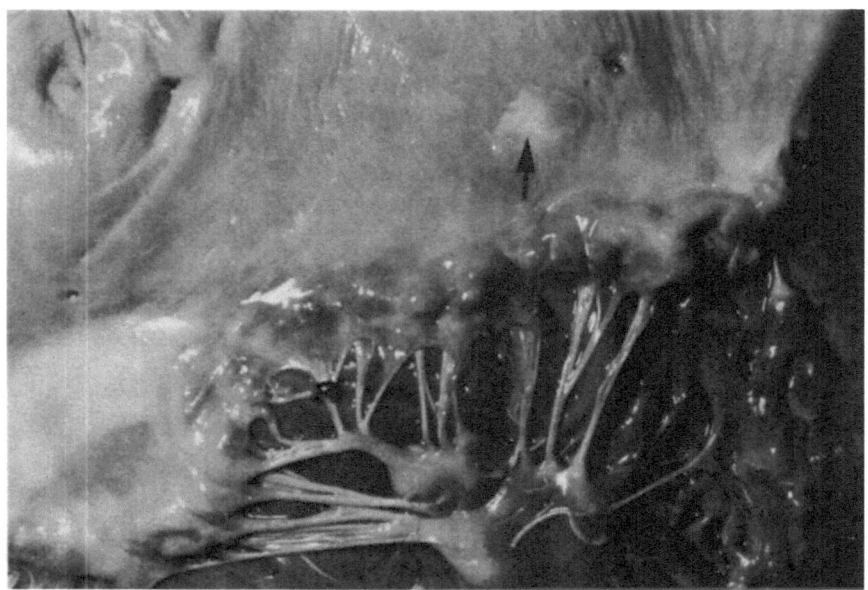

Figure 2.16. Mitral incompetence in early ring calcification. The posterior mitral cusp is
distorted by mild ring calcification, and a "jet lesion" (arrow) has formed on the
posterior atrial wall.

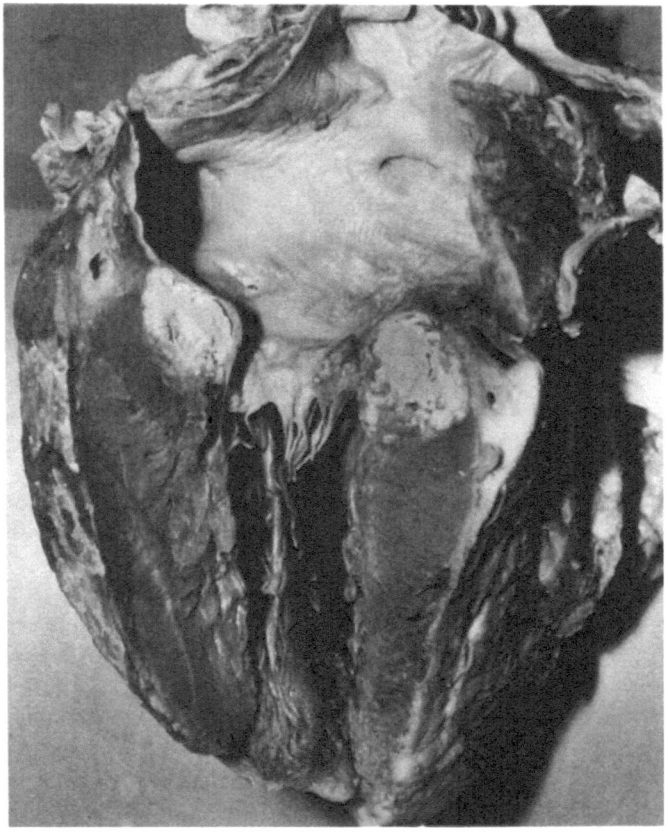

Fig. 2.17. "Caseation" in massive mitral ring calcification. Part of the posterior wall of the left atrium and ventricle have been cut away to show the large, soft, white mass involving the mitral ring and adjacent ventricular myocardium. (Specimen by courtesy of Dr. C.R. Tribe.)

spicules (Fig. 2.16) to transformation of the entire mitral ring to a rigid, calcified C-shaped bar that effectively prevents the normal systolic constriction of the mitral orifice. The earliest lesions are usually at the junction of medial commissure and ventricular wall, and in the middle of the posterior cusp attachment (Fig. 2.16). In the former site, they are in close relation to the bundle of His, and so may be associated with heart block. More extensive deposits frequently extend into the subvalve angle, often forming a prominent ridge over which the cusp is stretched and to which the chordae tendinae may

become adherent. Rarely, encroachment on the mitral orifice is sufficient to cause stenosis. Distortion and upward displacement of part of
the cusp by calcified spurs often occurs even in early or localized
calcification, and results in mitral incompetence (Fig. 2.16). Systolic
murmurs were noted in 73% of cases studied personally, and in one-
half to two-thirds of other large series (Fertman and Wolff 1946, Geill
1951, Simon and Liu 1954). Caseous softening of the calcified bar (Fig.
2.17) is not uncommon, and well-marked examples of this change may
be mistaken for tuberculomas or gummas. Calcified masses may erode
through the atrial surfaces of the valve cusps, but such erosion is
surprisingly infrequent, even with massive calcification. When it does

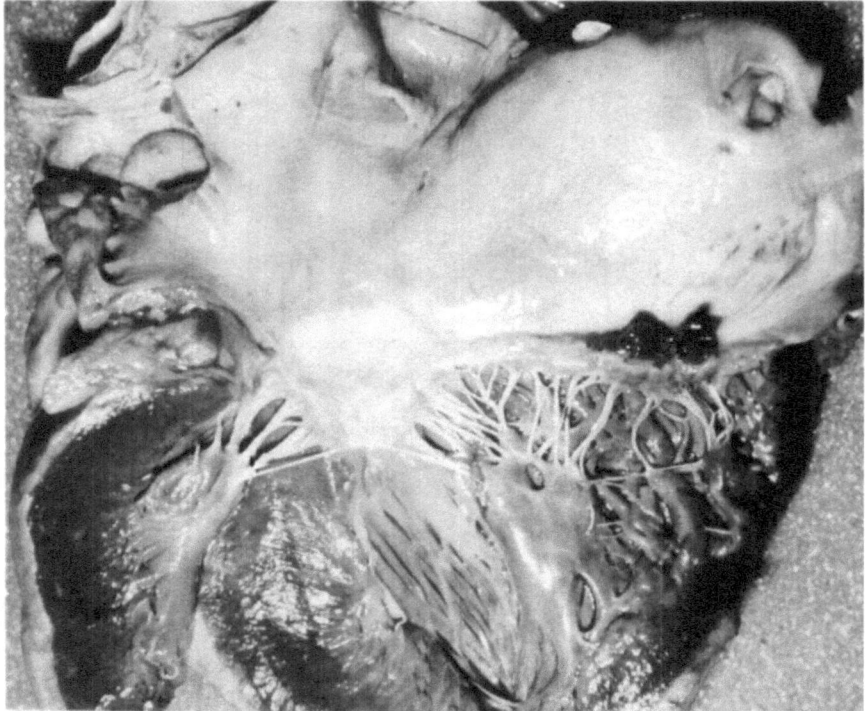

Fig. 2.18. Infective endocarditis (pneumococcal) on mitral ring calcification. The vegetations are over calcified masses extending from the ring through the atrial endocardium
of the posterior mitral cusp. From an 81-year-old woman, admitted with a clinical
diagnosis of bronchopneumonia and cerebral thrombosis. Autopsy also showed a
pneumococcal meningitis.

occur, however, the exposed masses of calcium provide sites for ready development of thrombotic vegetations and infection (Fig. 2.18).

Microscopically, the calcification appears as amorphous eosinophilic masses in decalcified sections, often with basophilic granular areas. Initially, these masses are confined to the fibrous ring, but when advanced they may extend deeply into the myocardium or into the subvalve angle. Thin-walled vessels and inflammatory cells are often seen at the margins of the calcified areas, and are not indicative of previous valvulitis. Marked inflammatory changes, foreign body giant cells, and palisaded fibroblastic reactions of "rheumatoid" type are occasionally seen, as are cartilage and bone.

The pathogenesis of mitral ring calcification seems unrelated to rheumatic fever, rheumatoid disease, or any known cardiac inflammatory process. An increased incidence has been noted in diabetes mellitus (Kirk and Russell 1969), osteitis deformans, (Harrison and Lennox 1948), and hypertension (Kirk and Russell 1969, Pomerance 1970), and the mitral ring is one of the sites affected by metastatic calcification. No abnormal calcium metabolism has been demonstrated in most cases, however, and the condition is generally accepted as an exaggeration of normal aging changes. The reason this should occur in only a minority of elderly patients and particularly in women remains obscure.

Mucoid Degeneration of Atrioventricular Valves

Recognition of this condition is comparatively recent (Fernex and Fernex 1958), and it is to be found in the literature under many names: Mucoid and myxomatous degeneration describe the microscopic features; floppy valve, the operative appearances; and ballooning, billowing, prolapse, and aneurysmal protrusion of the posterior mitral cusp, the gross pathological and cineangiographic appearances. The condition also seems to be responsible for many cases of the "late systolic murmur and click" syndrome (Jerasaty 1973).

Although the condition undoubtedly results in mitral incompetence, this incompetence is usually well tolerated, and many cases have been known to have murmurs for more than 20 years (Bittar and Sosa 1968, Davis et al. 1971, Allen et al. 1974). The disease clearly has a long natural history in the absence of complications. For most pathologists, therefore, isolated mucoid degeneration (i.e., degeneration unassociated with congenital cardiac or connective tissue disease) is mainly a disease of the elderly. The average age in 59 consecutive personally observed autopsy cases was 73.6 years. Several large clinical series

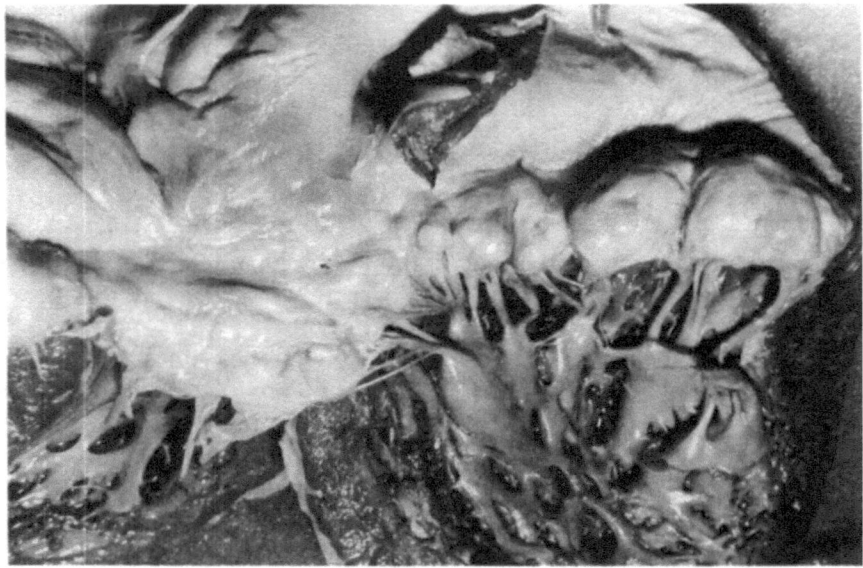

Fig. 2.19. Mucoid degeneration of mitral valve, most marked in the posterior cusp, which is expanded and resembles a partly deflated parachute or balloon. Note lack of commissural adhesions or contracted fused chordae tendinae. From a 68-year-old woman with a loud apical systolic murmur and thrill.

have now been published, but there are few pathological surveys, and the true incidence is difficult to assess. Personal experience (Pomerance 1969) and discussion with other pathologists suggest that potentially significant degrees of mucoid degeneration can be found in up to 7% of elderly hearts. Of 73 patients with mitral systolic murmurs recently reviewed, 27% showed this deformity (Denham et al. 1976).

Macroscopically (Figs. 2.19–2.22), the abnormality is usually confined to the mitral valve, the posterior cusp being affected more often and more severely than the anterior. The tricuspid valve may also be involved, but the changes are comparatively minor. The most striking feature is expansion of the affected cusp; the posterior leaflet may be up to twice the depth of the anterior, instead of the normal half to two-thirds. The cusps are voluminous, opaque, and white, resembling a partly collapsed parachute or deflated balloon. In systole they overshoot and prolapse into the atrium. Morphological evidence of mitral incompetence in the form of marked atrial dilatation and jet lesions of the atrial endocardium is often visible. The voluminous cusps are easily traumatized by normal valve movements, and small areas of ulceration and thrombus deposition on the atrial aspect are common. The chordae tendinae are long, and often taper from slightly thickened leaflet insertions. They are not fused or contracted, but may become adherent to areas of mural endocardial fibrosis that result from friction between chordae and posterior left ventricular wall when the normal anatomical relationships are altered. The combination of these

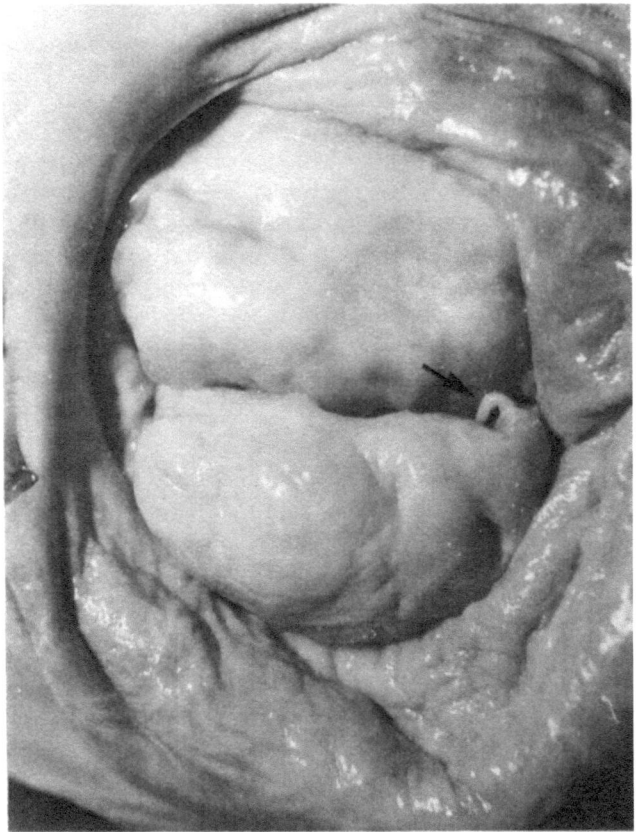

Fig. 2.20. Mucoid degeneration of mitral valve, seen from the left atrium. Both cusps are expanded, thick, and white, and prolapse into the atrial cavity. A ruptured chorda tendina can be seen (arrow). From an elderly man with "irregular heart" for 2 years, who died suddenly. Only minimal coronary atheroma was present.

friction lesions with clearly abnormal mitral cusps may lead to an erroneous diagnosis of rheumatic valve disease by those unfamiliar with mucoid degeneration. The two conditions are, however, quite distinct, both macroscopically and microscopically; the differentiating features are summarized in Table 2.1.

Microscopically, areas of loose, spongy tissue are seen replacing the normal dense collagen of the cusp fibrosa, and may also be seen in the chordae tendinae (Fig. 2.23). The anatomical layers of the cusp

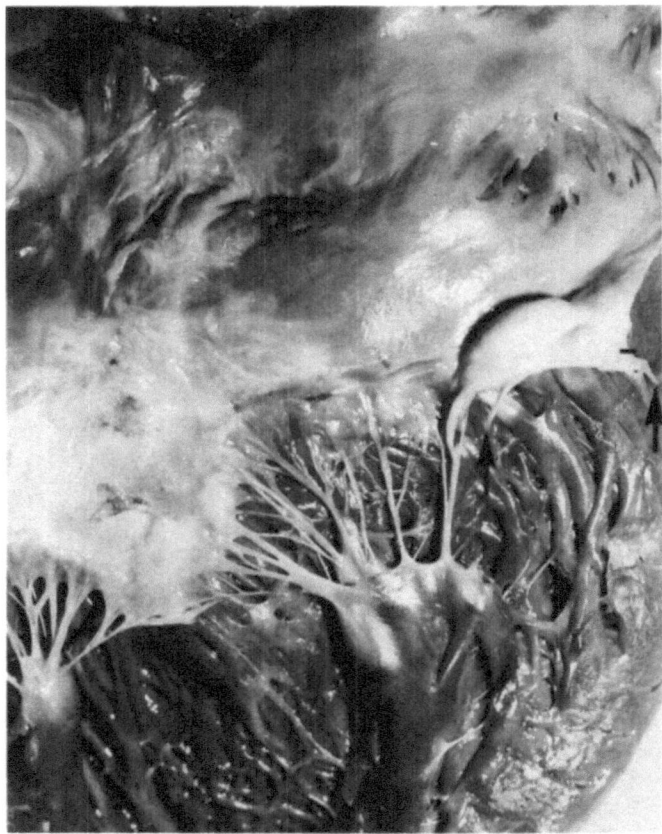

Fig. 2.21. Mucoid degeneration with rupture of chordae tendinae. The lateral half of the posterior mitral cusp shows ballooning deformity, and two chordae are ruptured (arrow). Well-marked jet lesions are present on the anterior mitral cusp and atrial septum.

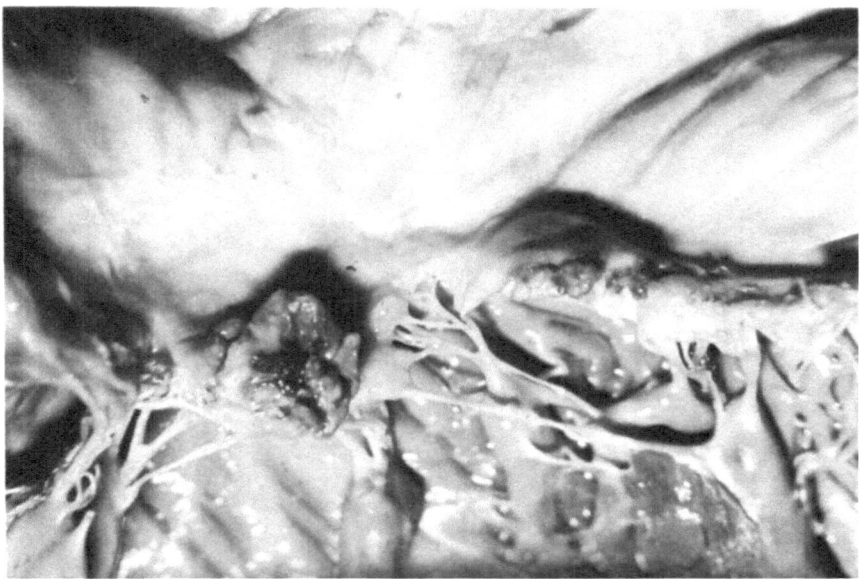

Fig. 2.22. Infective endocarditis (pyocyaneus) on mucoid degeneration. A large vegetation is present in the anterior mitral cusp, and a row of smaller vegetations on the posterior cusp, which also shows ballooning deformity. From a 73-year-old woman, admitted with congestive heart failure, a systolic murmur, and pyrexia following a dental abscess, who failed to respond to treatment.

TABLE 2.1. Features of Mucoid Degeneration Compared with Rheumatic Valve Disease

Mucoid degeneration	Chronic rheumatic valve disease
Degenerative process	Inflammatory process
Fibrosa affected only	All valve layers involved
Cusp expands (loss of density)	Cusp contracts (fibrosis following inflammation)
Commisures not adherent	Usually commissural adhesions
No calcification (apart from any coexistent mitral ring deposits)	Often calcified
Chordae thin, or showing friction changes only	Chordae usually thick, fused, contracted
Cusp anatomical layers remain distinct microscopically	Fibrous disorganization of cusp architecture microscopically
No vascularization	Vascularized cusps usual

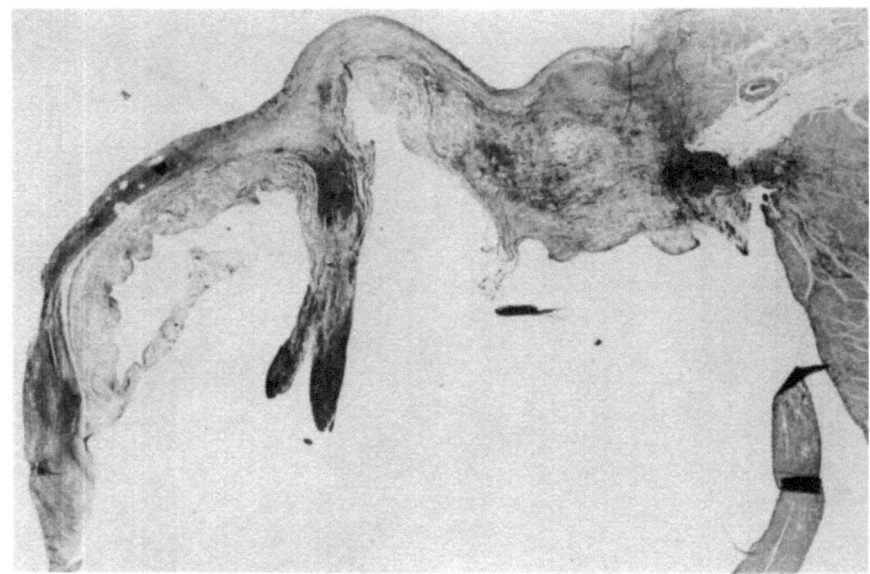

Fig. 2.23. Section through posterior mitral cusp from Fig. 17. Much of the normally dense collagen is replaced by loose connective tissue. The contrast between normal and degenerate collagen is well demonstrated in the central chorda tendina. (Hematoxylin and eosin, ×5.)

remain distinct, and there is no vascularization or other evidence of past inflammation. The loose tissue stains metachromatically, and histochemistry indicates that it is a complex mucoprotein or acid mucopolysaccharide. Ultrastructure studies have shown loss of the normal orderly arrangement and cross-banding of collagen fibers, and increased translucency of extrafibrillary ground substance (Kern and Tucker 1972). A variable, often marked degree of fibroelastic proliferation is seen on the atrial surface. Small areas of hemorrhage, ulceration, and thrombus are common, and are probably responsible for the susceptibility to infective endocarditis (Lachmann et al. 1975).

Rupture of the chordae tendinae (Figs. 2.20 and 2.21) is not uncommon, and death due to mucoid degeneration alone is usually attributable to this complication; this was the case in 8 of the 59 hearts personally examined. The exact mechanism is variable. Excessive tension resulting from the prolapse and loss of normal support from cusp apposition appears to be the only factor in some cases; in others, mucoid degeneration in the chordae is also present. The other comparatively frequent complication of mucoid degeneration is infective endocarditis (Fig. 2.22), which develops either on the affected cusps themselves or on mural or valvular jet lesions. Sudden death has also been reported in a few cases (see Jerasaty 1973), with no pathological basis for its occurrence.

The pathogenesis of mucoid degeneration is still unknown. Its

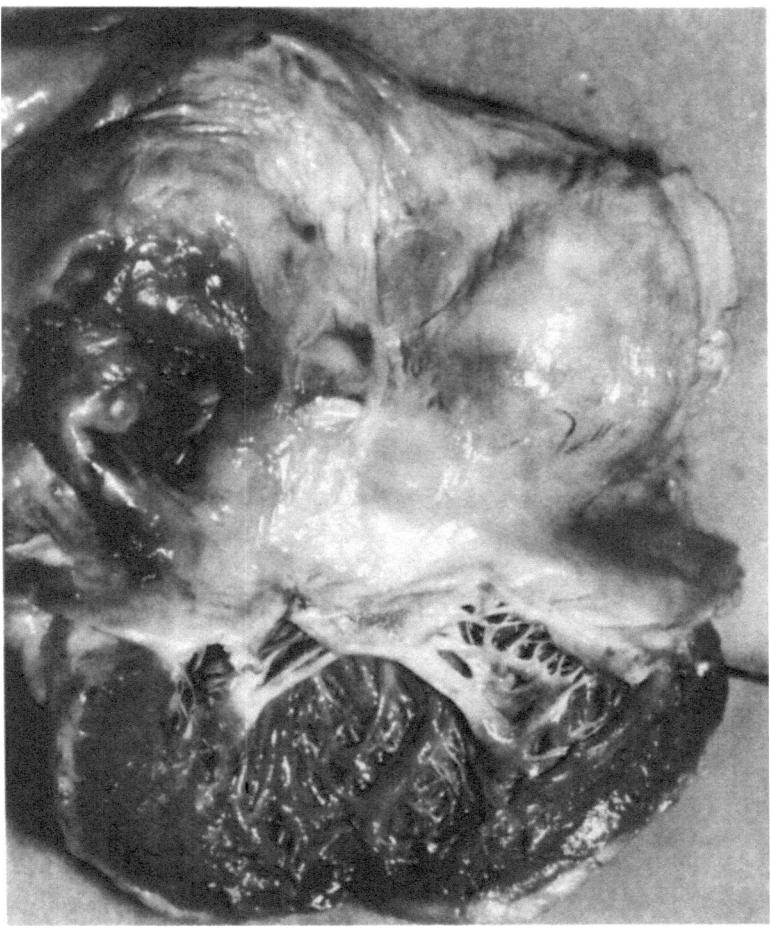

Fig. 2.24. Rheumatic mitral stenosis and incompetence. The mitral valve cusps are thick and contracted, the commissures mildly fused, and the chordae tendinae fused and contracted. Gross atrial dilatation is present. From an 85-year-old woman complaining of dysphagia and breathlessness for several years. She had chorea at 9 years of age.

similarity to the valve changes in the Marfan syndrome and occasional familial incidence in younger patients suggest that genetic factors may be concerned. The higher incidence in the elderly and the occurrence of a similar age-related lesion in dogs (see Whitney 1975) suggest that aging may be a factor. Lesser degrees of myxomatous change have been found in association with a variety of etiological processes in surgically excised valves (Kern and Tucker 1972). At present the most plausible hypothesis is that mucoid degeneration is a nonspecific change and may result from a number of causes, including aging.

Rheumatic Valve Disease

Rheumatic-type mitral deformities may be found in about 5% of elderly patients at autopsy (Bedford and Caird 1960, Pomerance 1965, Pomerance and Hodkinson 1976). The pathology does not differ fundamentally from that in younger patients, and ranges from minor cusp scarring and commissural adhesions to grossly thickened, distorted cusps with adherent, thickened, and contracted chordae tendinae (Figs. 2.24 and 2.25). Calcification is common, and usually involves the fused commissures. Microscopically, the normal valve

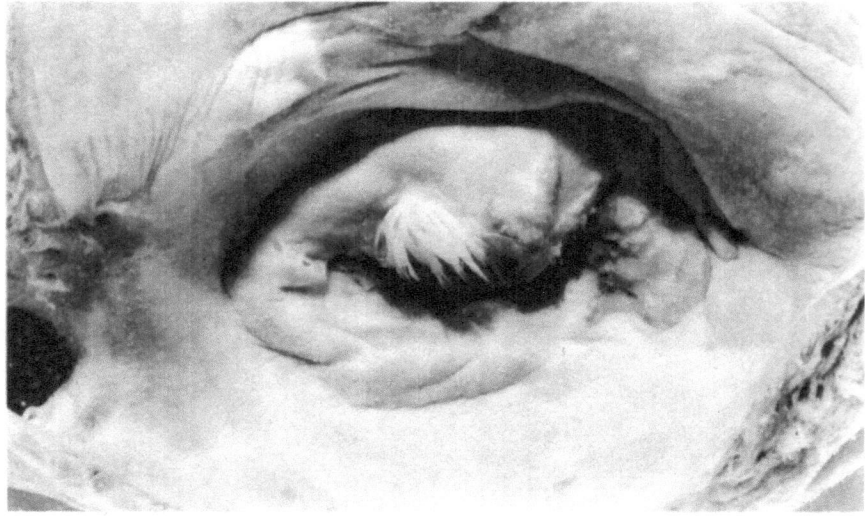

Fig. 2.25. Rheumatic mitral stenosis seen from left atrium. The commissures are fused, the anterior cusp contracted, and calcification is present in cusps and commissures. A large papillary "tumor" is present on the anterior cusp, and there are atrial jet lesions.

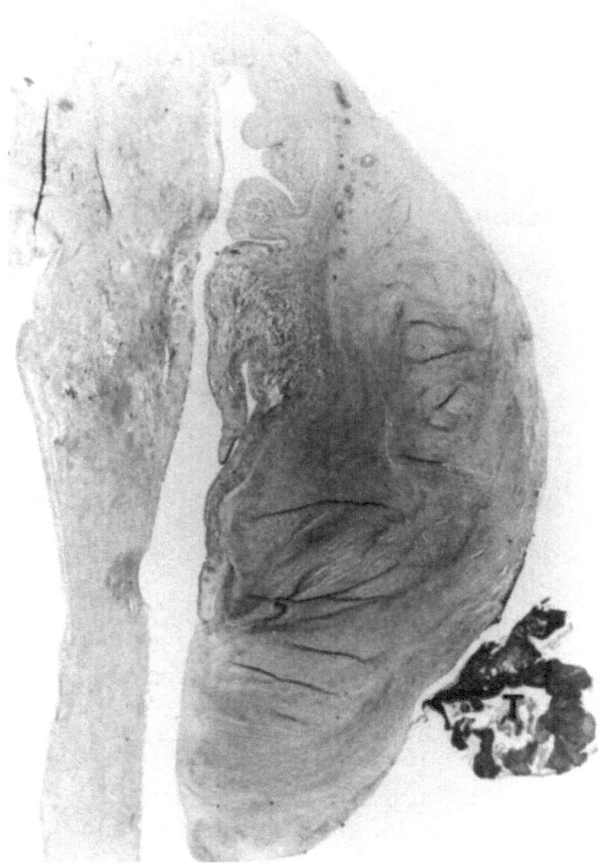

Fig. 2.26. Section of chronic rheumatic-type valve showing fibrous thickening, disorganization, and vascularization. A thrombus (T) is attached to the atrial surface. (Hematoxylin and eosin, ×10)

architecture is disorganized by irregular fibrosis affecting all layers of the cusp, and small, thick-walled vessels are usually present (Fig. 2.26). Small filiform fibroelastic structures (Lambl's excrescences) are common, and fibrin deposits in various stages of organization are generally seen on the surface. Progression of the valvular thickening and deformity is due to this continuing process of deposition of thrombus and its transformation to fibrous tissue, not to continuing inflammatory activity.

Although these macroscopic and microscopic appearances are widely accepted as pathognomonic of rheumatic valve disease, they are actually nonspecific sequelae of severe valvulitis and thrombus deposition, and their relationship to rheumatic carditis is now being increasingly questioned. It is well known that the proportion of patients with past histories of rheumatic fever is low in the elderly. A rheumatic history had been recorded in less than one-fifth of cases with rheumatic type mitral disease personally studied, and even in Bedford and Caird's (1960) careful clinical study a rheumatic history was obtained in only 38%, a similar figure to that of Limas (1972). Although poor memory may partly account for these figures, there is also increasing evidence for nonrheumatic origins in many cases. The decline in chronic rheumatic valve disease following the introduction of antibiotics has been in those cases with histories of rheumatic or scarlet fever (Vendsborg et al. 1968); those without rheumatic histories have not declined. Many infective agents are known to affect the myocardium and pericardium, and there seems to be no reason the valves should be peculiarly exempt. Indeed, routine sectioning of mitral valves from unselected autopsies not infrequently shows a mild focal valvulitis. In Britain and the U.S.A., Coxsackie B, ECHO, psittacosis, mycoplasma, and poliomyelitis are the most likely etiological agents (Lancet 1971, Burch et al. 1970), and all have been demonstrated in excised deformed valves (Ward and Ward 1974).

Infective Endocarditis

Following the introduction of antibiotics and the declining incidence of rheumatic fever, infective endocarditis has changed from a disease predominantly of young adults with rheumatic heart disease and is increasingly becoming a disease of elderly patients with no known previous valve pathology (Hughes and Gauld 1966, Lerner and Weinstein 1966, Lancet 1971, Applefeld and Hornick 1974, Thell et al. 1975). The changing pattern is due not only to antibiotics, but also to the survival of increasing numbers of patients to ages at which degenerative valve abnormalities and urogenital, biliary and gastrointestinal, and pulmonary diseases become common, and diagnostic and surgical procedures provoke bacteremia.

Figures for the incidence of infective endocarditis vary with the date of a study and the type of material. Reviews based on autopsies will inevitably include a greater proportion of elderly patients. Even with a high index of clinical suspicion, atypical presentation is likely to delay or obscure the diagnosis, and the infecting organism in this age group is likely to be a virulent one.

In the elderly, the organism is most likely to be a staphylococcus or enterococcus, although *Streptococcus viridans* is still isolated in a high proportion of cases. Fungal infections are increasing in frequency, usually associated with steroid therapy, long-term antibiotics, or treatment of malignant disease. In many cases, blood cultures are negative. The negative finding is often due to prior antibiotics, but uremia, prolonged infection, or inadequate bacteriological techniques may also be responsible (Tumulty 1967, Shinebourne et al. 1969).

Grossly, the characteristic pathological features are the vegetations, which consist of nodular masses of fibrin and red blood cells with varying numbers of inflammatory cells and microorganisms. They are usually found on the atrial surfaces of the mitral valve and the ventricular surfaces of aortic valves, along the lines of closure. Vegetations may also form on the mural endocardium at sites of jet

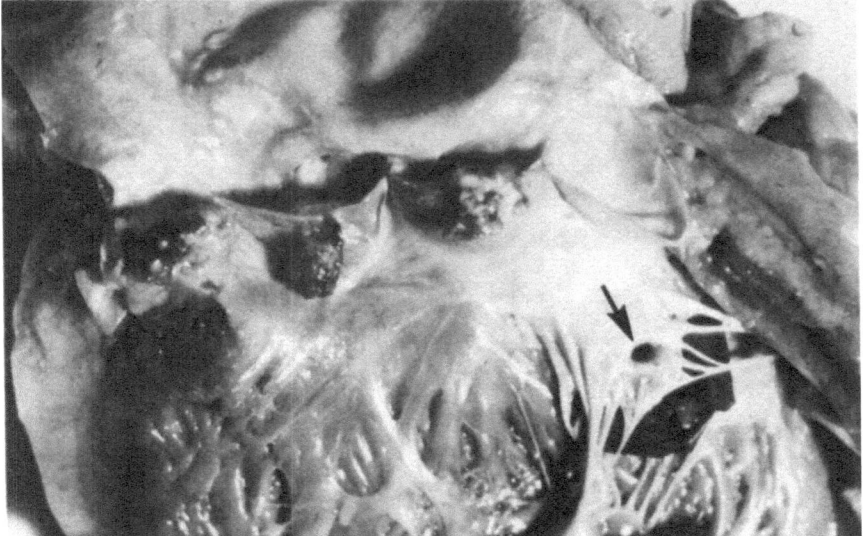

Fig. 2.27. Infective endocarditis (Staphylococcal) on previously normal valves. Vegetations are seen on the ventricular surfaces of three aortic cusps, and there is a perforation (arrow) through the anterior mitral cusp under a further vegetation. From a 76-year-old woman admitted in congestive cardiac failure with a pansystolic murmur, bundle branch block, but no pyrexia.

lesions. Endocarditis affecting the right side of the heart is uncommon in the elderly. The vegetations vary in size from pinhead to large friable masses almost obstructing the orifices. Very large vegetations are characteristic of fungal infections. Marked inflammatory changes and necrosis of the underlying valve are often present, and perforations of the cusps are not uncommon (Figs. 2.27 and 2.28). These findings are most often associated with *Staphylococcus pyogenes* and pneumococcal infections. Rupture of the chordae tendinae occurs if they become involved in the inflammatory process, and extension of infection into the valve rings will result in abscesses of the rings (Sheldon and Golden 1951) (Fig. 2.28). The myocardium frequently contains abscesses ranging from microscopic to several centimeters in diameter (Perry et al. 1952). Involvement of fibrous rings or upper interventricular septum is likely to result in heart block.

Infection may develop on rheumatic-type deformities, as in younger patients (Fig. 2.28), or on degenerative valve pathology (see Figs. 2.18 and 2.22), but most often no preceding abnormality is found (Pankey 1962, Uwaydah and Weinberg 1965, Burnside and De Sanctis

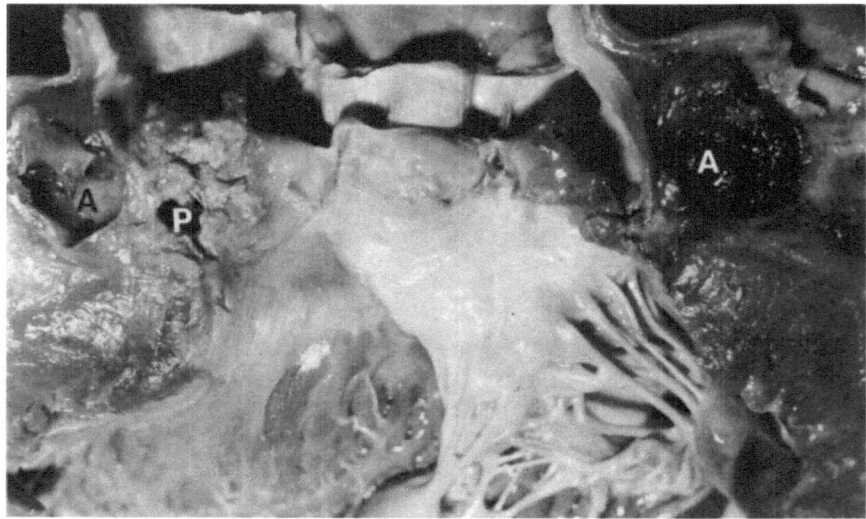

Fig. 2.28. Staphylococcal endocarditis on chronic rheumatic heart disease. There is a perforation (P) through an aortic cusp, and an abscess (A) of the aortic ring. There is moderate thickening and contraction of aortic and mitral cusps. From a 72-year-old woman with rheumatic fever in childhood and typical clinical signs of infective endocarditis.

1972, Applefeld and Hornick 1974, Thell et al. 1975). In 19 cases of bacterial endocarditis in patients over 65 examined personally, 3 had developed on rheumatic-type deformities, 4 on mitral ring calcification, and 3 on mucoid degeneration; 9 had apparently previously normal cusps. Minor postinflammatory changes can often be seen on careful inspection of infected valves, and it is possible that such changes may have been present but destroyed or overlooked in some valves described as normal. Even allowing for this possibility and the probability that mucoid degeneration was unrecognized in early studies, however, infective endocarditis in the elderly undoubtedly does arise on previously normal cusps in many cases. In such cases, present evidence suggests that predisposing valve pathology resulted from stress. Valvular swelling and edema can be induced experimentally by various stimuli, including surgery, infections, and hormones (Oka et al. 1968). Similar lesions can often be seen, as minute translucent nodules along the closure lines, on the mitral and aortic valves of patients dying in the hospital. The endocardium over these valves is easily damaged, and small nonbacterial thrombi form on the damaged areas. If bacteremia occurs, the thrombi are colonized and develop into bacterial vegetations. These stages in the evolution of infective endocarditis can also be observed in human valves.

Nonbacterial Thrombotic Endocarditis (NBTE)

This condition also appears in the literature as terminal, malignant, or marantic endocarditis; thrombendocardiosis; and degenerative verrucal endocardiosis. It is a frequent finding in the elderly because of its association with disseminated malignancy and other wasting diseases. It has most often been found in carcinoma of the pancreas, stomach, and lung (see Pomerance 1975 for detailed references).

Like infective endocarditis, NBTE is characterized pathologically by vegetations on the lines of closure of the mitral and aortic cusps (Fig. 2.29). These vary in size, color, and consistency, and are macroscopically indistinguishable from infective vegetations. Microscopically, they differ in that microorganisms and inflammatory reaction are absent. Vegetations are often endothelialized, and organization and calcification are occasionally seen. Minor postinflammatory scarring and rheumatic-type deformities are often present in the underlying valve; the reported incidence has ranged up to 85% (Eliakim and Pinchas 1966).

In most elderly patients, NBTE is a clinically unimportant aspect

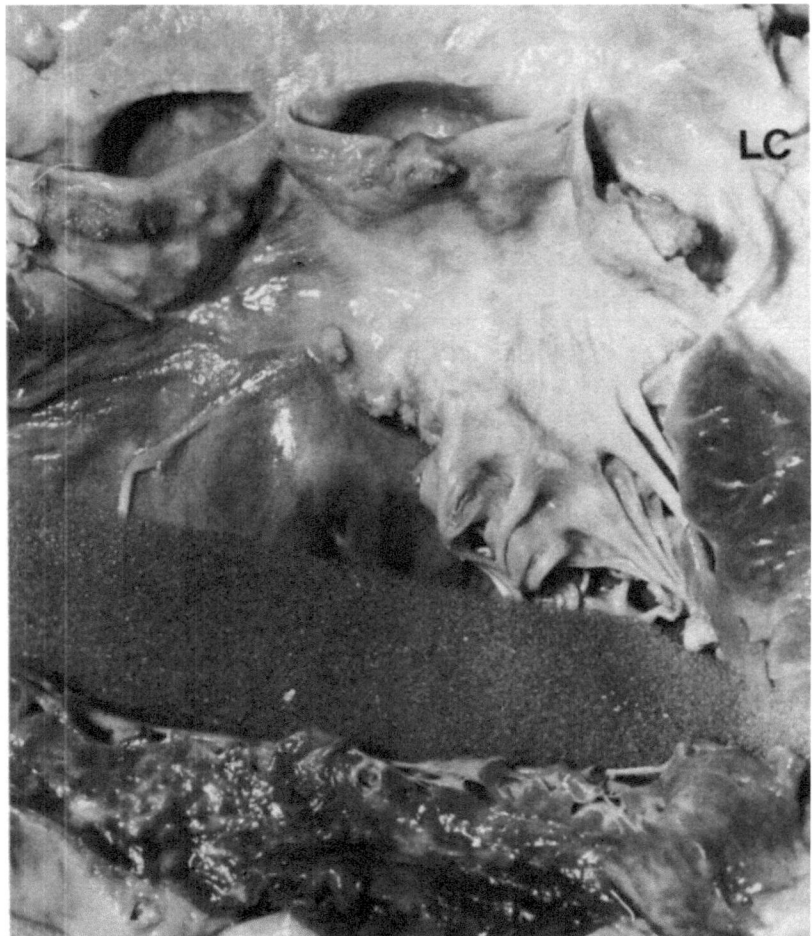

Fig. 2.29. Thrombotic endocarditis with multiple small myocardial infarcts. Thrombotic vegetations are present on the ventricular surfaces of all aortic cusps and on the aortic surface of the left coronary cusp (cut) LC, left coronary ostium. Multiple small areas of infarction are visible in the slice of left ventricle below. Marked degenerative valve calcification is distorting the aortic cusps and is seen in the mitral valve ring.

of terminal disease. Systemic emboli are common, however, and have been found in between 14 and 60% of reported series. The spleen, kidney, and brain are the organs most often affected, and NBTE is an important cause of cerebral symptoms in patients with malignant disease; indeed, its signs may be the first signs of carcinoma (Ashenhurst and Chertkow 1962, Bryan 1969). Coronary emboli are also frequent (Fig. 2.29), but as in infective endocarditis, macroscopic myocardial infarction can rarely be seen.

Valvular Pathology in Systemic Diseases and Isolated Aortic Incompetence

Rheumatoid Disease. In this disease, the heart valves, and in particular the aortic valve, are among the extraarticular sites affected (Fig. 2.30). Rheumatoid granulomas develop in the fibrous core and progress to fibrous thickening and contraction of the cusp (Carpenter et al. 1967). Thrombi are not a feature of the active lesion; thus, no commissural adhesions are formed, and functionally there is pure aortic incompetence.

Rarer collagen diseases with valvular involvement are ankylosing spondylitis (Graham and Smythe 1958, Bulkley and Roberts 1973) and Reiter's disease (Paulus et al. 1972). The aortic incompetence that may develop in both these conditions is due to degenerative changes in the aortic media; the valvular changes are secondary to the resulting dilatation of the aortic ring. The aortic valve cusps appear opaque and

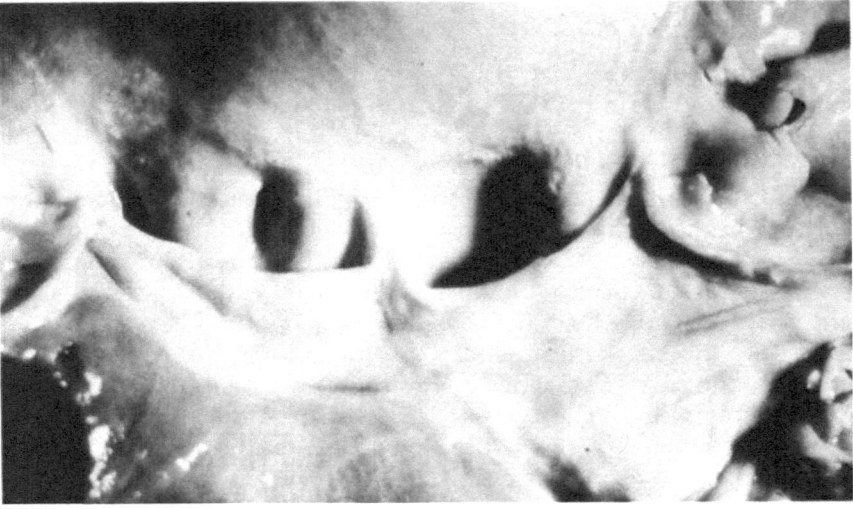

Fig. 2.30. Rheumatoid aortic incompetence. The aortic valve cusps are thickened and contracted, but without commissural adhesions. From a 67-year-old woman with severe rheumatoid disease who died of phenacetin nephropathy.

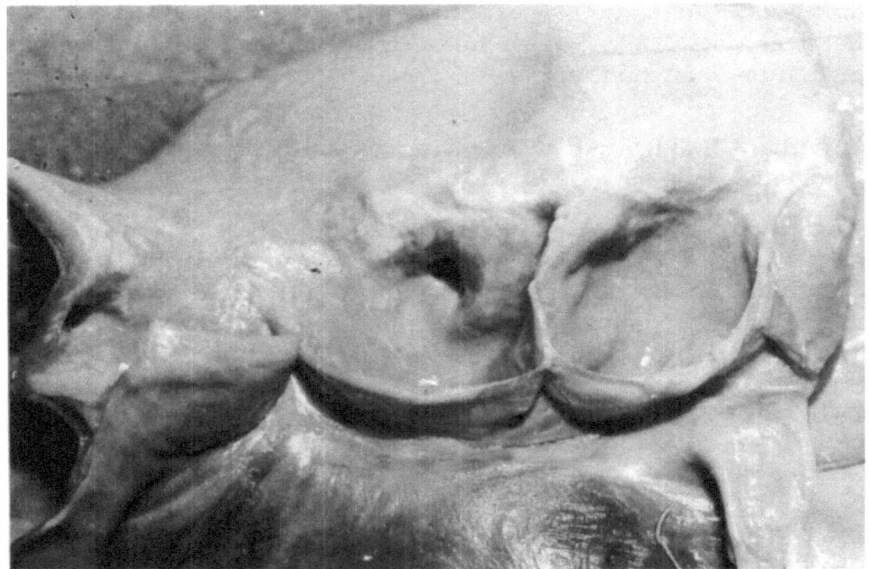

Fig. 2.31. Isolated aortic incompetence. The aorta and particularly the aortic sinuses are dilated, and the cusps show cordlike thickening of the free edges. From a woman of 77 known to have had aortic incompetence for 5 years.

contracted, the commissures are widened, and the free edges of the cusps show narrow cordlike thickening. Macroscopically and microscopically, the features closely resemble those of syphilitic aortitis, with endarteritis of vasa vasorum, focal fibrous scarring of aortic media, and superficial fibroelastic thickening without inflammatory changes in the aortic valve cusps.

Syphilitic Aortic Incompetence is now rare even in the elderly. The classic retracted cusps with rolled edges and widened commissures are now recognized as nonspecific changes—the first two merely reflecting the mechanical effects of dilatation of the ring, which stretches the cusps and allows the free edges to be traumatized by the regurgitant stream. The appearances once regarded as diagnostic of syphilis are more likely to be seen today in the collagen diseases described above or in nonspecific aortopathy.

Less extreme forms of the same valve pathology may be seen in the isolated aortic incompetence of the elderly (Fig. 2.31). This incompetence now seems to be a comparatively uncommon finding. It was found in less than 1% of approximately 300 geriatric autopsies reviewed over the past 5 years (Pomerance et al. 1976), in contrast to the 4.4% incidence in Bedford and Caird's study (1960). The underlying aortic pathology is probably multifactorial. In many cases, the aorta shows no distinctive features macroscopically, and the incompetence appears to be due to hypertension and dilatation of the aortic ring with aging (Gouley and Sickel 1943). Microscopically, there is only minor focal loss of elastica and small areas of cystic change. Other cases may show varying and sometimes extensive focal destruction and fibrous replacement of media, but without vasa vasorum changes (Fig. 2.32). Rarely, cystic medionecrosis and localized dissection involving the aortic ring may be responsible.

Uncommon Valve Abnormalities

Carcinoid Heart Disease affects the right-sided heart valves, which are thickened and contracted, with resulting stenosis and incompetence. Fibrous plaques may also be present in the right atrium and

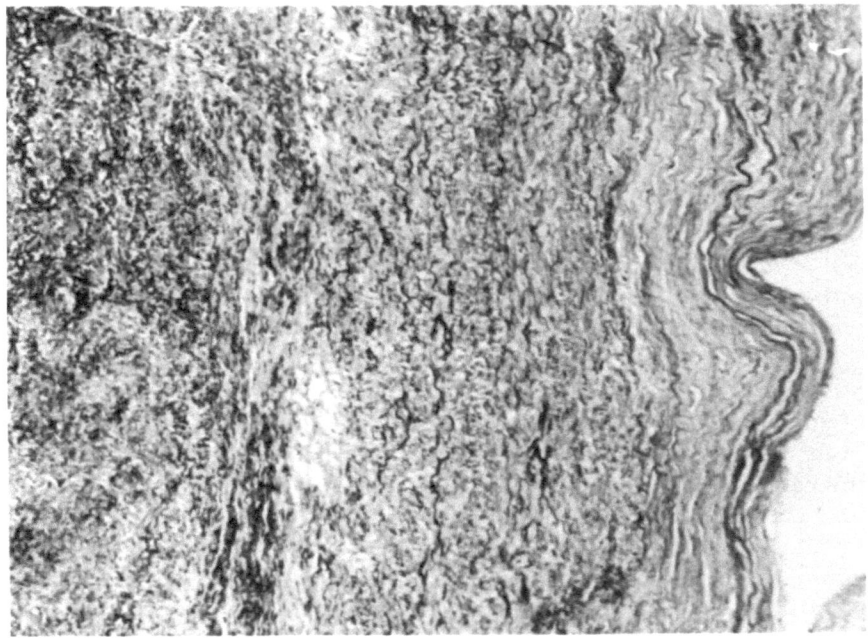

Fig. 2.32. Section of aorta from Fig. 2.31, showing fragmentation and destruction of elastic and small fibrous scars in aortic media. (hematoxylin and eosin, ×36)

extending on to the ventricular endocardium from the involved valve cusps. The microscopic appearances are distinctive, consisting of loose connective tissue applied to the surface of the affected cusps, from which it is sharply demarcated.

Papillary Endocardial Tumors (see Fig. 2.25) may be found on any valve, but are most commonly found on the aortic and mitral cusps. Reported cases and those seen personally have been mainly in elderly patients (Pomerance 1961, Nasser and Parker 1971). They are related to the filiform excrescences present on almost all elderly or damaged valves and are not true neoplasms. They are a common finding, but most examples are less than 2 mm in diameter; only occasionally do they reach 1 cm or larger. Most of these lesions are of no clinical importance, but occasionally they may be responsible for angina or sources of embolism.

Isolated Valvular Amyloid is a rare but striking pathological curiosity. Two of the three cases studied personally and the single recently reported case (Jacobovitz and Dustin 1974) were in patients over 70 years of age. The condition seems to be of no apparent clinical significance. The deposits are limited to the valve, appearing as nodular masses distorting the cusps, which are translucent on section.

Prosthetic Valve Pathology

With recent advances in cardiac surgery, increasing numbers of patients with prosthetic valves are reaching the geriatric age group; valve replacement in patients over 65 years of age is now also a common procedure. In this age group, the replacement valve is likely to be of the ball or disc-and-cage type, the main late complications of which are infection, thrombosis, and mechanical dysfunction.

Infective endocarditis in general has already been discussed. The artificial valve is a foreign body and thus predisposes to infection. The organism is often a fungus. Pathological examination shows thrombotic masses, usually growing on the margins of the ring or struts of the cage; histology shows that these masses contain microorganisms.

Thrombosis may occur on any type of prosthetic valve, and may result in emboli to the brain or the coronary circulation. Large amounts of thrombus may impede ball or disc movement, causing stenosis; rarely, the whole valve orifice becomes occluded by a pannus of thrombus. The recent introduction of cloth-covered prostheses has reduced the incidence of thrombosis.

Mechanical dysfunction can result from wear of the ball or disc, which may jam in either the open or the closed position, shrink, or fragment, with consequent sudden stenosis or incompetence. These complications are also becoming less frequent with continuing developments in prosthetic valve design.

ACKNOWLEDGMENTS

   The recent clinicopathological data included in this chapter were obtained from studies carried out with Drs. H. M. Hodkinson and M. J. Denham, geriatrics physicians at Northwick Park Hospital, who were financed by the British Heart Foundation.

References

Allen, H., Harris, A., and Leatham, A. (1974) *Br. Heart J.* **36**, 525.
Applefeld, M. M., and Hornick, R. B. (1974) *Am. Heart J.* **88**, 90.
Ashenhurst, E. M., and Chertkow, G. (1962) *Can. Med. Assoc. J.* **86**, 313.
Bedford, P. D., and Caird, F. I. (1960) *Valvular Disease of the Heart in Old Age*, J. A. Churchill, London.
Bittar, N., and Sosa, J. A. (1968) *Circulation* **38**, 763.
British Medical Journal (1971) **2**, 544.
Bryan, C. S. (1969) *Am. J. Med.* **46**, 787.
Bulkley, B. H., and Roberts, W. C. (1973) *Circulation* **48**, 1014.
Burch, G. E., Giles, T. D., and Colcolough, H. L. (1970) *Am. Heart J.* **80**, 556.
Burnside, J. W., and DeSanctis, R. W. (1972) *Ann. Intern. Med.* **76**, 615.
Carpenter, D. F., Golden, A., and Roberts, W. C. (1967) *Am. J. Med.* **43**, 922.
Davies, M. J. (1975) In Pomerance, A., and Davies, M. J. (eds.), *Pathology of the Heart*, Blackwell's Scientific Publications, Oxford and Edinburgh, pp. 413, 414.
Davies, M. J., and Pomerance, A. (1972) *Br. Heart J.* **34**, 150.
Davis, R. H., Schuster, B., Knoebel, S. B., and Fisch C. (1971) *Am. J. Cardiol.* **28**, 449.
Denham, M. J., Pomerance, A., and Hodkinson, H. M. (1976) *Postgrad. Med. J.* (in press).
Dewitsky, W. (1910) *Virchows Arch. Pathol. Anat. Physiol.* **199**, 273.
Di Giorgio, A. J. (1973) *Geriatrics* **28**, 131.
Eliakim, M., and Pinchas, S. (1966) *Isr. J. Med. Sci.* **2**, 42.
Fertman, M. H., and Wolff, L. (1946) *Am. Heart J.* **31**, 580.
Fernex, P. M., and Fernex, C. (1958) *Helv. Med. Acta* **25**, 694.
Fontana, R. S., and Edwards, J. E. (1962) *Congenital Cardiac Disease: A Review of 357 Cases Studied Pathologically*, W. B. Saunders Co.
Franklin, E. C., and Zucker-Franklin, D. (1972) *Adv. Immunol.* **15**, 249.
Geill, T. (1951) *Gerontologia* **6**, 327.
Gjol N. (1972) *Geriatrics* **27**, 126.
Glenner, G. G., Terry, W. D., and Isersky, C. (1973) *Semin. Hematol.* **10**, 1, 15.
Gore, I., and Saphir, O. (1947) *Am. Heart J.* **34**, 827.

Gouley, B. A., and Sickel, E. M. (1943) *Am. Heart J.* **26**, 24.

Graham, D. C., and Smythe, H. A. (1958) *Bull. Rheum. Dis.* **9**, 171.

Harrison, C. V., and Lennox, B. (1948) *Br. Heart J.* **10**, 167.

Haust, M. D., Rowlands, D. T., Garancis, J. C., and Landing, B. H. (1962) *Am. J. Pathol.* **40**, 185.

Hodkinson, H. M., and Pomerances, A. (1974) *Age and Ageing* **3**, 76.

Hodkinson, H. M., and Pomerance, A. (1976) (in preparation).

Hudson, R. E. B. (1965) *Cardiovasc. Pathol.* **2**, 1566.

Hudson, R. E. B. (1970) *Cardiovasc. Pathol.* **3**.

Hughes, P., and Gault, W. R. (1966) *Q. J. Med.* **35**, 511.

Jacobovitz, D., and Dustin, P. (1974) *J. Pathol.* **112**, 195.

Jeresaty, R. M. (1973) *Prog. Cardiovasc. Dis.* **15**, 623.

Kern, W. H., and Tucker, B. L. (1972) *Am. Heart J.* **84**, 294.

Kirk, R. S., and Russell, J. G. B. (1969) *Br. Heart J.* **31**, 684.

Kline, I. K. Kline, T. S., and Saphir, O. (1962) *Am. Heart J.* **65**, 446.

Korn, D., DeSanctis, R. W., and Sell, S. (1962) *N. Engl. J. Med.* **267**, 900.

Kristinsson, B., and Bentall, H. H. (1967) *Lancet* **2**, 693.

Lachman, A. S., Bramwell Jones, D. M., Lakier, J. B., Pocock, W. A., and Barlow, J. B. (1975) *Br. Heart J.* **37**, 326.

Lancet (1971) **1**, 897.

Lerner, P. I., and Weinstein, L. (1966) *N. Engl. J. Med.* **274**, 199, 259, 323, 388.

Limas, C. J. (1971) *Acta Cardiol. (Brux)* **26**, 249.

Limas, C. J. (1972) *Mod. Geriatrics* **2**, 165.

Linzbach, A. J., and Akuamoa-Boateng, E. (1973) *Klin. Wochenschr.* **51**, 164.

London, R. E., and London, S. B. (1965) *Circulation* **31**, 202.

McMillan, J. B., and Lev, M. (1959) *J. Gerontol.* **14**, 268.

McMillan, J. B., and Lev, M. (1962) *In* Shock, N. (ed.), *Biological Aspects of Ageing*, Columbia University Press.

McMillan, J. B., and Lev, B. (1964) *J. Gerontol.* **19**, 1.

Mönckeberg, J. G. (1904) *Virchows Arch. Pathol. Anat. Physiol.* **176**, 472.

Nassar, S. G. A., and Parker, J. C. (1971) *Arch. Pathol.* **92**, 370.

Oka, M., Belenky, D., Brodie, S., and Angrist, A. (1968) *Lab. Invest.* **19**, 113.

Page, D. L. (1970) *Hum. Pathol.* **1**, 151.

Pankey, G. A. (1962) *Am. Heart J.* **64**, 583.

Paulus, H. E., Pearson, C. M., and Pitts, W. (1972) *Am. J. Med.* **53**, 464.

Peery, T. M. (1958) *J. Am. Med. Assoc.* **166**, 1123.

Perloff, J. K., and Lindgren, K. M. (1974a) *Geriatrics* **29** (April), 94.

Perloff, J. K., and Lindgren, K. M. (1974b) *Geriatrics* **29** (August), 93.

Perry, E. L., Fleming, R. G., and Edwards, J. E. (1952) *Ann. Intern. Med.* **36**, 126.

Pomerance, A. (1961) *J. Pathol. Bacteriol.* **81**, 135.

Pomerance, A. (1965) *Br. Heart J.* **27**, 697.

Pomerance, A. (1967) *Br. Heart J.* **29**, 222.

Pomerance, A. (1969) *Br. Heart J.* **31**, 343.

Pomerance, A. (1970) *J. Clin. Pathol.* **23**, 354.

Pomerance, A. (1972) *Br. Heart J.* **34**, 569.

Pomerance, A. (1975a) *In* Pomerance, A., and Davies, M. J. (eds.), *Pathology of the Heart*, Blackwell Scientific Publications, Oxford and Edinburgh, pp. 359, 360.

Pomerance, A. (1975b) *Idem*, pp. 331, 334.

Pomerance, A. and Davies, M. J. (1975) *Br. Heart J.* **37**, 305.

Pomerance, A., and Hodkinson, H. M. (1976) (in preparation).

Pomerance, A., Slavin, G., and McWatt, J. (1976) *J. Clin. Pathol.* **29,** 22.

Roberts, W. C. (1970) *Am. J. Med.* **49,** 151.

Roberts, W. C., and Ferrans, V. J. (1975) *Hum. Pathol.* **6,** 287.

Robertson, W. B., and Strong, J. P. (1968) *Lab. Invest.* **18,** 538.

Rosai, J., and Lascano, E. J. (1970) *Am. J. Pathol.* **61,** 99.

Rosenthal, C. J., and Franklin, E. C. (1975) *J. Clin. Invest.* **55,** 746.

Salyer, W. R., and Hutchins, G. M. (1974) *Arch. Intern. Med.* **134,** 250.

Schenk, E. A., and Cohen, J. (1970) *Pathol. Microbiol.* **35,** 96.

Schwartz, P. (1970) Amyloidosis—*Cause and Manifestation of Senile Deterioration,* Ch. C. Thomas, Springfield.

Schwartz, C. J., and Mitchell, J. R. A. (1962) *Br. Heart J.* **24,** 761.

Sell, S., and Scully, R. E. (1965) *Am. J. Pathol.* **46,** 345.

Serentha, P., Baldoni, E., Bratina, G., and Galetti, G. (1973) *Gerontologia* **21,** 496.

Sheldon, W. H., and Golden, A. (1951) *Circulation* **4,** 1.

Shinebourne, E. A., Cripps, M. M., Hayward, G. W., and Shooter, R. A. (1969) *Br. Heart J.* **31,** 536.

Sievers, J. (1966) *Geriatrics* **21,** 125.

Simon, M. A., and Liu, S. F. (1954) *Am. Heart J.* **48,** 497.

Soyka, J. (1876) *Prager Med. Wochenschr.* **1,** 165.

Strehler, B. L., Mark, D. D., Mildvan, S. A., and Gee, M. V. (1959) *J. Gerontol.* **14,** 430.

Thell, R., Martin, F. H., and Edwards, J. E. (1975) *Circulation* **51,** 174.

Thung, P. J. (1957) *Gerontologia (Basel)* **1,** 234.

Tumulty, P. A. (1967) *Geriatrics* **22,** 122.

Uwaydah, M. M., and Weinberg, A. N. (1965) *N. Engl. J. Med.* **273,** 1321.

Van Tassel, R. A., and Edwards, J. E. (1972) *Chest* **61,** 104.

Vendsborg, P., Hansen, L. F., and Olesen, K. H. (1968) *Cardiologia (Basel)* **53,** 332.

Walford, R. L. (1969) *The Immunologic Theory of Ageing,* Munksgaard, Copenhagen.

Ward, C., and Ward, A. M. (1974) *Lancet* **1,** 755.

Whiting, R. B., Powell, W. J., Dinsmore, R. E., and Sanders, C. A. (1971) *N. Engl. J. Med.* **285,** 196.

Whitney, J. C. (1975) *In* Pomerance, A., and Davies, M. J. (eds.), *Pathology of the Heart,* Blackwell Scientific Publications, Oxford and Edinburgh, p. 592.

Wright, J. R., and Calkins, E. (1975) *J. Am. Geriatric Soc.* **23,** 97.

3

Pathology of the Conduction System

M. J. DAVIES

Introduction

Any review of the pathology of the conduction system in old age can only begin with the changes that are so universal as to be regarded as "normal." These changes are so striking in the conduction system that it seems likely they form the background to those age-related ECG changes that do not alter life expectancy recorded in clinical studies (Caird et al. 1974, Golden and Golden 1974).

Age Changes in the Conduction System

Sinus Node. This node lies in the anterior segment of the sinoatrial ring as the crest of the atrial appendage is crossed. In essence, it is an oval mass of small muscle fibers embedded in dense fibrous tissue (Fig. 3.1), arranged around a small central artery. With special stains, it is easy to show, in the young adult, that over 50% of the node is comprised of these muscle fibers, i.e., the P or pacemaking cells (James et al. 1966). With age, the number of P cells falls, this trend becoming pronounced by 60 years of age, and many patients over 75 years of age have less than 10% of P cells in the node (Fig. 3.2). These

M. J. DAVIES · Department of Histopathology, St. George's Hospital Medical School, University of London, Blackshaw Road, Tooting, London, SW17 0QT, England.

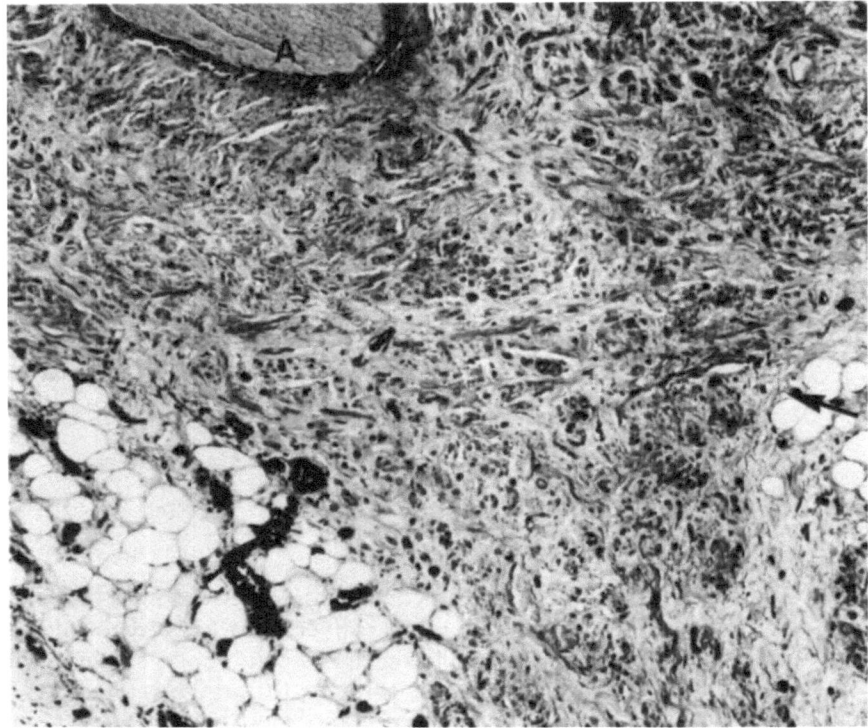

Fig. 3.1. Human sinoatrial node. The node (arrows) lies around the central artery (A) and consists of dense fibrous tissue containing small muscle fibers. Male, age 49, in sinus rhythm. (picro-Mallory)

data now seem to be incontrovertible; first noticed as a subjective assessment by Lev (1954), they were quantified by Davies and Pomerance (1972) and Sims (1972), with more recent confirmation by Théry (1975). The loss of P cells with age must be a significant factor in the ease with which atrial arrhythmias occur in geriatric patients. The cause of this loss remains conjectural, but no vascular basis has ever been demonstrated.

    Internodal Atrial Myocardium. The question of aging changes in this area is more controversial. Difficulty arises in morphological studies, because even if these paths are electrophysiologically specialized, they do not have any specific histological features (Janse and Anderson 1974). If the atrial myocardium in the interatrial septum is examined histologically, however, the amount of fibrous tissue increases with age, and the number of muscle fibers decreases (Davies and Pomerance 1972). In addition, considerable amounts of adipose tissue infiltrate between and separate the muscle fibers (Prior 1964). A further factor is the occurrence of small deposits of amyloid within the atrial septum in a proportion of geriatric patients (Pomerance 1975).

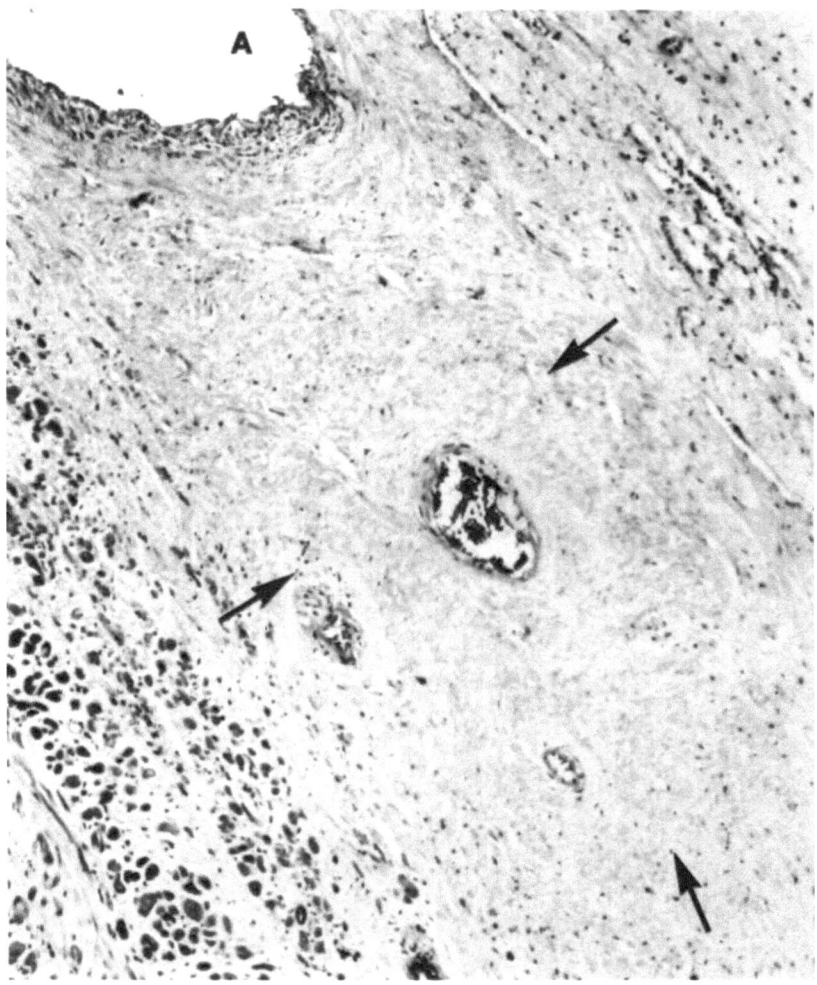

Fig. 3.2. Human sinoatrial node. The node (arrows) is recognizable as a mass of fibrous tissue around an artery (A). The fibrous tissue contains virtually no muscle fibers. Female, age 79, in atrial fibrillation. (picro-Mallory)

A-V Nodal Area. Recent embryological and anatomical studies
have somewhat altered views on this area (Anderson et al. 1975). The
node lies just beneath the right atrial endocardium, immediately
anterior to the coronary sinus, and posterior to the membranous
interventricular septum as it is crossed by the insertion of the
tricuspid valve. The node has a deep portion with two components, a
mitral and a tricuspid branch, separated by the nodal artery. A more
superficial transitional or junctional area of node overlies the deep
portion. Atrial fibers sweep down the septum to join the superficial
portion and to some extent the posterior aspect of the deep node. The
deep node gives rise to the bundle of His, and when completely
enclosed within the central fibrous body, the penetrating main bundle
is regarded as beginning. The main bundle passes through the central
fibrous body to reach the upper border of the muscular interventricular septum and is normally the only electrophysical connection between atria and ventricles. The arrangement of muscle fibers in the A-
V node is characteristically that of an interweaving mass of small
fibers (Fig. 3.3). This arrangement passes into the more parallel

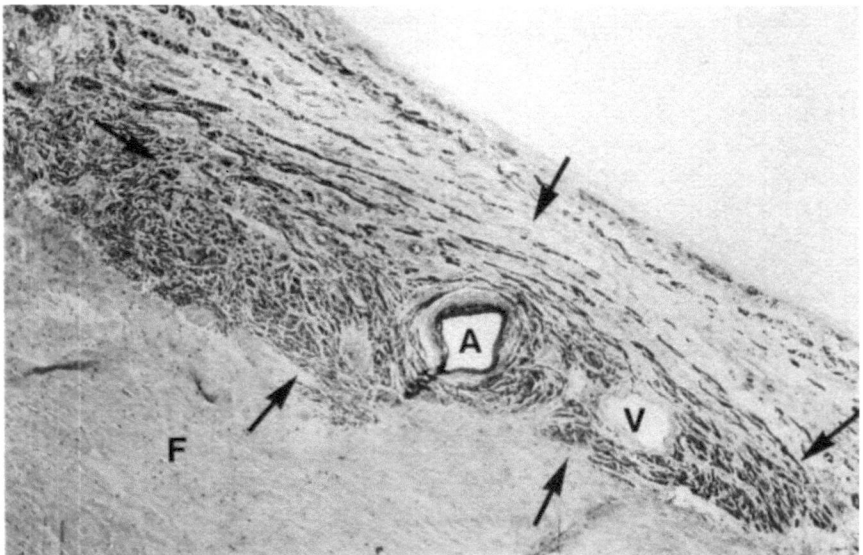

Fig. 3.3. Human A-V node. The node (arrows) consists of interweaving small fibers
adjacent to the central fibrous body (F). An artery (A) and vein (V) are present.
(hematoxylin and eosin)

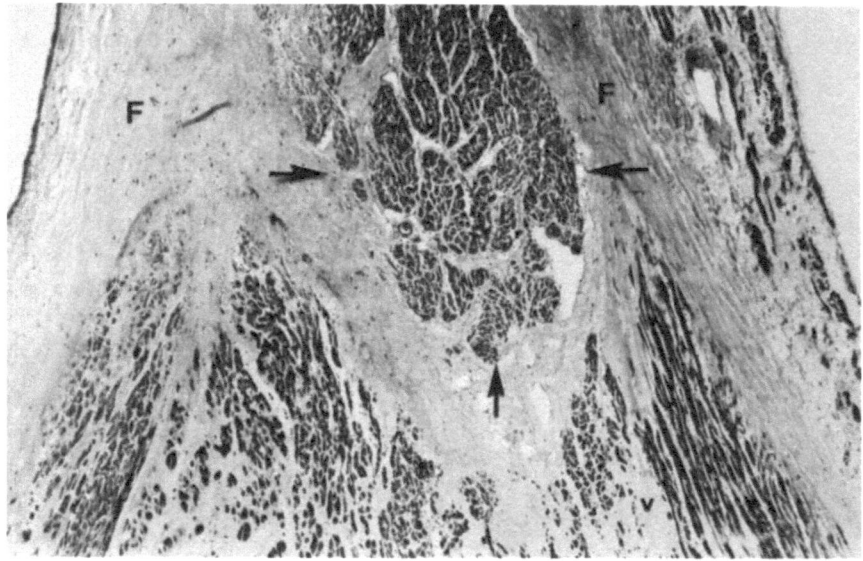

Fig. 3.4. Human penetrating main bundle in transverse section (arrows). The bundle lies within the central fibrous body (F) and consists of bundles of parallel muscle fibers. (hematoxylin and eosin)

arrangement of the main bundle (Fig. 3.4). Normally, the A-V node is completely separated from the ventricular muscle by the dense collagen of the central fibrous body. In children, some accessory muscle bundles (Mahaim tracts) often cross this zone, but are almost inevitably obliterated in the adult, and certainly by geriatric age.

Age-related changes in the A-V node are not pronounced and not recorded. Some attenuation of connections between the atrial muscle and superficial node is often apparent, especially when fatty infiltration is marked (Prior 1964). Sclerosis of the collagen of the central fibrous body occurs, but appears to have no real effect on the node or penetrating bundle.

Anatomy of the Bundle of His and Its Branches

The main bundle first gives rise to the numerous small branches (fascicles) of the left branch (Fig. 3.5), and then continues as the more solid and discrete right branch (Fig. 3.5). The main bundle here is referred to as the bifurcating bundle of His. Anatomical relations are important: the bifurcating bundle lies on the crest of the muscular

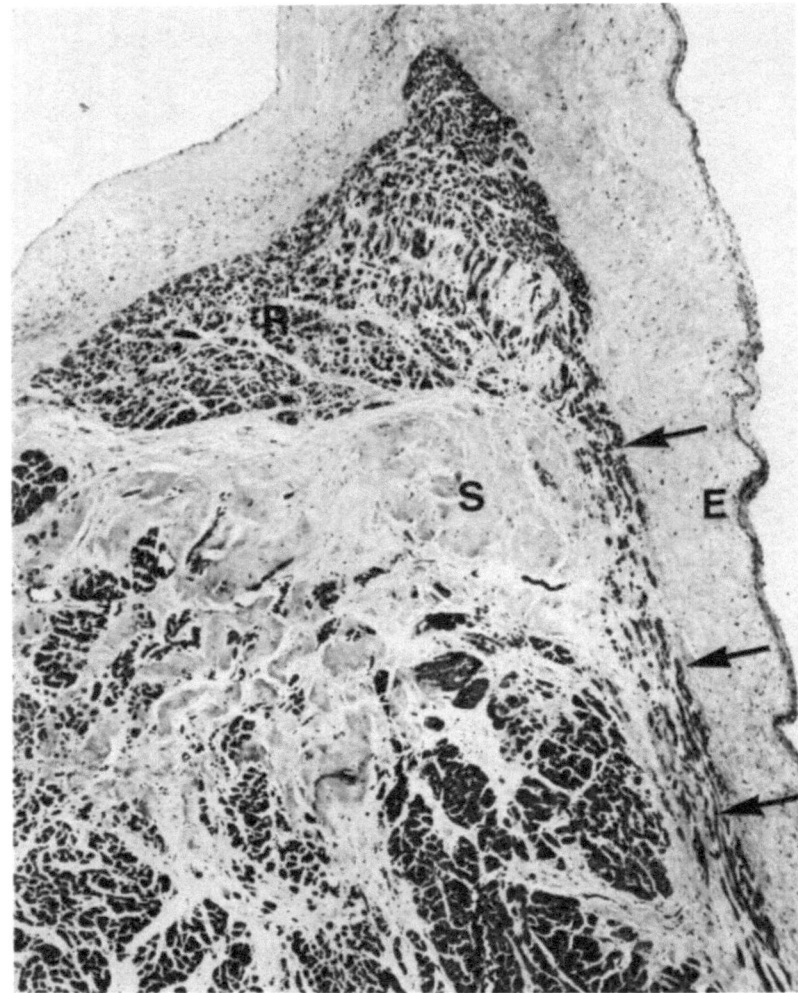

Fig. 3.5. Human bifurcating bundle. The right branch (R) is a solid muscle bundle; one of the anterior left fascicles (arrows) runs between the endocardium of the LV outflow (E) and the apex of the upper IV septum (S). Considerable fibrosis of the upper septum is present. (hematoxylin and eosin)

interventricular septum at the inferior border of the membranous interventricular septum; thus, the anterior cusp of the mitral valve and the noncoronary cusp of the aortic valve are very close. As the left bundle branch fascicles leave the main bundle, they run in a narrow cleft between the collagen of the upper interventricular septum and

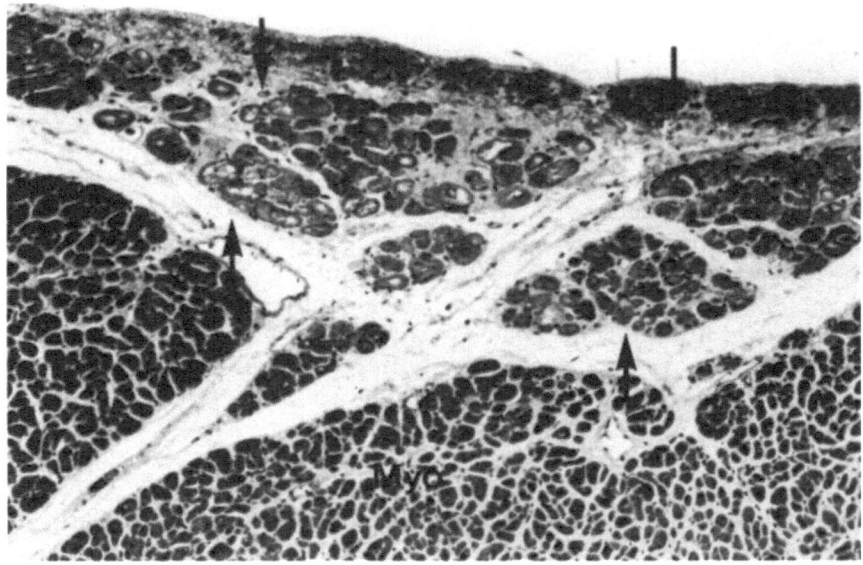

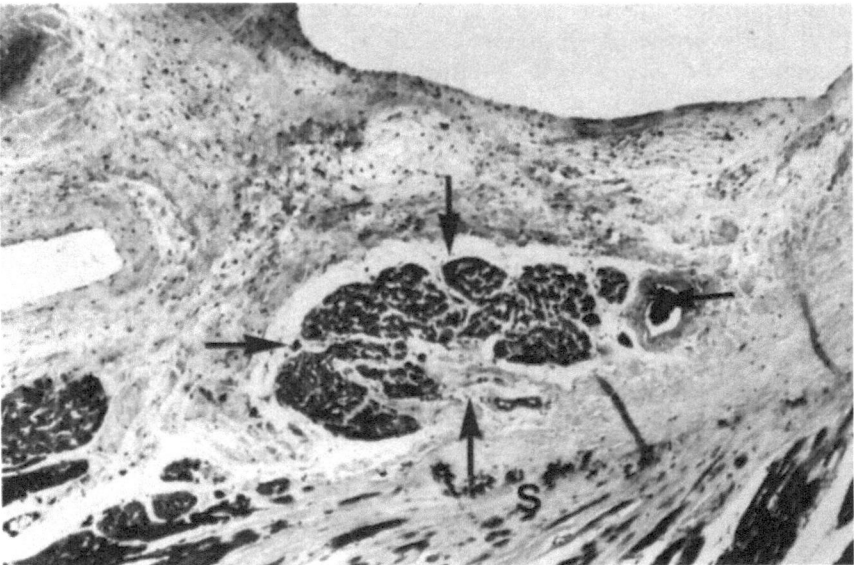

Fig. 3.6. (Top) Human left bundle branch in the septum (mid third). The fibers cut in cross section (arrows) are larger and more vacuolated than contractile fibers (Myo). (Bottom) Human right branch in upper septum (arrows). The branch is a single muscle bundle. Calcification due to aging in adjacent fibrous tissue (S). (hematoxylin and eosin)

the endocardium of the left ventricular outflow. They pass down in the septum immediately beneath the endocardium.

There is considerable controversy over the anatomy of the left bundle branch in the ventricular septum. Rosenbaum (1970) has claimed the left branch to be bifascicular, with an anterior and posterior division. The concept is based on gross dissection, however, and actual reconstruction at the histological–microscopic level by Demoulin and Kulbertus (1972) and Kulbertus (1975) has shown considerable variation from subject to subject. The left branch is a complex network in which a middle segment is frequently present, in addition to anterior and posterior divisions. Personal study suggests the branch to be multifascicular, with free communication between anterior and posterior fascicles by fibers running transversely in the septum.

In the middle and lower third of the septum, the conduction fibers of the left branch become larger, with a pale vacuolated appearance on light microscopy (Fig. 3.6). These cells are the closest morphological equivalent in man to the very much larger pale cells in the bundle branch of the pig described by Purkinje (e.g., see Matousek and Posner 1969). Ultrastructural studies (Benscome et al. 1969) show these fibers to have very scanty myofibrillary contractile elements and specialized intercellular connections to allow rapid conduction. There is no certain knowledge of the connections between Purkinje cells and the contractile myocardium, although a steady transition between the two fiber types has some electrophysiological and morphological evidence for its support (Mendez et al. 1969, Truex and Smythe 1964).

The right bundle branch runs as a single muscle strand down the septum to reach the base of the anterior papillary muscle of the right ventricle. In animals, but very rarely in man, it crosses the cavity of the ventricle in the outflow tract in the moderator band. From the base of the papillary muscle, the bundle branches into an anastomotic network of conduction fibers throughout the ventricle immediately beneath the endocardium.

Age-Related Changes in the Bundle of His

Bifurcating Main Bundle. Distinct age-related changes occur in this region. Loss of a proportion of the left bundle fascicles at their origin is universal over 60 years of age, and loss of over 50% of fibers not unusual (Fig. 3.7A,B). The mechanism of this loss has been the subject of some interest. Lev suggests that mechanical strain on the area of the upper interventricular septum produces increasing fibrosis, followed by sclerosis and microcalcification, and the left fascicles are subject to compression and distortion as they run through this area (Lev 1964, Lev et al. 1974). He has termed this process "sclerosis of the left side of the cardiac skeleton" and considers any cause of left ventricular hypertrophy, particularly hypertension to accelerate the process. In addition, the blood supply of the bifurcating bundle is by arteriolar vessels running in the main bundle; any degree of arteriosclerosis would potentiate the damaging effect of mechanical strain (Van der Hauwaert et al. 1972, Lev et al. 1974).

Distal Bundle Branches. These branches in the ventricles show some increase in fine fibrous tissue and elastic with increasing age. Detailed morphometry by Demoulin and Kulbertus (personal communication) has shown that, in addition, a small but real decrease in the number of conduction fibers occurs with age.

The age related changes occurring in the conduction system can therefore be summarized as (1) a loss of P cells in the sinus node, and (2) loss of the proximal connections of a proportion of the left fascicles to the main bundle.

Less morphologically striking but still demonstrable changes occur in the internodal atrial myocardium, in the atrial/A-V nodal junction, and in the distal conduction networks in the left ventricle. All these changes thus involve a loss of conduction and nodal specialized tissue that cannot definitely be ascribed to any pathological process, but appears to be simply an expression of age.

Blood Supply of the Conduction System

The sinus node is arranged around a small central artery, from which arterioles run into the node itself. The nodal artery is the termination of the main arterial supply to the atria; it is derived from the proximal right coronary in 50–60% of subjects and from the left circumflex in the remainder (Romhilt et al. 1968).

The artery to the A-V node is constantly derived from the origin of the posterior descending coronary artery, this being from the right in 90% and from the left circumflex coronary artery in 10% of normal subjects (Romhilt et al. 1968). There is no relationship between the blood supply of the two nodes. The A-V nodal artery passes in an anterior direction through atrial muscle without any branching before supplying arterioles to the node itself. It then penetrates the central

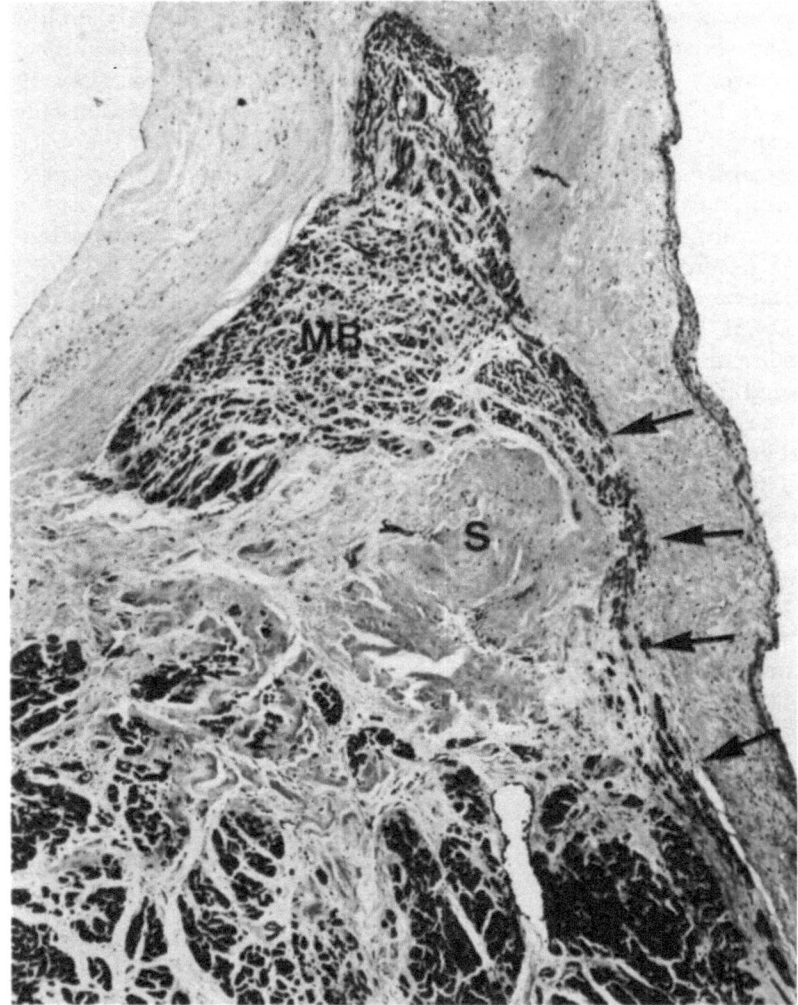

Fig. 3.7.A. The bifurcating main bundle (MB) gives rise to one left fascicle, which is bowed (arrows) across a mass of fibrous tissue in the upper septum (S).

fibrous body to reach and supply a small segment of the upper portion of the muscular interventricular septum. The main bundle is supplied by parallel arterioles running in the long axis of the bundle from the node (Clarke 1965, Kennel and Titus 1972, Van der Hauwaert et al. 1972).

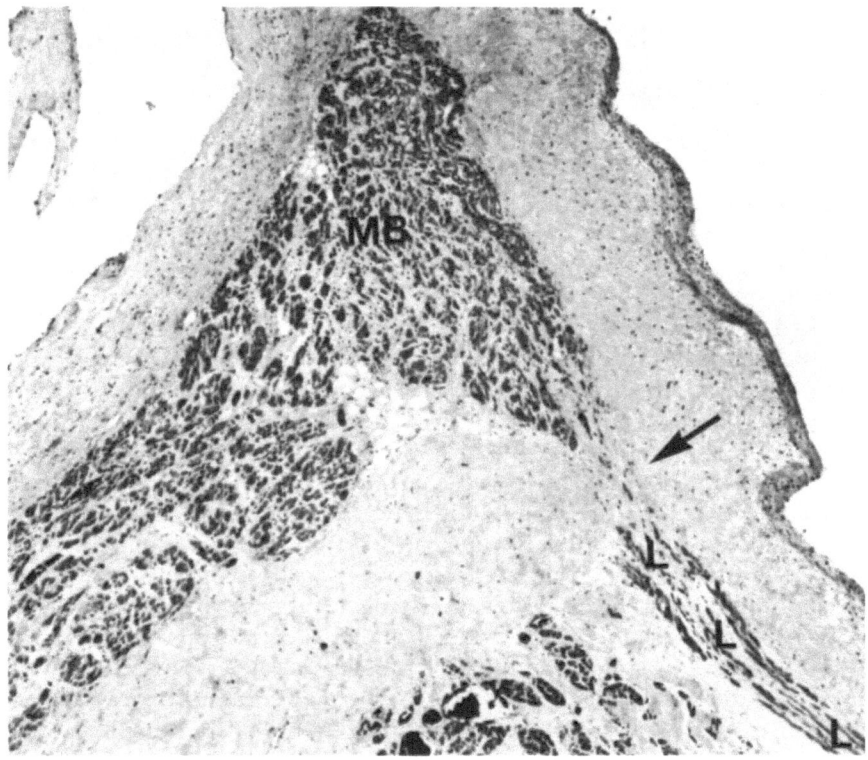

Fig. 3.7.B. A section more anterior to Fig. 3.7.A. Here, there is loss of continuity between the main bundle (MB) and left branch (L) at the area marked by the arrows.

The bundle branches receive arterioles from long, penetrating septal branches of the left anterior descending coronary artery, and there is a "watershed" where this supply abuts onto the long arterioles running in the main bundle. A small portion of the posterior aspect of the left bundle branch in the midseptum receives blood from the short, penetrating septal branches of the posterior coronary artery.

With age, hyalinization and fibrosis of the media of arteries and arterioles within the nodes and the main bundle becomes almost universal. Some authorities regard these changes as being responsible in part for the loss of conduction tissue with age. Microradiographic studies have not supported these views, showing that loss of luminal filling is not present (Kennel et al. 1973).

Pathology of Specific Conduction Abnormalities in Old Age

Atrial Arrhythmias

The pathology of sino-atrial disease, including sinus bradycardia, sinus arrest, and sinoatrial block, remains a poorly explored field, and electrophysiological studies of nodal function in life have far outstripped conventional morphological studies at autopsy. Clinical study of living patients (Rasmussen 1971; Shaw, personal communication) reveals very little of etiological significance, but does confirm a marked geriatric bias in these arrhythmias.

Pathological studies have shown that occasional cases of sino-atrial disease are due to vascular occlusion of the nodal artery (Lippestad and Marton 1967), but two series (Warembourg et al. 1974, Théry 1975, Brownlee et al. 1975) comprising 16 cases in all emphasize that the usual picture is a severe partial or even total loss of muscle fibers and P cells in the sinus node. The sinus node may be very small and distorted, or completely replaced by fibrous tissue, suggesting a process of exaggerated aging atrophy, possibly superimposed on congenitally small sinus nodes. A small number of cases result from amyloid replacing the sinus node. Detailed postmortem angiography down to small vessels (Brownlee et al. 1975) shows no vascular basis for nodal destruction. It is therefore probable that clinically significant cases of sino-atrial disease represent the extreme end of a spectrum of muscle-fiber loss occurring with age. Patients who have a congenitally small node or who suffer any condition in life producing loss of conduction cells, such as diphtheria, may reach the threshold for clinical symptoms even earlier.

Atrial Fibrillation

Transient atrial fibrillation is often associated with dilatation of the atria following pulmonary embolism or with pericarditis. The latter affects the sinus node area because of its subepicardial location.

Established atrial fibrillation is usually associated with varying combinations of P cell loss in the sinus node, fibrosis of internodal atrial myocardium, and chronic atrial dilatation (Davies and Pomerance 1972, Sims 1972, Théry 1975). The natural aging changes are already advanced in this direction, and any condition accelerating these factors—such as ischemic disease, chronic rheumatic valve disease, or senile cardiac amyloid—will precipitate fibrillation in geriatric patients.

TABLE 3.1. Common Causes of Chronic A-V Block: Autopsy Study of 177
Cases

Idiopathic bilateral bundle branch fibrosis	69	(33.3%)
Ischemic (coronary artery disease)	30	(16.8%)
Cardiomyopathy	25	14.0%)
Calcific A-V block	17	(9.5%)
All other causes	36	(20.3%)
	177	

Chronic A-V Block

Clinical studies of chronic A-V block confirm the marked geriatric
bias of this conduction abnormality. Of 177 patients with chronic A-V
block personally autopsied, 68% were over 65 years old. Personal
study of this large autopsy series shows the common causes to be four
disease entities (Table 3.1), of which two—idiopathic bilateral bundle
branch fibrosis and calcific A-V block—have a marked predilection for
old age. The major anatomical site of damage to the conduction system
lies in the bifurcating main bundle and bundle branches (Table 3.2).

Idiopathic Bilateral Bundle Branch Fibrosis. This name is a cumber-
some yet descriptive one for an entity characterized by slowly progressive loss of conduction fibers in the bundle branches without demonstrable myocardial or vascular disease. The loss of conduction fibers
leads to replacement fibrosis, thus marking the original outline of the
bundle branches.

TABLE 3.2. Site of Anatomical Destruction of Conduction
System in Chronic A-V Block: Autopsy Study of 177
Cases

Prenodal	3	(1.7%)
A-V node	12	(6.8%)
Node/penetrating bundle	11	(6.2%)
Penetrating bundle	32	(18.1%)
Bifurcating bundle/LBB	31	(17.5%)
RBB/LBB	88	(49.1%)
	177	

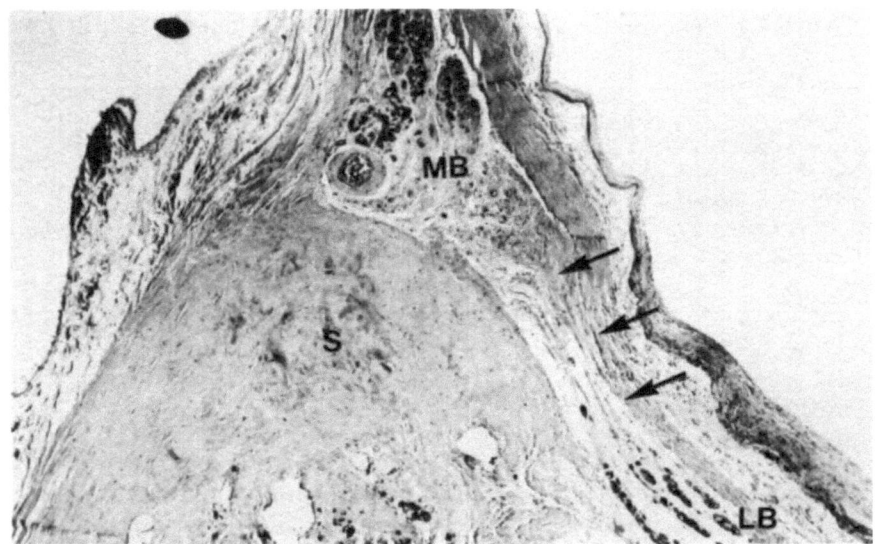

Fig. 3.8. Lev type bundle branch fibrosis. Female, age 78, with complete A-V block. The main bundle (MB) contains very scanty muscle fibers only at the upper pole. No fibers remain in the left branch over a long area (arrows) until lower in the septum (LB). Very extensive fibrosis of the upper septum (S) with early calcification.

The entity has been known for many years, being well described by both Aschoff and Mönckeberg, but has come to be appreciated as far from rare only with the advent of cardiac pacing. Within the disease complex, two distinct forms are highlighted in the literature. Lev (1964) has emphasized a type in which loss of conduction fibers in the proximal left bundle and adjacent bifurcating bundle occurs (Fig. 3.8). Damage to the distal branches is minimal, and he stresses the very focal nature of the conduction damage. In contrast, Lenégre (1964) describes a diffuse disease affecting the middle and distal portions of both bundle branches (Fig. 3.9A,B). While both authors describe entities that appear pathologically different and have evoked use of the terms "Lev's disease" and "Lenégre's disease," our own studies of sex incidence, age incidence, and pathology suggest considerable merging of the two disease patterns. Our own autopsy series of 69 cases of bundle branch fibrosis shows a mean age of 70 at death overall, with a mean age for the Lev form of 74 and for the Lenégre form of 67. The Lev form is more common in women; the Lenégre form, in men.

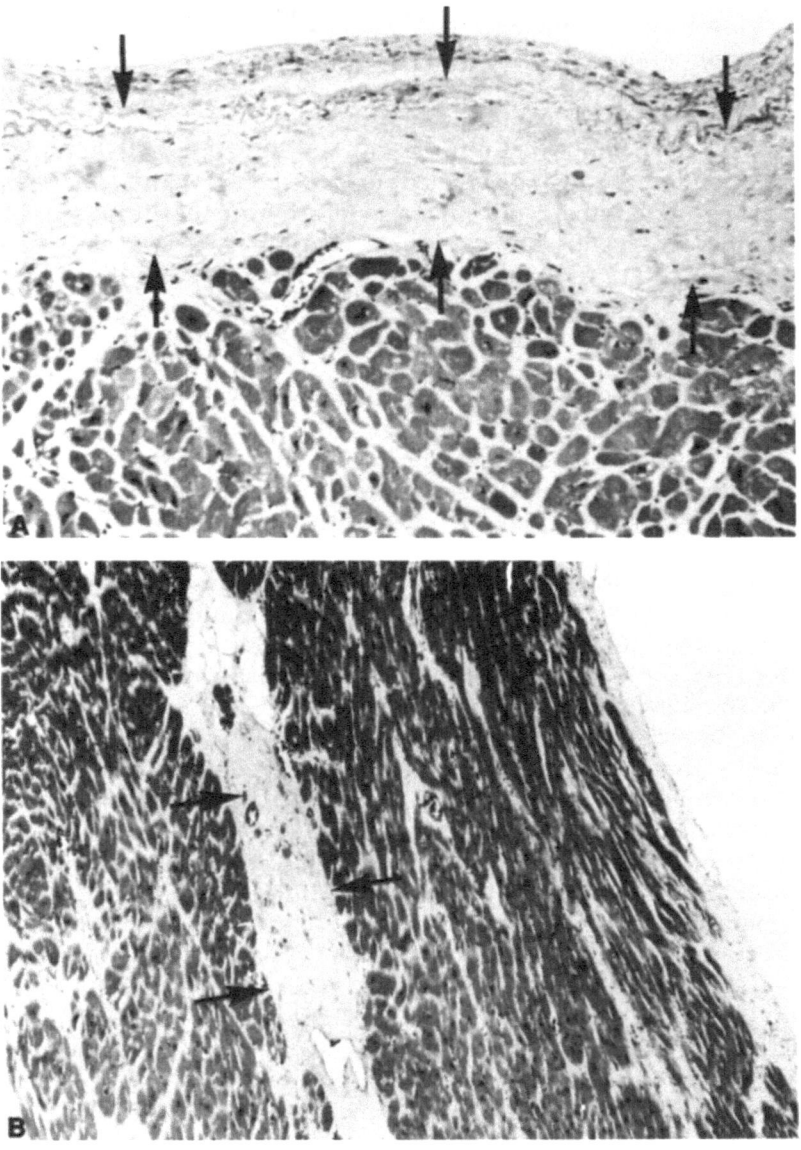

Fig. 3.9. (A) Left branch (arrows) in Lenégre form bundle branch fibrosis. The section, which is an identical plane and site to Fig. 6 and shows virtual complete loss of conduction fibers while adjacent contractile myocardium is unremarkable. (B) Right branch (arrows) in Lenégre bundle branch fibrosis. No conduction fibers are present, and only a fibrous strand of tissue remains. Adjacent myocardium normal.

Views on the etiology and pathogenesis of the damage to the conduction system in idiopathic bundle branch fibrosis are diverse. It seems unlikely that the condition is a homogeneous entity; it probably represents the end-stage of several processes or of a combination of processes. Lev emphasizes the very focal destruction of the bifurcating main bundle as an exaggerated or accelerated aging change. He describes the sclerosis and microcalcification of the fibrous tissue of the upper interventricular septum that occurs with age as extending into the bifurcating bundle. Two factors are ascribed in the pathogenesis of this process—mechanical strain and arteriosclerosis of the long vessels running from the node through the main bundle to the bifurcating bundle.

In contrast, no such simple explanation can fit the diffuse peripheral conduction fiber loss of the Lenégre form. Lenégre himself considered the disease a primary degeneration or cardiomyopathy of condution fibers, but this hardly explains the disease at a cellular level. Demonstration of antibodies with specificity against Purkinje fibers in patients with bundle branch fibrosis and an association of A-V block with other autoimmune diseases may point to a possible pathogenetic mechanism (Fairfax, personal communication).

Previous myocarditis has been evoked as a possible etiological factor (Hudson 1965), with diphtheria the most common form considered. The demonstration of age-related loss of conduction fibers in the bundle branches (Demoulin and Kulbertus, personal communication) suggests that patients with a lower reserve of conduction tissue, perhaps following severe diphtheria, could become symptomatic in the seventh decade of life.

Coronary atherosclerosis of major epicardial arteries has never been clearly implicated, and detailed autopsy analysis, including angiography, confirms the normality of the coronary artery tree in most cases of bundle branch fibrosis (Davies 1971). Small-vessel disease at the arteriolar level has been implicated (James 1967, Knierium 1974), but is difficult to prove short of complex injection and microradiographic techniques, which have rarely been performed. In addition, arteriosclerosis is almost universal at the age range being studied. It seems likely that decreasing arteriolar blood supply in the main bundle plays a contributory role in some cases of the Lev form of bundle branch fibrosis, but small-vessel disease remains otherwise unproved as an important pathogenetic mechanism (Kennel et al. 1973).

Whatever the etiology and pathogenesis of bundle branch fibrosis, it can be seen as the end-stage of a slowly progressive process culminating in A-V block in patients mainly over 65 and often over 75 years of age. The pathology runs a spectrum from only very focal destruction of the bifurcating bundle to widespread loss of conduction fibers in the Purkinje networks of the ventricles. Our own experience suggests that no clear distinction between the ends of the spectrum is possible clinically.

Myocardial function is usually good in patients with bundle branch fibrosis, but in the group overall, diffuse myocardial scarring is more pronounced than in control subjects (Davies 1971, Knierium 1974). In addition, considerable left ventricular hypertrophy is seen, although this condition may simply reflect a response to the slow heart rate; cardiac failure does occur often, however, without other discernible cause. Our own data suggest this to be more common toward the Lenégre end of the spectrum, and an occasional case of this type of bundle branch fibrosis culminates in frank congestive cardiomyopathy.

Destruction of the Penetrating–Bifurcating Bundle by Large Calcific Masses. This is the second common cause of chronic A-V block associated with old age. In contrast to the microcalcification of Lev's disease, these calcific masses are visible on screening of the heart in life, and can be easily seen by the naked eye at autopsy. The calcific masses arise in the mitral valve ring or from the aortic valve sinuses and involve the main bundle because of its close anatomical relationship. Senile mitral valve ring calcification is relatively common, occurring to some degree in up to 10% of patients over 50 years of age. When calcific deposits are massive, they may extend into the membranous septum, compressing and then transecting the main bundle (Fig. 3.10A,B). The association of massive mitral ring calcification with A-V block was well documented by Rytand and Lipsitch (1946), with subsequent series by Korn et al. (1962) and Pomerance (1970) confirming the association. Senile aortic ring and sinus calcification with or without stenosis extends into the septal area less commonly, but may do so (Table 3.3). Nongeriatic causes of aortic calcification, such as bicuspid calcific aortic stenosis, are also associated with the occasional occurrence of chronic A-V block. Paget's disease of bone in old age is described as a potentiating factor in massive mitral ring calcification, inducing A-V block (King et al. 1969).

Other Causes of Chronic A-V Block. Many other causes of chronic A-V block may be seen in old age, but are equally or even more commonly seen in younger subjects. *Cardiomyopathies* of the conges-

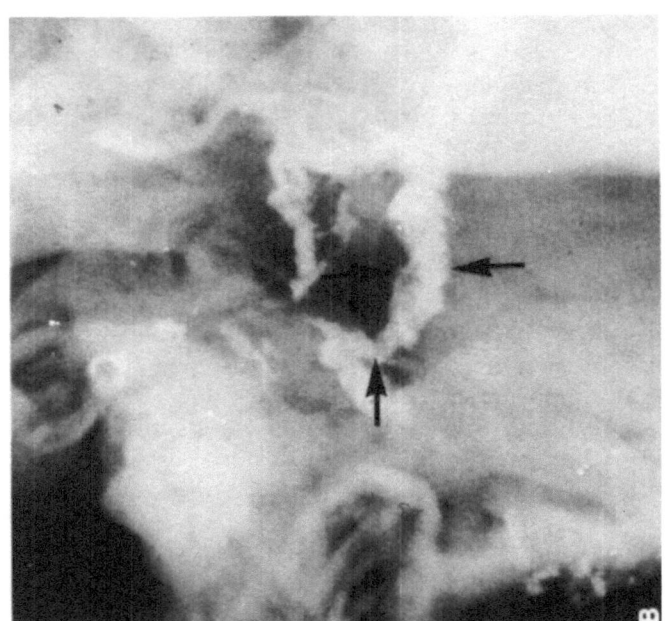

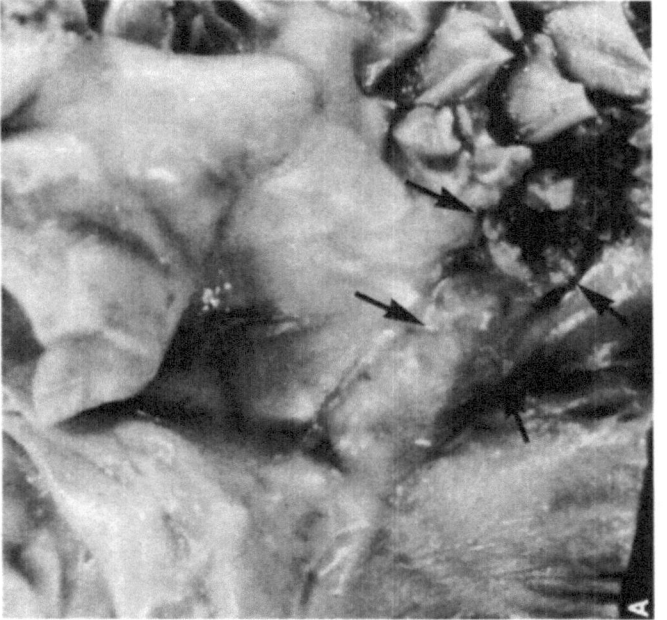

Fig. 3.10. (A) Calcific A-V Block in a male, age 82. A mass of calcium (arrows) extends into the membranous septum from the mitral valve. (B) Plain X-ray of heart. The calcific mass (arrows) lies at the border of the muscular and membranous interventricular septum, transecting the main bundle.

TABLE 3.3. Calcific Chronic A-V Block: 17 Cases at
Autopsy

Aortic stenosis	Bicuspid	4
	Senile tricuspid	3
	Rheumatic	1
Aortic sclerosis	Senile	4
Massive mitral ring calcification	Senile	4
	Senile + Paget's disease of bone	1

tive form are associated with an incidence of chronic A-V block, heavy involvement of the left bundle branch in the disease process usually being the striking feature at autopsy. Hypertrophic obstructive cardiomyopathy has very little association with A-V block. Primary amyloidosis involving the heart is associated with A-V block, as is an occasional case of senile cardiac amyloid. Amyloid is deposited within the internodal atrial myocardium, both nodes and main bundle, rather than the bundle branches, and atrial arrhythmias are more common than A-V block.

Ischemic heart disease produced chronic A-V block when the conduction system is destroyed within areas of old myocardial infarction. The most common morphological picture is destruction of both bundle branches in an extensive anteroseptal infarct or series of anteroseptal infarcts over a period of time. Rarely, a posterior infarct extends sufficiently forward into the septum to destroy the bundle branches; even more rarely, posterior infarction is associated with thrombosis extending into the nodal artery itself with infarction of the A-V node. The pattern of ischemic disease producing chronic A-V block is essentially similar, whatever the patient's age.

Congenital A-V block due to absence of a focal segment of the conduction system either at the atrial–A-V node junction or the main bifurcating bundle (Carter et al. 1974, Lev 1972) is usually regarded as a disease of children or young adults. Clinical studies do show, however, the remarkably good prognosis of this condition (Campbell and Emanuel 1967), and we have encountered an occasional example in our autopsy series running into the age-65 group.

Other rare causes of chronic A-V block include both primary benign tumors, such as the mesothelioma of the A-V node (Davies 1975, Kaminsky et al. 1967); malignant primary sarcomas arising in the right atria; and the occurrence of secondary deposits in, or adjacent to, the A-V node or main bundle. Carcinoma of the bronchus is most common, although isolated case reports record virtually every primary site in association with A-V block.

When the heart is involved, collagen diseases are frequently associated with chronic A-V block, due to the rich connective tissue support of the conduction system. Ankylosing spondylitis with an aortitis and aortic regurgitation is associated with a very high incidence of A-V block (Buckley and Roberts 1973, Liu and Alexander 1969), reflecting the proximity of the node to the aortic root. Rheumatoid granulomata may transect the main bundle (Hoffman and Leight 1965, Gallagher and Gresham 1973). The small-vessel "arteritic" component of polyarteritis and disseminated lupus erythematosus appears responsible for conduction disturbances in these conditions (James 1967).

Posttraumatic and postsurgical A-V block (Davies and Pomerance 1975) play little role in the geriatric age group.

Acute A-V Block Accompanying Acute Myocardial Infarction
(Sutton and Davies 1968)

There is no essential difference in this association in geriatric as compared with younger subjects. Two distinct pathophysiological entities exist. In posterior (inferior) infarction, the A-V node is temporarily inhibited either by anoxia or by metabolites diffusing from adjacent dead muscle. Pathological study shows actual structural damage to be very rare. The arterial occlusion always lies proximal to the origin of the A-V nodal artery, but the time course of onset of block occurring as it does on the second or third day is rarely consistent with a simple vascular–anoxia mechanism. Experimental reproduction of the situation in dogs suggests diffusion of K^+ ions to suppress the node. In anterior infarction associated with A-V block, in contrast, major structural damage to the middle and proximal bundle branches is often present. Here also, however, considerable recovery of conduction may occur, suggesting that inhibition of conduction tissue adjacent to dead muscle also occurs. The prognosis of posterior infarction with A-V block is significantly better, and the incidence of residual block low. Anterior infarcts with block, in contrast, have a poor prognosis and high residual conduction defect risks.

Left Axis Deviation and Left Bundle Branch Block

Rosenbaum has been largely responsible for the concept that lesions of the anterior radiation of the left bundle branch are responsible for marked left axis deviation and that "left anterior hemiblock" is an acceptable term (Rosenbaum *et al.* 1970). Detailed morphological studies (Demoulin and Kulbertus 1972, 1973) suggest, however, that while the ECG appearances designated as left anterior hemiblock do represent damage to the left bundle branch, this damage can rarely be localized exactly and solely in the anterior division of the bundle branch.

The aging changes in the origin of the left fascicles from the bifurcating bundle discussed earlier involve varying degrees of loss of continuity between the main bundle and left ventricular conduction networks. This loss cannot usually be localized as involving only the anterior or posterior division, but occurs in scattered foci throughout the left branch origins. The process often involves over 50% of the left fascicles in otherwise normal hearts of subjects over 65 years of age (Davies 1971). As emphasized by Lev, the process is essentially one of mechanical wear and tear with age, although it is potentiated by hypertension; by atherosclerosis of the left anterior descending coronary artery, which ultimately supplies arterioles to the left branch; and by arteriosclerosis of these arterioles. This loss of conduction fibers is responsible for a spectrum of changes ranging from simple left axis deviation through left bundle branch block to the Lev form of bundle branch fibrosis with complete A-V block. These hearts will be macroscopically normal, apart, perhaps, from left ventricular hypertrophy, and are predominantly seen in patients over 65 years of age. Aortic stenosis is also often associated with marked destruction of the left fascicles at their origin, as in hypertension. Anteroseptal myocardial infarction will involve varying proportions of the left branch, depending on the degree of extension into the septum. Damage occurs in the proximal and middle third of the branch, and in patients over 65 is superimposed on the aging changes described above (Grayzel and Neyshaboori 1975).

Right Bundle Branch Block

Right bundle branch block is much less related to age than left, and epidemiological studies suggest that right ventricular hypertrophy in cor pulmonale and ischemic heart disease are important factors (Edmunds 1966). Morphological studies have shown destruction of the right branch in areas of old infarction, but the cause of right bundle branch block following severe right ventricular hypertrophy is still obscure (Lev et al. 1961).

Preexcitation Syndromes

The classic view of the conduction system until recent years held that the only electrical connection between atria and ventricles was by the main bundle of His, and that the collagen of the central fibrous body and the mitral and tricuspid valve rings separated atria and ventricles at all other sites. Recent work (Anderson et al. 1974, Anderson et al. 1975, Davies and Anderson 1975) has shown defects in the central fibrous body and valve rings, and the existence of remnants of nodal tissue in both mitral and tricuspid rings of normal adult hearts. This tissue probably represents persistence of parts of the ring of nodal fibers normally found in fetal hearts at these sites. These nodal remnants are clearly the "accessory bundles" seen by Kent (e.g., see Anderson et al. 1974). Numerous pathological studies have now shown accessory conduction pathways in the right atrium–right ventricle to be responsible for Type B Wolff–Parkinson–White (WPW) syndrome, and accessory pathways on the left for Type A. Abolition of the ECG abnormality by transection of the accessory path at operation is now well established.

That the ECG appearances of the WPW syndrome and its variants are not excessively rare is now being recognized, and many patients are not symptomatic. While preexcitation syndromes are usually considered as diseases of younger subjects, the good prognosis of some patients means examples will be found in old age. The problem of the pathology of the preexcitation syndromes is now not whether accessory paths exist, but why they function only in some subjects and what factors precipitate clinical symptoms after many years. The onset of atrial fibrillation associated with aging changes in the atria may be one such factor.

References

Anderson, R. H., Davies, M. J., and Becker, A. E. (1974) *Eur. J. Cardiol.* **2**, 219.

Anderson, R. H., Becker, A. E., Brechenmacher, C., Davies, M. J., and Rossi, L. (1975) *Eur. J. Cardiol.* **3**, 11.

Benscome, S. A., Trillo, A., Alanis, J., and Benitez, D. (1969) *J. Electrocardiography* **2**, 27.

Brownlee, W. C., Evans, R. C., and Shaw, D. B. (1975) *Br. Heart J.* **37**, 779.

Buckley, B. H., and Roberts, W. C. (1973) *Circulation* **48**, 1014.

Caird, F. I., Campbell, A., and Jackson, T. F. M. (1974) *Br. Heart J.* **36**, 102.

Campbell, M., and Emanuel, R. (1967) *Br. Heart J.* **29**, 577.

Carter, J. B., Blieden, L. C., and Edwards, J. E. (1974) *Arch. Pathol.* **97**, 51.

Clarke, J. A. (1965) *Br. Heart J.* **27**, 879.

Davies, J. M. (1971) *In: Pathology of Conducting Tissue of the Heart*, Butterworth, London.

Davies, J. M. (1975) *In* Pomerance, A., and Davies, M. J. (eds.), *Pathology of the Heart,* Blackwell Scientific Publications, Oxford and Edinburgh.

Davies, M. J., and Anderson, R. H. (1975) *In* Pomerance, A., and Davies, M. J. *Pathology of the Heart,* Blackwell Scientific Publications, Oxford and Edinburgh.

Davies, M. J., and Pomerance, A. (1972) *Br. Heart J.* **34,** 150.

Davies, M. J., and Pomerance, A. (1975) *In* Pomerance, A., and Davies, M. J. (eds.), *Pathology of the Heart,* Blackwell Scientific Publications, Oxford and Edinburgh.

Demoulin, J. C., and Kulbertus, H. E. (1972) *Br. Heart J.* **34,** 807.

Demoulin, J. C., and Kulbertus, H. E. (1973) *Am. Heart J.* **86,** 712.

Edmands, R. E. (1966) *Circulation* **34,** 1081.

Gallagher, P. J., and Gresham, G. A. (1973) *Br. Heart. J.* **35,** 110.

Golden, G. S., and Golden, L. H. (1974) *J. Am. Geriatr. Soc.* **22,** 329.

Grayzel, J., and Neyshaboori, M. (1975) *Am. Heart J.* **89,** 419.

Hoffman, F. G., and Leight, L. (1965) *Am. J. Cardiol.* **16,** 585.

Hudson, R. E. B. (1965) *In* Arnold, E. (ed.), *Cardiovascular Pathology,* London.

James, T. N. (1967) *Am. J. Cardiol.* **20,** 679.

James, T. N., Scherf, L., Fine, G., and Morales, A. R. (1966) *Circulation* **34,** 139.

Janse, M. J., and Anderson, R. H. (1974) *Eur. J. Cardiol.* **2,** 117.

Kaminsky, N. I., Killip, T., Alonso, D. R., and Hagstrom, J. W. C. (1967) *Am. J. Cardiol.* **20,** 248.

Kennel, A. J., and Titus, J. L. (1972) *Proc. Mayo Clinic* **47,** 562.

Kennel, A. J., Titus, J. L., McCallister, B. D., and Pruitt, R. D. (1973) *Am. Heart J.* **85,** 593.

King, M., Huang, J. M., and Glassman, E. (1969) *Am. J. Med.* **46,** 302.

Knierium, H. J. (1974) *In: Fortschritte der Morphologischen Pathologie—A-V Block,* Urban and Schwarzenberg, Munich.

Korn, D., de Sanctis, R. W., and Sell, S. (1962) *N. Engl. J. Med.* **267,** 900.

Kulbertus, H. E. (1975) *British Heart Foundation: First European Symposium, Abstracts 9.*

Lenégre, J. (1964) *Progr. Cardiovasc. Dis.* **6,** 409.

Lev, M. (1954) *J. Gerontol.* **9,** 1.

Lev, M. (1964) *Progr. Cardiovasc. Dis.* **6,** 317.

Lev, M. (1972) *Progr. Cardiovasc. Dis.* **15,** 145.

Lev, M., Unger, P. M., Lesser, M. E., and Pick, A. (1961) *Am. Heart J.* **61,** 593.

Lev, M., Unger, P. M., Rosen, K. M., and Bharati, S. (1974) *Circulation* **50,** 479.

Lippestad, C. T., and Marton, P. F. (1967) *Am. Heart J.* **74,** 551.

Liu, S. M., and Alexander, C. S. (1969) *Am. J. Cardiol.* **23,** 888.

Matousek, M., and Posner, E. (1969) *Br. Heart J.* **31,** 718.

Mendez, C., Mueller, W. J., Meredith, J., and Moe, G. K. (1969) *Circ. Res.* **24,** 361.

Pomerance, A. (1970) *J. Clin. Pathol.* **23,** 354.

Pomerance, A. (1975) *In* Pomerance, A., and Davies, M. J. (eds.), *Pathology of the Heart,* Blackwell Scientific Publications, Oxford and Edinburgh.

Prior, J. T. (1964) *Arch. Pathol.* **78,** 11.

Rasmussen, K. (1971) *Am. Heart J.* **81,** 38.

Romhilt, D. W., Hackel, D. B., and Estes, E. H. (1968) *Am. Heart J.* **75,** 279.

Rosenbaum, M. B. (1970) *Mod. Concepts Cardiovasc. Dis.* **39,** 141.

Rosenbaum, M. B., Elizari, M. V., and Lazzari, J. O. (1970) *The Hemiblocks,* Tampa Tracings Oldsmar.

Rytand, D. A., and Lipsitch, L. S. (1946) *Arch. Intern. Med.* **78,** 544.

Sims, B. A. (1972) *Br. Heart J.* **34,** 336.

Sutton, R., and Davies, M. J. (1968) *Circulation* **38,** 987.

Théry, C. (1975) *British Heart Foundation: First European Symposium, Abstracts 11.*
Truex, R. C., and Smythe, M. Q. (1964) *Ann. N.Y. Acad. Sci.* **127,** 19.
Van der Hauwaert, L. G., Stroobandt, R., and Verhaeghe, L. (1972) *Br. Heart J.* **34,** 1045.
Warembourg, H., Théry, C., Leikieffre, J., Delbecque, H., and Gosselin, B. (1974) *Arch. Mal. Coeur Vaiss.* **67,** 787.

4

Cardiac Output in Old Age

TORE STRANDELL

Cardiac Output at Rest

To date, the effect of aging on cardiac output has only been estimated from cross-sectional studies. The first determinations at rest with the direct Fick principle, i.e., measurements of oxygen uptake and oxygen difference between arterial and mixed venous blood, were made by Cournand et al. (1945); after catheterization of the right auricle or ventricle, these workers measured the cardiac output in 17 normal males 21–58 years old, and found a definite decrease with rising age.

A more extensive study was performed by Brandfonbrener et al. (1955), who applied the dye dilution technique with bolus injections of Evans blue dye through a short catheter in an antecubital vein and rapid sampling from a brachial artery. Their material consisted of 67 ambulatory male patients 19–86 years old. All had normal electrocardiograms and none had signs or symptoms of cardiovascular disease. Some were convalescing from respiratory infections or awaiting discharge after admission for orthopedic conditions. A linear decrease in cardiac output and cardiac index with age, averaging 1.0% and 0.8% per year, respectively, was found at rest in the supine position (Fig. 4.1).

These findings by Brandfonbrener et al. were reinforced when Granath et al. (1961, 1964) studied 17 healthy male volunteers 61–83 years old with pulmonary artery catheterization and measurements of cardiac output according to the direct Fick principle. These values were compared with data similarly obtained from 25 young men

TORE STRANDELL · Department of Clinical Physiology, St. Eriks Sjukhus, S-112 82 Stockholm, Sweden.

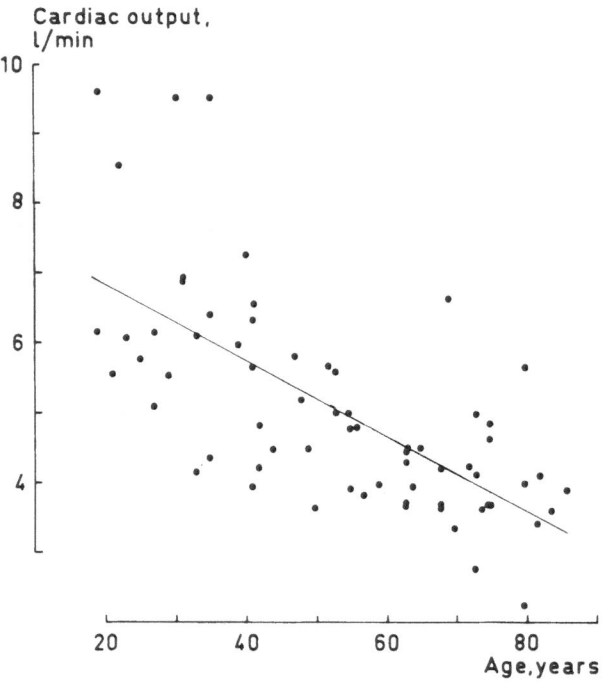

Fig. 4.1. Cardiac output at rest in recumbent position in relation to age in 67 "basal" males without circulatory disorder. From Brandfonbrener et al. (1955).

(mean age 23 years) previously studied in the same laboratory by Bevegård et al. (1960) and Holmgren et al. (1960). The 17 elderly men were invited from a previous Health Survey of the city of Stockholm, from the Labour Exchange, from old age homes, and from gymnastic groups for the aged, and were probably more physically fit than the average healthy subject of the same age. At a mean age of 71 years, their average cardiac output, at rest in a recumbent position, of 5.8 liters/min was 1.8 liters/min, or about 25%, lower than the corresponding value in the 23-year-old males.

Slightly lower cardiac outputs were observed by the same technique in 55 male patients, 60–86 years old, studied before prostatectomy (Renck 1969). Not all these patients had normal hearts, however; some had heart or lung diseases, or both.

Other studies by the direct Fick, or dye dilution techniques—by Foster et al. (1964) on 16 normal males 16–51 years old, by Malmborg (1965) on 11 males 39–55 years old, by Julius et al. (1967) on 54 sedentary males and females 18–68 years old, and by Hansson et al. (1968) on 75 normal males 20–49 years old—have failed to show any significant effect of age on resting cardiac output in the supine position. The reason for this finding may be at least partly that the age ranges studied were too narrow. It is evident from Fig. 4.1 that the interindividual variation in cardiac output is large, and that age accounts for only a minor part of this variation. Unless the number of subjects studied and their age range are large, therefore, this decrease with age will not be shown. Another possibility is that the decrease in cardiac output with age is not linear, as Fig. 4.1 would suggest, but that the most marked changes occur after, for example, 50 years of age.

There is no reason to believe that the decrease in cardiac output with age is different in women than in men, but sufficient data for proof are not available.

In the sitting position at rest, no significant difference in cardiac output was observed between old and young men (Granath et al. 1961, 1964; Julius et al. 1967), and no age change was recorded in the standing position (Hansson et al. 1968). This lack of differences with age is explained by the less marked decrease in cardiac output of elderly compared to young subjects when changing from the supine to the upright position, the decrease being 0.5 liters/min and 2.0 liters/min, respectively (Granath et al. 1961, 1964; Bevegård et al. 1960).

Cardiac Output During Exercise

During exercise in the supine position, the increase in cardiac output with increasing work load and oxygen uptake has been found to be the same in old and young (Figs. 4.2 and 4.3). At a given oxygen uptake, the cardiac output was thus lower in the old men, both at rest and during exercise, the average difference being 2.0 liters/min. With narrower age spans, no significant age differences in cardiac output during supine exercise were observed (Foster et al. 1964, Malmborg 1965).

During exercise in the sitting position, the increase in cardiac output with increasing work load and oxygen uptake was also found to be the same in old and young (Fig. 4.3). At all levels of oxygen uptake the cardiac output, like that in the supine position, was lower in the old men, the average difference during exercise being 1.3 liters/min. Because the old men had lower maximal oxygen uptakes than the young men, the calculated maximal cardiac output with exercise was also lower in old age. Less regular or insignificant effects of age have

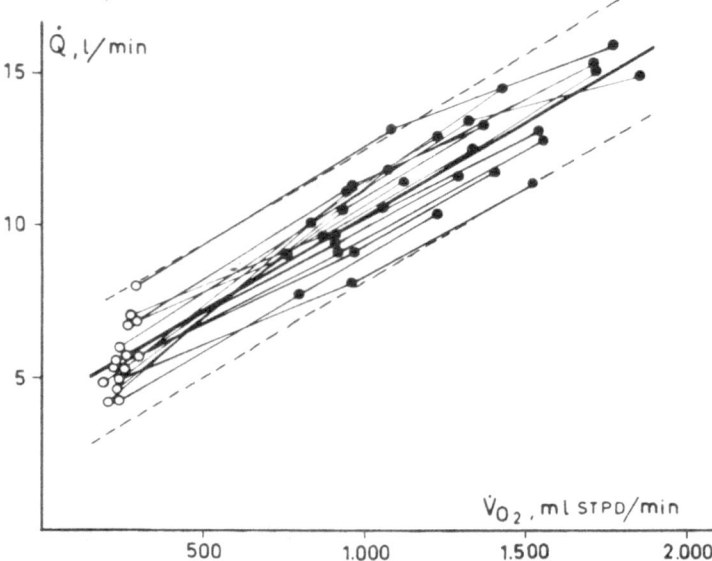

Fig. 4.2. Cardiac output ($\dot{Q}$) at rest (open circles) and during exercise (solid circles) in recumbent position in relation to oxygen uptake in 16 men 61–83 years old. From Granath et al. (1964).

also been reported (Hansson et al. 1968, Julius et al. 1967, Hartley et al. 1969). With the nitrous oxide method, higher cardiac outputs were observed with exercise in the elderly men and women studied (Becklake et al. 1965); in view of the data derived from more direct methods previously mentioned, methodological errors or differences in material may be assumed to explain these findings.

There is thus evidence from cross-sectional studies that cardiac output in elderly men is lower than in young men, both at rest in the supine position and during exercise in both the sitting and supine positions.

Causes of Reduced Cardiac Output in Old Age

The exact mechanisms that lead to the decrease in cardiac output with age are not yet completely understood. In some way, however, this decrease is related to the structural changes that occur with advancing age. These changes include increase in thickness and rigidity of the walls of the larger arteries and veins due to increased

collagen–elastin ratio, cross-linking, degenerative and sclerotic lesions in the endocardium, and increase of the elastic tissue in the
myocardium (see Bourne 1961). There is also a progressive increase of
coronary artery sclerosis with age (Lober 1953). These structural
changes will not be discussed in detail, but it should be noted that it
is impossible to distinguish clearly between degenerative changes and
"normal" physiological alterations with age. Naturally, the reduced
vascular distensibility affects the reflex mechanisms that regulate
cardiovascular function by means of stretch receptors, but the influence of age on these functions is not yet sufficiently studied.

With increasing age, there is a decrease in lean body mass (Shock
et al. 1953), with a reduction of the muscle mass and the number of
cells in the parenchymatous organs. This change is reflected in a
progressive decrease in basal metabolic rate with age, which reduces
the need for circulatory transport of oxygen. This decrease, however,
does not seem to account for more than about half the decrease in

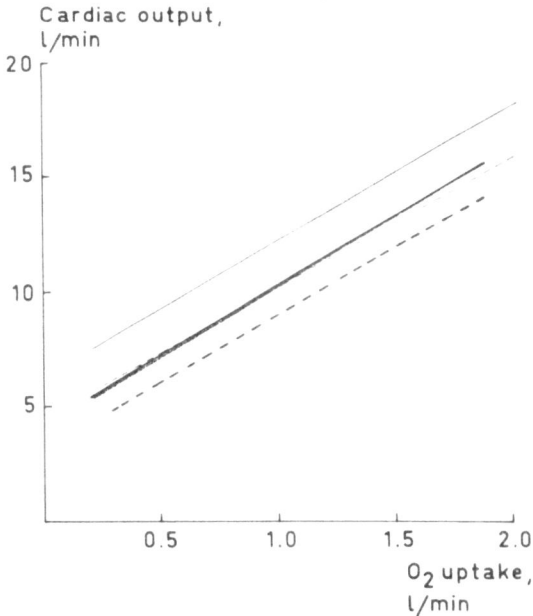

Fig. 4.3. Regression lines for cardiac output on oxygen uptake in 16 old men (mean age
71 yr, heavy lines) and 25 young men (mean age 23 yr, light lines) in recumbent (solid
lines) and sitting (dashed lines) position. From Granath et al. (1964), Bevegård et al.
(1960), and Holmgren et al. (1960).

cardiac output with age, as judged by the estimates of Landowne et al. (1955) and the observations by Granath et al. (1961, 1964).

Heart Rate

The hypokinetic circulation in elderly subjects with low values for cardiac output both at rest and during exercise could be due to reduction in heart rate or stroke volume, or in both. No significant changes with age, however, have been observed in heart rate at rest or during submaximal work loads, either in cross-sectional studies of subjects with similar degrees of physical activity (Robinson 1938, Åstrand 1960, König et al. 1961, Hollman 1963, Strandell 1964a) or in longitudinal studies (Dill and Consolazio 1962).

The maximal heart rate during exercise (Fig. 4.4) on the other hand, has always been found to decrease with age (Robinson 1938, Åstrand 1960, König et al. 1961, Hollman 1963, Strandell 1964b). In all these studies, the variability of the maximal heart rate was the same within the various age groups, and this variation has been found to be closely related to the level of heart rate at rest and during submaximal work (Strandell 1964b); i.e., subjects who have low heart rates at rest and during exercise also have low maximal heart rates.

The reason for this inability to reach high heart rates during exercise in old age is not clear. It cannot be due to inability of the

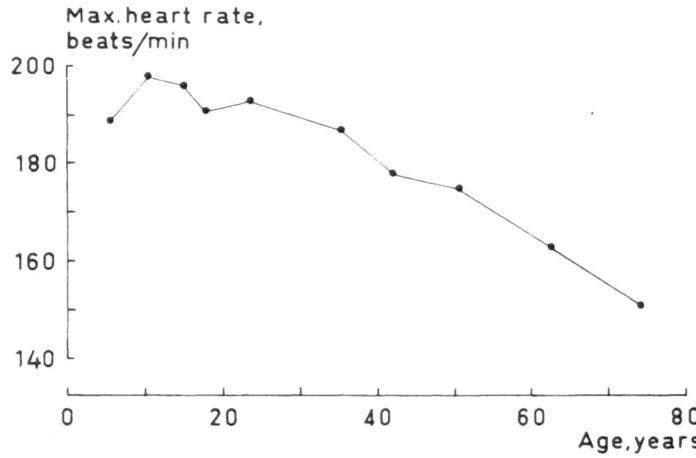

Fig. 4.4. Maximal heart rate during upright exercise in relation to age in 81 normal nonathletic males. From Robinson (1938).

heart to beat fast, however, because heart rates far above the maximal can be recorded during exercise in some apparently healthy old subjects during short bursts of paroxysmal supraventricular tachycardia during and after exercise (Strandell 1963).

It has long been known that the heart in old subjects reacts with a smaller rate increase on standing than in younger subjects (Norris et al. 1953). This finding, however, does not necessarily mean a changed sensitivity of the heart to sympathetic stimulation. A decline with age of the sympathetic drive to the heart during exercise has been suggested, however, by Conway et al. (1971), who observed a smaller effect of propranolol on heart rate and cardiac output during exercise in older than in younger subjects. This age difference needs further study, however, because it seemed to be present only at the highest work loads and only in the male group.

Stroke Volume

The decrease in cardiac output with age at rest and during submaximal exercise is thus entirely due to a reduction of stroke volume (Brandfonbrener et al. 1955, Granath et al. 1961, 1964). On the other hand, the decrease in the maximal cardiac output with age is more marked, and also due to the decrease in maximal heart rate during exercise. The smaller increase in stroke volume in old compared to young men on changing from rest in the sitting position to rest in the supine position or to exercise is evident from Fig. 4.5.

The magnitude of the stroke volume is influenced both by factors related to diastolic filling and initial fiber length, such as filling pressures and ventricular distensibility, and by factors related to systolic ejection, such as arterial pressures and myocardial contractility.

The systolic pressure load of the left ventricle, the systolic arterial pressure, is the best studied of these variables. Due to the increase in the rigidity of the walls of the aorta and the larger arteries with age the function of these vessels as a compression chamber is reduced, and the arterial pulse pressure increases with age, as does the resistance of the systemic circulation (Master et al. 1950, Landowne et al. 1955). The rise during exercise in systolic and mean arterial pressure has been found to be greater in old than in young subjects (Abboud and Huston 1961, König et al. 1962, Granath et al. 1961, 1964). The higher systolic pressure load of the left ventricle in old compared to young subjects is therefore still more marked during exercise than at rest.

The distensibility of the pulmonary artery also decreases with

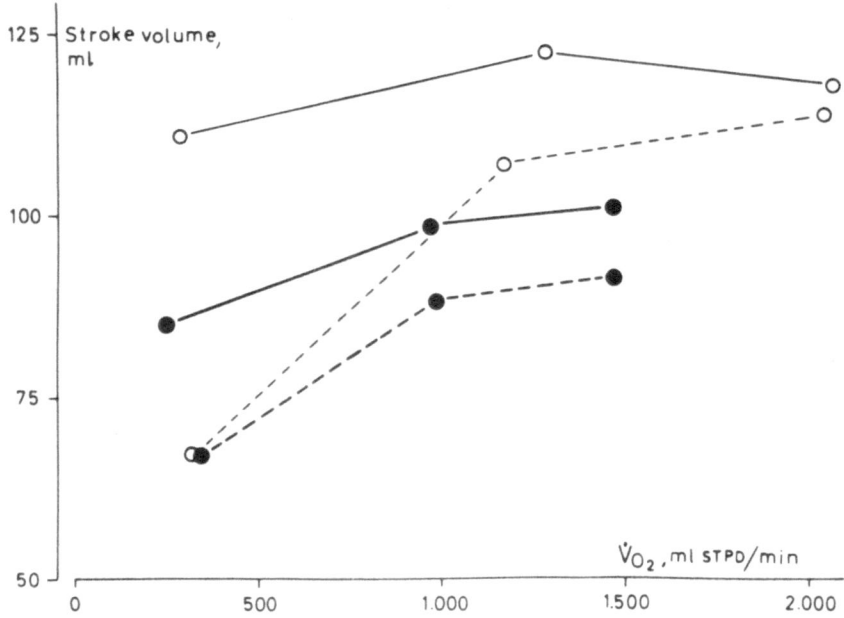

Fig. 4.5. Mean stroke volumes in relation to oxygen uptake at rest and during exercise in old (solid circles) and young men (open circles) in recumbent (solid lines) and sitting (dashed lines) position. From Granath et al. (1964), Bevegård et al. (1960), and Holmgren et al. (1960).

increasing age (Harris et al. 1965). The pulse pressure at rest is accordingly increased with age; this increase, however, is due not to an increase in the pulmonary artery systolic pressure, but to a slight decrease in the diastolic pressure (Granath et al. 1961, 1964; Gloger 1972). During exercise in both the supine and sitting positions, the systolic and mean pressures in the pulmonary artery increased about 10 mm Hg more in old than in young subjects (Table 4.1), indicating an increased flow resistance in the pulmonary vascular bed (Granath et al. 1961, 1964; Emirgil et al. 1967; Gloger 1972).

Thus, in old age, there is evidence, both at rest and still more during exercise, of increased impedance to systolic ejection by both the left and the right ventricle, which could contribute to a decrease in stroke volume or an increase in filling pressure.

The filling pressures at rest of both the left and the right ventricle, as judged by the pulmonary capillary venous pressure and the right ventricle end-diastolic pressure, were found to be the same in old and young subjects (Granath et al. 1961, 1964). During exercise, however,

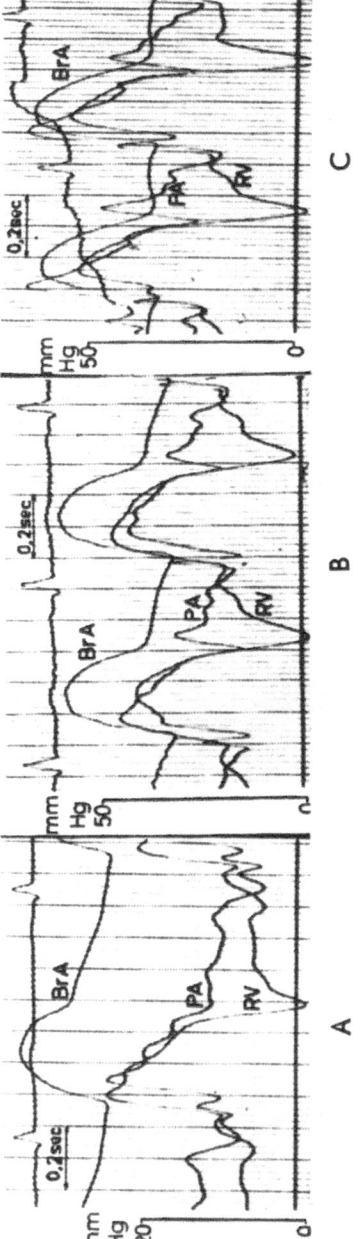

Fig. 4.6. Marked early-diastolic dip in pressure tracing from the right ventricle (RV) during recumbent exercise in a 75-year-old healthy man. (A) At rest, heart rate 81 beats/min, stroke volume 71 ml; (B) at 300 kpm/min, heart rate 104 beats/min, stroke volume 88 ml; (C) at 600 kpm/min, heart rate 125 beats/min, stroke volume 103 ml. From Granath et al. (1964).

TABLE 4.1. Pressures (mm Hg) at Rest and During Supine Bicycle Exercise in 17 Healthy Elderly Men Compared to Similar Data in 25 Young Men

Group	Oxygen uptake (liters/min)	Heart rate (beats/min)	Pulmonary capillary venous	Pulmonary artery			Right ventricle		
				Systolic	Diastolic	Mean	Systolic	End diastolic	Initial diastolic
Old men[a]									
Rest	0.26	67	9.9	24.3	10.1	15.9	25.8	8.1	3.1
Work I	0.96	104	22.0	45.3	19.9	31.6	48.1	13.5	4.3
Work II	1.46	130	22.1	45.7	21.3	32.4	51.4	13.1	2.9
Young men[b]									
Rest	0.29	70	12.5	23.3	12.3	17.2	27.6	9.3	3.1
Work I	0.96	97	15.4	33.3	16.9	24.5	37.6	9.3	3.7
Work II	2.06	157	15.6	35.3	15.1	23.5	46.6	6.2	−2.4

[a] Mean age, 70.5 yr (Granath et al. 1964).
[b] Mean age, 23.3 yr (Bevegård et al. 1960, Holmgren et al. 1960).

these pressures increased significantly more in the 60–83-year-old males than in the young ones, with average values about 7 mm Hg higher in the group of old men (Table 4.1). With a normal distensibility of the ventricular walls, these increased filling pressures during exercise in old age would cause a substantial increase in myocardial fiber length and stroke volume. There was evidence of reduced heart wall compliance, however, since in some cases the right ventricular pressure tracings during exercise showed very marked early diastolic dips (Fig. 4.6), as have been described in conditions with increased rigidity of the heart wall, such as constrictive pericarditis and endocardial or myocardial fibrosis. The high filling pressures observed during exercise may therefore be related to increased rigidity of the heart wall in old age, rather than to myocardial insufficiency requiring an increased length and tension of the myocardial fibers (Strandell 1964c).

The increased incidence of myocardial fibrosis in old age might contribute to this heart wall rigidity. Thus, the old men with the highest filling pressures during exercise were those with the most marked left axis deviation in the frontal plane ECG (Granath and Strandell 1964) and signs of left anterior fascicular block, which is most often related to myocardial fibrosis (Grant 1956). Another possibility might be the greater rigidity of the intercellular collagenous connective tissue that has been observed in old compared to young hearts (Kohn and Rollerson 1959). A stiffer heart wall would also increase the internal friction during contraction, which would affect unfavorably the relationship between useful and total ventricular work.

The high filling pressures during exercise observed in old age thus seem to be an adjustment to a reduced distensibility of the heart wall, which probably also increases the internal frictional losses, and to an increased impedance to ejection (Strandell 1964c). The decrease in stroke volume with age may be related both to the changes mentioned above and to a decrease in the myocardial contractility. This last factor is difficult to measure exactly, but can be evaluated indirectly.

It can be argued that the finding of a hypokinetic circulation with low cardiac output and stroke volume in old age combined with high filling pressures during exercise indicates myocardial insufficiency. Many facts, however, contradict such a view. Within the group of healthy elderly men studied by cardiac catheterization thus far, there was no relationship between high filling pressures and large heart volumes or the degree of S-T depression in the exercise ECG (Strandell 1964c). Nor were the lowest values of stroke work observed in the subjects with the largest hearts and the most marked electrocardiographic abnormalities, as is the case in patients with arterial hypertension (Varnauskas 1955). On the contrary, the healthy old men with the highest pulmonary capillary venous pressures during exercise had the most marked simultaneous increases in cardiac output in relation to oxygen uptake (Granath and Strandell 1964). They also had the most marked increases of stroke volume on exercise and the most marked simultaneous increases in pulse pressure in both the brachial and pulmonary arteries. The higher filling pressures during exercise were thus related to a higher stroke work. In addition, those who were physically most active had the highest filling pressures during exercise.

These healthy elderly men were thus quite different from those patients with myocardial insufficiency due to previous infarction or angina pectoris studied with heart catheterization by Malmborg (1965). His patients with the highest pulmonary capillary venous pressures during exercise had the lowest cardiac outputs, the smallest increases of cardiac output with increasing oxygen uptake, and the lowest exercise tolerance. Thus, high filling pressures seem to be a prerequisite for an effective response of the central circulation during exercise in physically fit healthy elderly men; in coronary artery disease and myocardial insufficiency, on the other hand, high filling pressures were a compensatory mechanism in the most disabled patients, who had poor responses of the central circulation to exercise.

Within the group of elderly men studied, there were also significant relationships between the filling pressures of the heart and pulmonary ventilation; the lowest pressures during exercise were observed in the subjects in whom the highest values for airway resistance could be expected (Granath and Strandell 1964).

Effect of Digitalization

In order to evaluate further the possibility of myocardial insufficiency in old age, 5 healthy men 66–80 years old were studied by right heart catheterization at rest and at two work loads in the supine position (Strandell 1970). Thereafter, they were digitalized with 1.6 mg deslanoside (Cedilanid) i.v., and the study was repeated 1½ h later. At rest, the subjects had after digitalization a slightly lower average stroke volume and a higher heart rate, but unchanged cardiac output, and slightly lower filling pressures in both the left and the right ventricle. All these changes, however, could be related to the effect of the previous exercise. During exercise, the heart rate, stroke volume, and cardiac output were the same before and after digitalization. The filling pressures of the left and right ventricles during exercise were somewhat lower at the first work load after digitalization, but less so at the second. It was not possible to state whether or not the slightly lower filling pressures during mild exercise with unchanged stroke volume were an effect of digitalization or of the previous exercise period. In some of the healthy elderly men, however, the high filling pressures during exercise did not decrease after digitalization.

Thus, although the pumping capacity of the heart decreases with age, there are no indications that this decrease is related in healthy subjects to subclinical coronary artery disease or myocardial insufficiency.

Effect of Physical Activity

The effect of short-term physical training on the central circulation in old age is not well known. In the group of 61–83-year-old men, the recent degree of physical activity, as recorded in the case history, was positively related to the ability to increase the stroke volume during an increase in work load in the supine position (Granath and Strandell 1964). A positive relationship was also observed between the degree of physical activity and the pulmonary capillary venous pressure during exercise in the supine position. Thus, the physically active men had the largest stroke volumes and the highest pulmonary capillary venous pressures during exercise. Three of these men took part in intense physical training for 3–4 weeks; they increased their maximal oxygen uptake by 10% and reduced their heart rates at submaximal loads accordingly. When these men were again studied by right heart catheterization, no change in the relationship between cardiac output and oxygen uptake was observed, but the average stroke volume during sitting exercise and the stroke volume at the highest work load in the supine position were about 10% higher than before the training period. At the same time, the average pulmonary capillary venous pressures and pulmonary artery pressures were about 5 mm Hg higher at the work load in the supine position.

These changes after training are in agreement with the previous findings, and indicate that the effect of physical activity and training on the central circulation, with an increase in stroke volume during exercise and in the maximal cardiac output, was connected in large part with regulation of the distribution of the blood volume, and presumably with the ability to increase the central blood volume during exercise. Simultaneously, the heart volume in the supine position increased after training by an average of about 10%.

The findings in these elderly men were thus similar to observations in young men, among whom active athletes have higher filling pressures during exercise than ordinarily trained men (Bevegård et al. 1963).

Dye dilution studies on the effect of short-term physical training in men 38–55 years old (Hartley et al. 1969) have shown, as in the group of elderly men studied, that the increase in maximal oxygen uptake was due solely to an increase in stroke volume, not to a simultaneous increase in the arteriovenous oxygen difference, as occurs in young men. They therefore suggested that changes in the distribution of blood flow by training are minimized by the aging process.

The effect on cardiac output of long-term intense physical training and aging was studied by dye dilution in 9 active athletes 44–55 years old by Grimby et al. (1966). Higher cardiac outputs in relation to oxygen uptake were observed at rest and during exercise, in comparison to young athletes and to untrained men. Apart from somewhat low hemoglobin concentrations, which might have been compensated for by an increased cardiac output, no explanation of these high cardiac outputs has thus far been found.

From the cross-sectional studies mentioned and the longitudinal ones of Hollman (1965) and Dill et al. (1967), it is quite clear that the maximal cardiac output and maximal oxygen uptake decrease less with increasing age in physically active than in sedentary subjects. Regular physical activity of suitable intensity and type should therefore be a good way of maintaining physical working capacity into old age.

Distribution of Cardiac Output in Old Age

The distribution of cardiac output at rest and during exercise in young subjects has been extensively described by Wade and Bishop (1962). Exactly how the reduction in cardiac output with age affects the various regional blood flows is less well known, but in all organs studied the regional flow resistance increases with age.

Davies and Shock (1950) observed a progressive decrease with age in *renal blood flow*, measured as diodrast clearance. The decrease of flow between the fourth and ninth decades was about 55%, or 0.6 liters/min; it is most probably related to the decrease with age in the number of active nephrons.

The *cerebral blood flow* has also been found to decline with age. Fazekas et al. (1952), using a modification of Kety's nitrous oxide method, compared groups of men between the ages of 34 and 68, and observed a decrease of about 20% with a slightly greater decrease in cerebral oxygen uptake.

The effect of aging on the *splanchnic blood flow*, which is the major regional flow in the body, is not known in detail. No major decrease with age has been observed, but it is likely that the blood flow to the metabolically active liver decreases at least in proportion to the decrease with age in the basal metabolic rate, or about 15% between 25 and 65 years of age.

No reports on the effect of age on the *coronary blood flow* in healthy subjects are available, because of the methodology involved. No major effects are to be expected, however, since Holmberg et al. (1971) showed the coronary blood flow at rest and during moderate exercise to be the same in patients with coronary heart disease and slightly younger control patients without coronary heart disease. Only during severe exercise were the coronary blood flow and the myocardial oxygen consumption lower than in the control group. When only such slight differences can be observed between patients with and without proven coronary artery stenosis, change with age in apparently healthy subjects is probably slight, except for the expected decrease of the maximal flow capacity.

Changes in total *skeletal muscle blood flow* are difficult to assess, but no significant decline with age in calf blood flow at rest was found by venous occlusion plethysmography by Allwood (1958). In his groups of healthy males, ages 18–24 and 70–82, respectively, the average values were, however, lower in the calf in the older group, and the vascular resistance was significantly higher in the old compared to the young group.

Like the renal circulation, the *skin blood flow* has functions other than to satisfy the metabolic needs of the tissues, and the arteriovenous oxygen difference is high. Since the skin blood flow is an integrated part of the thermoregulatory system of the body, the range of normal flow levels is wide even during standard conditions. Although a somewhat lower average value of the foot blood flow at rest was obtained in men 70–82 years old, compared to men 18–24 years old, the difference was not significant (Allwood 1958). Low skin temperatures are a well-known clinical finding in old age even in healthy subjects, however, and this finding indicates a low skin blood flow. In some healthy elderly men with low cardiac outputs, the reduction in blood flow to the lips, nose, and hands can lead to clearly visible cyanosis, especially in the erect position, when sympathetic tone is high. Thus, cyanosis of these parts in old age can be a simple effect of the normal reduction in cardiac output, and need not signify cardiac decompensation.

The effect of age on the *distribution of cardiac output during exercise* has not yet been studied in detail. That the rise in cardiac output in relation to oxygen uptake was the same in old (Granath et al. 1961, 1964) and young men (Bevegård et al. 1960, Holmgren et al. 1960), in both the supine and the sitting position, favors the idea of a similar distribution in old and young. Some studies are available of leg blood flow, which constitutes a major part of the increase in cardiac output during exercise. No differences in femoral venous oxygen saturation at rest or during bicycle exercise with one leg were observed by Carlson and Pernow (1961) between groups of healthy male volunteers 20–37 and 48–56 years old, indicating no significant change in leg blood flow with age. In a group of 7 healthy, well-trained, athletic men 52–59 years old, the same leg blood flow at rest was found by Wahren et al. (1974) as in a group of 8 physically fit, healthy men 25–30 years old (Jorfeldt and Wahren 1971). In both studies, the same constant-rate intra-arterial indicator infusion technique was applied. During exercise, however, the increase in leg blood flow was less in the middle-aged athletes, and was largely compensated for by a larger arteriovenous oxygen difference. It cannot be stated at present whether this difference in leg blood flow during exercise is due to age or to the exceptionally high degree of physical fitness of the older group, which had more than 10 years' participation in cross-country running and an average maximal oxygen uptake of 3.5 liters/min. Because muscle blood flow measured with the ^{133}Xe-clearance method has been found to be lower at a given work load in trained subjects than in untrained ones (Grimby et al. 1967), it is still an open question whether or not age per se reduces muscle blood flow during exercise.

Limiting Factors for Physical Work Capacity in Old Age

In parallel with the decrease with age in the maximal heart rate and stroke volume during exercise, and thus in the maximal cardiac output, physical performance is reduced. The decrease with age observed in cross-sectional studies of the maximal oxygen uptake (Fig. 4.7), however, is for various reasons less marked than the decrease in longitudinal studies (Hollman 1965, Dill et al. 1967). It has also been shown that the decrease in maximal oxygen uptake is more marked in

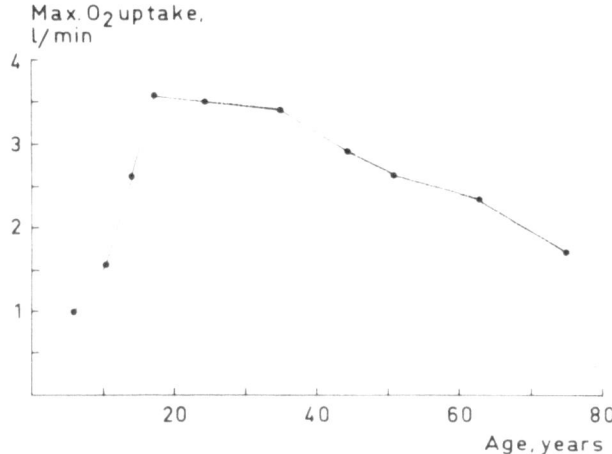

Fig. 4.7. Maximal oxygen uptake during upright exercise in relation to age in 81 normal nonathletic males. From Robinson (1938).

sedentary than in physically active subjects (Hollman 1965, Dill et al. 1967). The question then arises whether or not the reduced maximal cardiac output in old age is the main cause of the reduced physical work capacity. As age changes occur simultaneously in other organs, such as skeletal muscle and the lungs, the limitation might well be found outside the central circulation. In young subjects, both the physical work capacity (Kjellberg et al. 1949, Åstrand et al. 1963) and the stroke volume during exercise (Holmgren et al. 1960) are closely related to cardiovascular dimensions such as heart volume, total hemoglobin, and blood volume, suggesting that the work capacity is limited mainly by central circulatory factors (Sjöstrand 1960). Among 26 healthy men 61–83 years old (Strandell 1964b), however, there was no correlation of even probable significance between maximal work capacity and circulatory dimensions. Within the group of 17 of these old men (Granath and Strandell 1964) who were studied by right heart catheterization, the maximal work capacity was not related to any data on pressure and flow, except slightly to stroke volume at the highest work load. This relationship was lost, however, when the influence of age on the maximal work capacity was eliminated. Thus, there are no indications of a close relationship between maximal work capacity and central circulatory factors in old age. Nor were there any relationships in the group of 26 elderly men between maximal work capacity and lung volumes or measurements of pulmonary ventilatory function obtained by static and dynamic spirometry. Ventilatory factors, therefore, do not significantly limit the capacity for this type of physical exercise, but pulmonary limitation may be present in some subjects. In none of these subjects, however, were signs of pulmonary insufficiency present during maximal working intensity when arterial oxygen and carbon dioxide tensions were studied.

The closest relationship observed was the negative one between the maximal work capacity and the lactate concentration in arterial blood at a given submaximal work load. The maximal work capacity, representing the aerobic capacity, thus varied with the ability of the subjects to avoid accumulation of metabolites from anaerobic metabolism, and this ability could be assessed at submaximal work loads. The maximal physical work capacity was accordingly related to peripheral factors (Strandell 1964c), as has been suggested earlier in young subjects (Åstrand 1952, Cobb and Johnson 1963), and may have been associated with the muscular mass engaged in the exercise, the distribution of muscle blood flow, the diffusion of oxygen from the capillaries into the muscle cell, and cellular metabolic factors. The increased oxygen extraction by well-trained muscles has been related to the marked increase in the activity of oxidative mitochondrial enzymes and in the number and size of the mitochondria after physical training (Morgan et al. 1969). To date, however, these factors have not been studied in detail in old age.

References

Abboud, F. M., and Huston, J. H. (1961) *J. Clin. Invest.* **40**, 933.

Allwood, M. J. (1958) *Clin. Sci.* **17**, 331.

Åstrand, I. (1960) *Acta Physiol. Scand.* **49**, Suppl. 49.

Åstrand, P. O. (1952) *Experimental Studies of Physical Working Capacity in Relation to Sex and Age*, Munksgaard, Copenhagen.

Åstrand, P. O., Engström, L., Eriksson, B. O., Karlberg, P., Nylander, I., Saltin, B., and Thoren, C. (1963) *Acta Paediatr. Scand. Suppl.* **147**.

Becklake, M. R., Frank, H., Dagenais, G. R., Ostiguy, G. L., and Guzman, C. A. (1965) *J. Appl. Physiol.* **20**, 938.

Bevegård, S., Holmgren, A., and Jonsson, B. (1960) *Acta Physiol. Scand.* **49**, 279.

Bevegård, S., Holmgren, A., and Jonsson, B. (1963) *Acta Physiol. Scand.* **57**, 26.

Bourne, G. H. (1961) *Structural Aspects of Ageing*, Pitman Medical Publishing Co. Ltd., London.

Brandfonbrener, M., Landowne, M., and Shock, N. W. (1955) *Circulation* **12**, 557.

Carlson, L. A., and Pernow, B. (1961) *Acta Physiol. Scand.* **52**, 328.

Cobb, L. A., and Johnsson, W. P. (1963) *J. Clin. Invest.* **42**, 800.

Conway, J., Wheeler, R., and Sannerstedt, R. (1971) *Cardiovasc. Res.* **5**, 577.

Cournand, A., Riley, R. L., Breed, E. S., Baldwin, E. de F., and Richards, D. W. (1945) *J. Clin. Invest.* **24**, 106.

Davies, D. F., and Shock, N. W. (1950) *J. Clin. Invest.* **29**, 496.

Dill, D. B., and Consolazio, C. F. (1962) *J. Appl. Physiol.* **17**, 645.

Dill, D. B., Robinson, S., and Ross, J. C. (1967) *J. Sports Med. Phys. Fitness* **7**, 4.

Emirgil, C., Sobol, B. J. Campodonico, S., Herbert, W. H., and Mechkati, R. (1967) *J. Appl. Physiol.* **23**, 631.

Fazekas, J. F., Alman, R. W., and Bessman, A. N. (1952) *Am. J. Med. Sci.* **223**, 245.

Foster, G. L., Reeves, T. J., and Meade, J. H. (1964) *J. Clin. Invest.* **43**, 1758.

Gloger, von K. (1972) *Z. Kreislaufforsch.* **61**, 728.

Granath, A., Jonsson, B., and Strandell, T. (1961) *Acta Med. Scand.* **169**, 125.

Granath, A., Jonsson, B., and Strandell, T. (1964) *Acta Med. Scand.* **176**, 425.

Granath, A., and Strandell, T. (1964) *Acta Med. Scand.* **176**, 447.

Grant, R. P. (1956) *Circulation* **14**, 233.

Grimby, G., Häggendal, E., and Saltin, B. (1967) *J. Appl. Physiol.* **22**, 305.

Grimby, G., Nilsson, N. J., and Saltin, B. (1966) *J. Appl. Physiol.* **21**, 1150.

Hansson, J. S., Tabakin, B. S., and Levy, A. M. (1968) *Circulation* **37**, 345.

Harris, P., Heath, D., and Apostolopoulos, A. (1965) *Br. Heart J.* **27**, 651.

Hartley, L. H., Grimby, G., Kilbom, Å., Nilsson, N. J., Åstrand, I., Bjurö, J., Ekblom, B., and Saltin, B. (1969) *Scand. J. Clin. Lab. Invest.* **24**, 335.

Hollman, W. (1963) *Höchst- und Dauerleistungsfähigkeit des Sportlers*, Johann Ambrosius Barth, München.

Hollman, W. (1965) *Körperliches Training als Prävention von Herz-Kreislauf-Krankheiten*, Hippokrates Verlag, Stuttgart, West Germany.

Holmberg, S., Serzysko, W., and Varnauskas, E. (1971) *Acta Med. Scand.* **190**, 465.

Holmgren, A., Jonsson, B., and Sjöstrand, T. (1960) *Acta Physiol. Scand.* **49**, 343.

Jorfeldt, L., and Wahren, J. (1971) *Clin. Sci.* **41**, 459.

Julius, S., Amery, A., Whitlock, L. S., and Conway, J. (1967) *Circulation* **36**, 222.

Kjellberg, S. R., Rudhe, U., and Sjöstrand, T. (1949) *Acta Radiol.* **31**, 113.

Kohn, R. R., and Rollerson, E. (1959) *Circ. Res.* **7**, 740.

König, K., Reindell, H., Mosshoff, K., Roskamm, H., and Kessler, M. (1961) *Arch. Kreislaufforsch.* **35**, 37.

König, K., Reindell, H., and Roskamm, H. (1962) *Arch. Kreislaufforsch.* **39**, 143.

Landowne, M., Brandfonbrener, M., and Shock, N. W. (1955) *Circulation* **12**, 567.

Lober, H. (1953) *A.M.A. Arch. Pathol.* **55**, 357.

Malmborg, R. O. (1965) *Acta Med. Scand. Suppl.* **426.**

Master, A. M., Dublin, L. I., and Marks, H. H. (1950) *J. Am. Med. Assoc.* **143**, 1464.

Morgan, T. E., Short, F. A., and Cobb, L. A. (1969) *Am. J. Physiol.* **216**, 82.

Norris, A. H., Shock, N. W., and Yiengst, M. J. (1953) *Circulation* **8**, 521.

Renck, H. (1969) *Acta Anaesthesiol. Scand. Suppl.* **34.**

Robinson, S. (1938) *Arbeitsphysiologie* **10**, 251.

Shock, N. W., Yiengst, M. J., and Watkin, D. M. (1953) *J. Gerontol.* **8**, 388.

Sjöstrand, T. (1960) *In: Clinical Cardio-pulmonary Physiology*, Grune and Stratton, Inc., New York, p. 201.

Strandell, T. (1963) *Acta Med. Scand.* **174**, 479.

Strandell, T. (1964a) *Acta Physiol. Scand.* **60**, 197.

Strandell, T. (1964b) *Acta Med. Scand.* **176**, 301.

Strandell, T. (1964c) *Acta Med. Scand. Suppl.* **414.**

Strandell, T. (1970) *Symposium on Incipient Cardiac Insufficiency*, Sandoz Ltd., Basel, p. 203.

Varnauskas, E. (1955) *Scand. J. Clin. Lab. Invest.* **7**, Suppl. 17.

Wade, O. L., and Bishop, J. M. (1962) *Cardiac Output and Regional Blood Flow*, Oxford, Blackwell Scientific Publications.

Wahren, J., Saltin, B., Jorfeldt, L., and Pernow, B. (1974) *Scand. J. Clin. Lab. Invest.* **33**, 79.

5

Blood Pressure and Its Regulation

R. H. JOHNSON

Introduction

This chapter is concerned with blood pressure regulatory mechanisms in the elderly and the conditions in which they are disturbed. It is not intended to be a general review of circulatory physiology and the disorders that affect it. A full account of the normal circulation is that of Folkow and Neil (1971); clinical disorders affecting circulatory regulation are described by Johnson and Spalding (1975). Hypertension in old age is considered in detail in Chapter 7, and is therefore mentioned only briefly here.

The ability to adjust the activity of the heart and peripheral circulatory resistance as stresses affect the circulation is maintained throughout life:

> "You are old, Father William," the young man said,
>   "And your hair has become very white;
> And yet you incessantly stand on your head—
>   Do you think, at your age, it is right?"
>
> "In my youth," Father William replied to his son,
>   "I feared it might injure the brain;
> But now that I'm perfectly sure I have none,
>   Why, I do it again and again."

R. H. JOHNSON · University Department of Neurology, Institute of Neurological Sciences, Southern General Hospital, Glasgow, G51 4TF, Scotland.

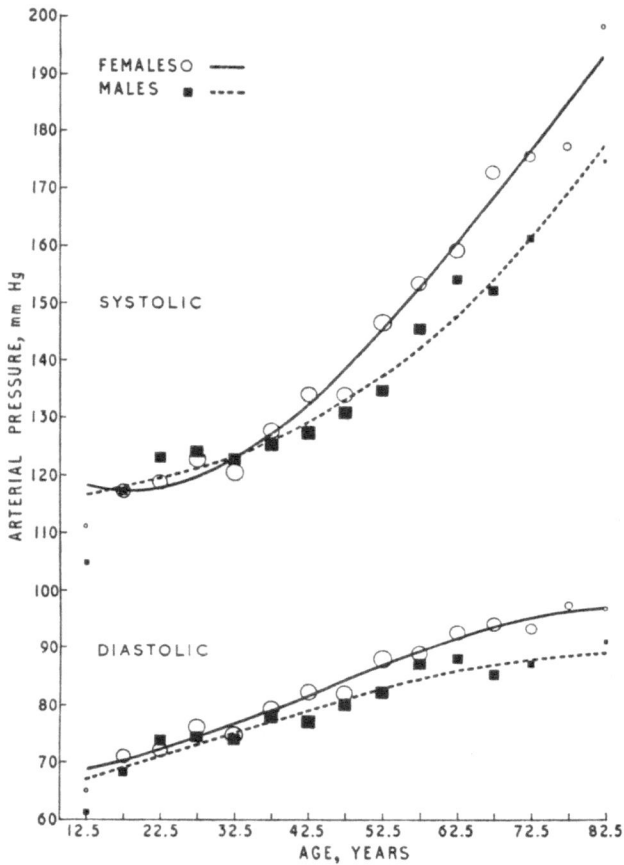

Fig. 5.1. Systolic and diastolic blood pressures for females and males. The area of each circle or square is proportional to the number of subjects in each 5-year age group (Hamilton et al. 1954). There is a wide range of systolic pressure in the elderly, but the range of diastolic pressure is much less.

Normal Blood Pressure in the Elderly

The normal range of arterial blood pressure between systolic and diastolic pressures increases with age (Hamilton et al. 1954). Elderly subjects without disease may therefore have blood pressures that would be unacceptable in younger age groups (Fig. 5.1). Systolic blood pressure ranges particularly widely (Master et al. 1958; Anderson and Cowan 1959, 1972; Caird 1963). The effect of aging on diastolic pressure is much less unless weight gain also occurs (Ulrych et al. 1973). In a study of 114 elderly people over 70 years of age in the community, it was found that diastolic pressures were not significantly greater in the older subjects in the series (Martin and Millard 1973). There was a statistically significant increase in electrocardiographic abnormalities when the diastolic pressure was 100 mm Hg or more, and this figure may therefore be regarded as the acceptable upper limit in elderly subjects. This conclusion is in agreement with the conclusions of other workers (Gavey 1949; Master et al. 1958; Anderson and Cowan 1959, 1972).

Arterial blood pressure shows a diurnal rhythm (Richardson et al. 1964); it also alters widely in relation to exertion (Humphreys and Lind 1963, Lind and McNicol 1967a,b). It has been suggested that variability of blood pressure should be considered in the genesis of vascular accidents, particularly since blood pressure fluctuations are greater in subjects with hypertension (Zulch and Hossmann 1967). A series of men with ischemic cerebrovascular disease were therefore studied by means of automatic blood pressure monitoring over 24 h (Gross and Marshall 1970). Supportive evidence was obtained that variance of blood pressure was related to the height of blood pressure. It did not appear, however, that there was any difference between those with definite evidence of cerebral infarction and those who had had transient ischemic attacks.

The arterial blood pressure depends primarily on the cardiac output and the peripheral resistance. It is kept within due bounds by a number of mechanisms, particularly the baroreceptor reflex (Heymans and Neil 1958). The chief baroreceptors are in the carotid sinus near the bifurcation of the carotid arteries and in the arch of the aorta. The afferent nerve supply for the carotid sinus is in the ninth cranial nerve; for the arch of the aorta, it is in the vagus. Afferent impulses reach the cardiovascular centers in the brain stem, eliciting motor responses that tend to keep the blood pressure constant. The efferent pathways are parasympathetic through the vagi that slow the heart, and sympathetic through fibers to peripheral vessels, thus altering peripheral resistance. Sympathetic fibers also innervate the heart (Mitchell 1953). Animal experiments have suggested that other vascular baroreceptor reflexes may exist in the venous or arterial circulation, or that different central pathways are involved (Sarnoff and Yamada 1959, Beacham and Kunze 1969, Andrews et al. 1971). Nevertheless, there is no good evidence at present for effective baroreceptor reflexes except from the carotid sinus and the arch of the aorta.

The baroreceptor reflexes are called into play when the circulation is stressed, as when one stands. When a healthy subject stands, the blood pressure usually changes little. The systolic pressure may fall 10–15 mmHg; the diastolic pressure may rise or fall 5 mmHg (Currens 1948). Change of posture from the horizontal to the vertical results in a fall in cardiac output to 75–80% of the output when supine (Bickel- mann et al. 1961, Folkow and Neil 1971). The maintenance of blood pressure on standing is also associated with an increase in heart rate, which is usually greater in the young than in the old. In young people, the increase is about 20 beats/min, whereas in old age the increase is 10–15 beats/min (Hellström 1961, Strandell 1964). This difference illustrates that baroreceptor activity diminishes with age (Bristow et al. 1969), and details are therefore given below. Any disruption of the baroreflex arc results in failure of blood pressure homeostasis, and cerebral perfusion is not maintained. This review therefore continues with details of cerebral blood flow regulation. Failure of cerebral blood pressure regulation results in the development of symptoms, begin- ning with graying of vision. The subject then feels dizzy and will lose consciousness if the fall in blood pressure is not corrected. Such episodes may occur intermittently and transiently—"syncope"—or may develop whenever the subject stands—postural hypotension. This review therefore concludes with a discussion of disorders in which there is failure of regulation. The first part of the concluding section describes causes of syncope in the elderly; the second part considered chronic causes of failure of blood pressure homeostasis, which results in orthostatic hypotension.

Baroreceptor Reflex Sensitivity

One method of assessing baroreceptor reflex sensitivity is to record blood pressure through an intra-arterial cannula and to give intravenous injections of a pressor agent such as angiotensin (0.25–2.0 μg) or the α-stimulating agent phenylephrine (50–200 μg) (Pickering et al. 1968, Smyth et al. 1969, Sleight et al. 1971). These drugs cause a transient rise in blood pressure and reflex bradycardia. The systolic pressures of successive arterial pulses are plotted against heart rate (or pulse intervals), and the relationship of change in heart rate to the alteration in blood pressure is an index of activity of baroreceptor reflexes from both the carotid sinus and the aorta. This test depends, on the efferent side, on vagal control of heart rate, and ignores changes in peripheral vascular resistance. It has been shown, how- ever, that direct stimulation of the nerve supplying the carotid sinus produces similar effects on heart rate and on peripheral resistance

(Carlsten et al. 1958). The test also requires that aortic baroreceptor activity be similarly affected, and although no evidence is available in man, some studies in animals point to this being so (James 1972).

The baroreceptor sensitivity increases during sleep (Pickering et al. 1968; Bristow et al. 1969b) and after β-adrenergic blockade at rest, but not during exercise (Sleight et al. 1971). These findings suggest that normally at rest, β-adrenergic sympathetic sensitivity modifies bradycardia induced by the baroreceptor reflex. Baroreceptor sensitivity is decreased in exercise in subjects with high arterial pressure and as age increases, at least up to the age of 65 (Fig. 5.2) (Bristow et al. 1969a, Bristow et al. 1969c, Sleight et al. 1971, Gribbin et al. 1971). The change in sensitivity may be due to decreased distensibility of the arterial wall at the baroreceptor site (Bristow et al. 1969a,c, Sleight 1971), as distensibility of the sinus is essential for the baroreceptors to be stimulated (Hauss et al. 1949). Studies on necropsy specimens from the carotid artery have substantiated that its arterial wall and that of the carotid sinus are less distensible with increasing age (Fig. 5.3) (Winson et al. 1974).

The effect of baroreflex activity may also be examined by studying the effect of *Valsalva's maneuver* (1707) on blood pressure and heart rate. In this maneuver, an acute rise in intrathoracic pressure is obtained by asking the subject to take a deep inspiration and then to

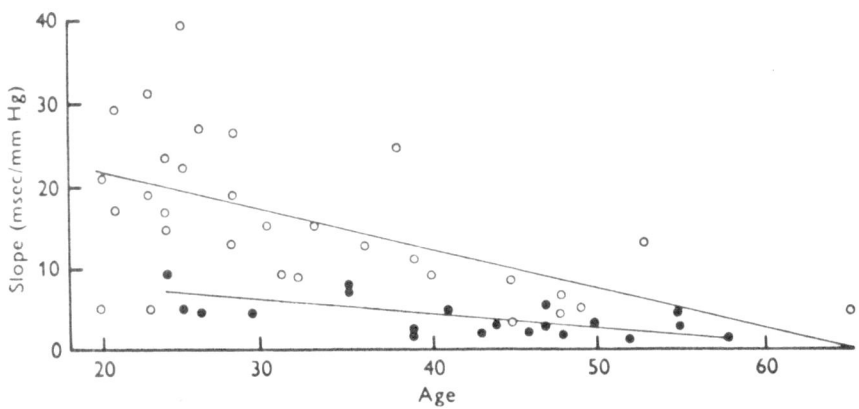

Fig. 5.2. Baroreflex sensitivity pulse interval related to change in blood pressure (msec/mmHg) related to age in normotensive subjects (O) and subjects with hypertension (mean arterial blood pressure above 100 mm Hg (●) (Bristow et al. 1969a). Baroreceptor sensitivity is reduced with increasing age and with hypertension.

LOAD (g)

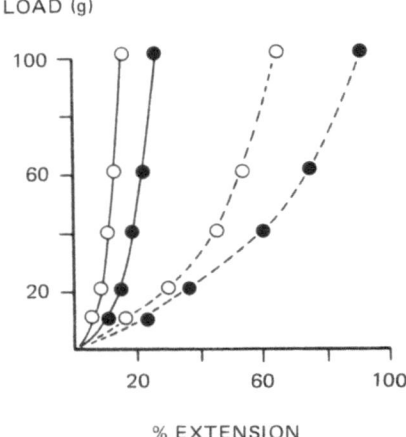

Fig. 5.3. Circumferential extensibility of the right carotid sinuses (O) and right common carotid arteries (●) in a 27-year-old man (– – –) and a 75-year-old woman (———) (Winson et al. 1974). The carotid sinus is more rigid than the common carotid artery in both subjects, and the vessels of the older subject are more rigid than those of the younger.

% EXTENSION

attempt to expire forcibly for at least 7 sec, keeping his nose and mouth closed. There is an initial rise in blood pressure (Fig. 5.4, phase I), and then the raised intrathoracic pressure inhibits venous return to the heart and the blood pressure falls (phase II). After about 5 sec in a normal subject, the blood pressure levels off and begins to rise (phase III); this rise is attributed to reflex vasoconstriction. When the intrathoracic pressure is released, the blood pressure rises and, in normal subjects, exceeds the original levels because of the persistence of vasoconstriction (phase IV). The rise in blood pressure causes bradycardia through the baroreceptor reflex. The changes of heart rate and blood pressure at different stages of the maneuver have been extensively examined and are reviewed by Johnson and Spalding (1974). A relationship has been suggested between the fall in arterial pulse pressure during the maneuver and the maximum rise in diastolic pressure in the seconds after the maneuver (Sharpey-Schafer 1955, Sharpey-Schafer and Taylor 1960), and it has been suggested that this relationship is affected by age (Appenzeller and Descarries 1964, Gross 1970). This method of assessing the cardiovascular effects of the maneuver has not been altogether satisfactory (Corbett 1969, Johnson and Spalding 1974). Alternative criteria indicating impairment of circulatory reflexes (Corbett 1969, Johnson and Spalding 1974) are (1) Absence of a systolic blood pressure overshoot in phase IV, (2) lower heart rate in phase II than in phase IV, (3) a fall in mean blood pressure in phase II below 50% of the resting mean arterial pressure.

Cerebral Blood Flow in the Elderly

Although it has been suggested that the cerebral blood flow and cerebral metabolic rate of elderly patients are the same as those of young healthy controls (Dastur et al. 1963), the consensus is that as age increases, both cerebral blood flow and cerebral metabolic rate fall (Fazekas et al. 1952, Purves 1972, Schieve and Wilson 1953, Wang and Busse 1975). The density of cortical neurons is also reduced with advancing age (Fig. 5.5) (Brody 1955, Kety 1956, Purves 1972). It is not known, however, whether the explanation of the reductions with age is that blood flow is adjusted to metabolic requirements or that

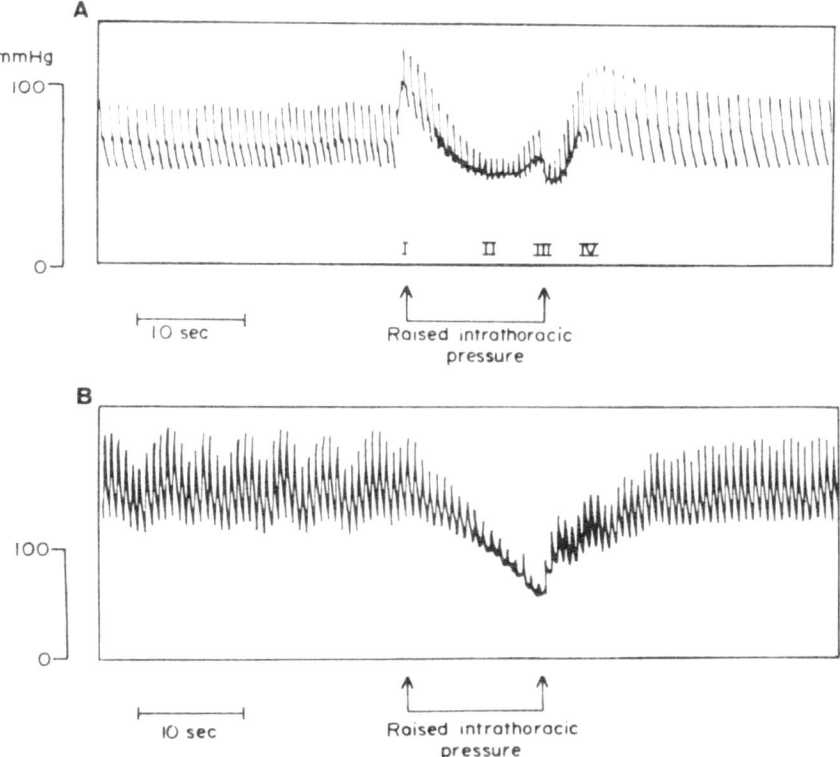

Fig. 5.4. Blood pressure in a normal subject (A) and a patient with orthostatic hypotension (B) before, during, and after Valsalva's maneuver (Johnson and Spalding 1974). The four phases of the blood pressure response are described in the text. The patient's response is blocked.

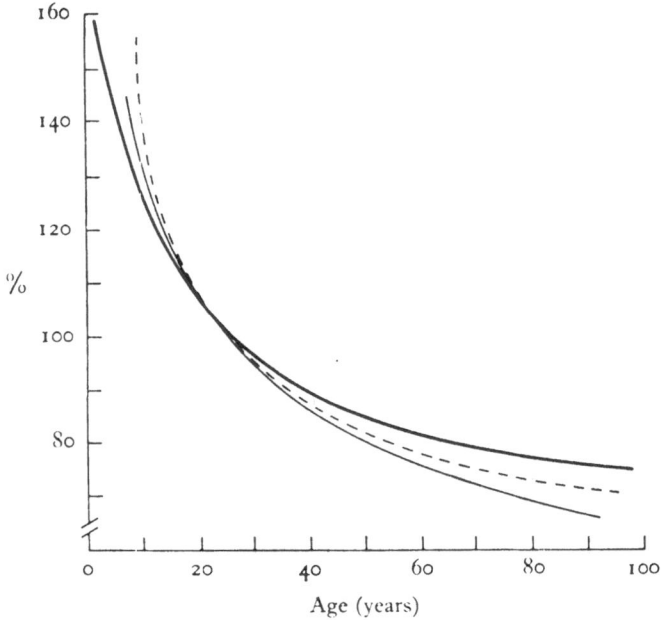

Fig. 5.5. The changes with advancing age of cerebral blood flow (----), cerebral oxygen consumption (———), and density of cortical neurons (———) related to mean values at the age of 25 years (Kety 1956).

cerebral metabolism is regulated by the rate of cerebral perfusion. Some authors have concluded that there is an inverse relationship between total cerebral blood flow (and metabolic rate) and the degree of dementia (Freyham et al., 1951; Fazekas et al., 1953; Lassen et al., 1957). Reduction in cerebral blood flow in elderly patients appears to be related to the severity of cerebrovascular disease (Yoshida et al. 1975). Subjects with low blood flow through the gray matter of the brain have lower scores on intellectual testing, especially of performance (Table 5.1) (Wang and Busse 1975). Lower blood flow through the gray matter was found in subjects with lower mean arterial blood pressure (Table 5.2). It may be that the elevation of blood pressure in the normal range found with old age (see Fig. 5.1) is related to the maintenance of adequate cerebral blood flow. This maintenance may in turn allow cerebral metabolism to continue normally and intellectual function to be retained. The change in cerebral blood flow may be a consequence rather than a cause of cerebral cell loss, however, depending on the nature of the disease.

The cerebral blood flow changes with hyper- or hypocapnia are reduced with advancing age (Fazekas et al., 1952; Schieve and Wilson 1953). In a study of three groups of elderly subjects (a) normotensive but with arteriosclerosis, (b) hypertensive without arteriosclerosis, and (c) hypertensive with arteriosclerosis, it was found that the first group had a smaller response of cerebral blood flow to hypercapnia than the other two groups (Novack et al., 1953). It was concluded that these responses are related to the extent of vascular disease.

Failure of Blood-Pressure Regulation in the Elderly

Any fall in blood pressure may result in failure of normal cerebral perfusion and the development of symptoms associated with cerebral hypoxia. If the fall is slight, the patient experiences dizziness or visual blackout, and there may be altered consciousness. If the fall is rapid and considerable, the patient loses consciousness. It is useful to consider disorders that may present with episodic loss of consciousness—*syncope*—because this is a clinical problem, and also to consider conditions in which there is a more continuous failure to maintain blood pressure, particularly in response to the upright posture— *orthostatic hypotension*. There is overlap between such classifications, however, since patients with orthostatic hypotension may present with syncope.

TABLE 5.1. Comparison of Intellectual Test Results[a] in 24 Elderly Subjects with High and 24 with Low Gray Matter Cerebral Blood Flow

Intellectual scores	Gray matter blood flow (ml/100 g per min)	
	High flow	Low flow
Verbal	60.3±20.9	52.5±21.3
Performance	31.8±13.7	23.7±11.4[b]
Full	92.1±33.7	76.9±32.2

[a] Wechsler tests: means±SD.
[b] There was a significantly lower performance scale in those with low flows ($P < 0.05$). (Wang and Busse 1975)

TABLE 5.2. Relationship between Mean Arterial Blood Pressure and Mean Gray Matter Blood Flow (±SD) in Elderly Patients[a]

	Mean arterial blood pressure (mm Hg)		
	94 or less	95–114	115 or more
Number of patients	10	29	9
Gray matter blood flow (ml/100 g per min)[b]	42.3±4.4	47.5±10.0	52.5±11.5

[a] Wang and Busse (1975).
[b] Mean gray matter blood flow is significantly greater in the highest than in the lowest blood pressure group ($P < 0.02$).

Causes of Syncope

An important differential diagnosis is epilepsy, and it is not uncommon for such patients to present at a neurological clinic for investigations of attacks of unconsciousness or convulsions, or both. The cardiac causes of syncope (Fig. 5.6) are considered in detail in other chapters. It may also develop with overactivity or paralysis of the reflex arc from baroreceptors subserving blood pressure regulation. Those that are particularly likely to occur in the elderly due to active reflexes are described below. Others, such as emotional fainting and reflex hypotension from visceral stimulation, although they may occur in any age group, usually occur in younger people. Such conditions are reviewed in detail by Johnson and Spalding (1974). Disorders related to paralyzed reflexes from baroreceptors are discussed in the later section on orthostatic hypotension.

Cough Syncope. Loss of consciousness after coughing (Charcot 1876) was not widely recognized until recently (Whitty 1943, Baker 1949). In adults, it has usually been reported in those who smoke. After a bout of coughing, there may be momentary loss of consciousness, in which the subject falls to the ground and may twitch. Less severe symptoms are dizziness and temporary mental clouding. These symptoms are circulatory in origin, due to an acute reduction of supply pressure of blood to the brain (Sharpey-Schafer 1953a,b) similar to the changes that accompany Valsalva's maneuver (see Fig. 5.4). Venous return is impeded, and the cardiac output and arterial blood pressure fall. The reflex response is an increase in peripheral vascular resistance, which results in an overshoot of arterial blood pressure when the paroxysm stops. Some patients cough intermittently and repeatedly, and in them another factor enters into the syncope. The coughing produces large pressure transients within the chest, which are transmitted to the aorta and thence along major arteries. These arterial pressure transients stimulate baroreceptors and result in a reflex fall in peripheral vascular resistance, and hence in arterial blood pressure (Sharpey-Schafer 1953a,b; Gastaut et al. 1959). Treatment depends on reducing or stopping coughing; in particular, the patient should give up smoking. Although the circulatory explanation probably accounts for most cases, it may be that some are epileptic (Whitty 1943).

Carotid Sinus Syncope (or Syndrome). This condition occurs in middle-aged or elderly patients, usually men who suffer from symptoms due to a hypersensitive carotid sinus reflex (Weiss and Baker

Cardiopulmonary disease	Arrhythmias
	Paroxysmal tachycardia
	Ventricular fibrillation
	Atrioventricular block
	Sinoatrial block
	Stokes–Adams attacks
	Coronary artery disease
	Angina pectoris
	Myocardial infarction
	Obstructive disease
	Congenital cyanotic heart disease
	Myxoma and ball valve thrombus
	Hypertrophic obstructive cardiomyopathy
	Pulmonary hypertension
	Pulmonary embolism
Reflex circulatory disorders	Active reflexes
	Emotional fainting
	Voluntarily induced syncope
	Micturition syncope
	Cough syncope
	Carotid sinus syncope
	Reflex from viscera, eyeballs, or swallowing
	Paralyzed reflexes
	Neurogenic causes of orthostatic hypotension (see Fig. 5.8)
	Alcohol and drug toxicity
Other	Hypoglycemia
	Hyperventilation
	Anemia

Fig. 5.6. Causes of syncope.

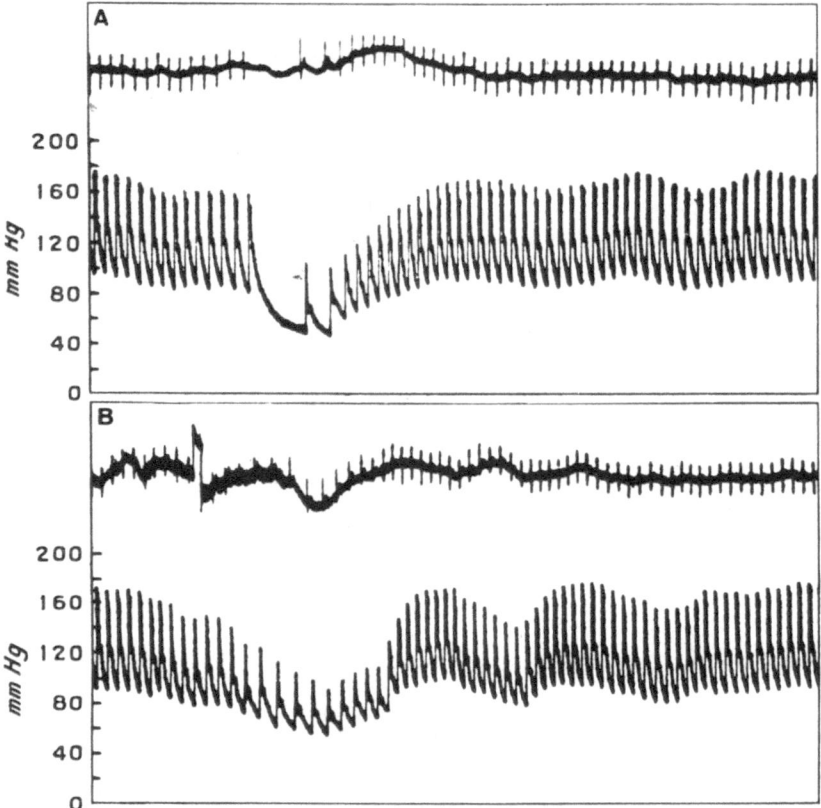

Fig. 5.7. (A) Effect of carotid sinus stimulation on heart rate and arterial blood pressure;
(B) the same study carried out in the same patient after atropine (1 mg) intravenously
(Hutchinson and Stock 1960). Carotid sinus stimulation caused asystole and hypotension. The degree of hypotension was similar after atropine, implying a vasodilator
component of the reflex.

1933, Hutchinson and Stock 1960, Heron et al. 1965). The condition
has been called carotid sinus syncope, but only about a third lose
consciousness, though some of those have convulsions. Other major
symptoms are vertigo, mental confusion, and focal disturbances such
as unilateral sensory symptoms or clonic movements of a limb (Hutchinson and Stock 1960). The focal symptoms have been attributed to
concomitant cerebrovascular disease. An attack may be provoked by
turning the head to one side, particularly with a tight collar; tying a
tie; or exertion. Part of the mechanism underlying the attacks was
described by Parry (1799), who noted slowing of the heart rate on

pressure on one of the carotid arteries. Stimulation of the carotid sinus by external pressure in these patients produces not only cardiac slowing via vagal activity, but also peripheral vasodilatation (Fig. 5.7).

The tendency for carotid sinus syncope to occur mainly in elderly men may be related to a greater severity and frequency of bradycardia in response to carotid sinus stimulation in old men (Mankikar and Clark 1975). The diagnosis may be assisted by pressure over the carotid sinus and observation of the heart rate. It is essential to listen to the heart or watch an ECG and to cease stimulation as soon as bradycardia begins (Arenberg et al. 1971), for death can occasionally occur with carotid pressure (Nelson and Mahru 1963). Although it has been recommended that the test should not be carried out on patients over 75 years of age (Lown and Levine 1961), Mankikar and Clark (1975) found the investigation safe in their 386 patients, of whom 248 were 80–104 years old. Treatment consists of atropine by mouth to block the vagal effects of the reflex. Spontaneous remission may occur, but if attacks persist, even with medical treatment, denervation of the carotid sinus may be considered (Hutchinson and Stock 1960).

Micturition Syncope. This condition (Proudfit and Forteza 1959) is said to occur in patients who faint at the end of or soon after micturition. It is particularly likely to be misdiagnosed as epilepsy (Coggins et al. 1964), and it is a disorder predominantly of men of all

---

Cerebrovascular disease
Idiopathic orthostatic hypotension

    Multiple-system degeneration, including Parkinsonism, postganglionic
    autonomic degeneration, deficient catecholamine release

Parkinson's disease (idiopathic paralysis agitans)
Spinal Cord Lesions
Tabes Dorsalis
Polyneuropathy

    Acute polyneuropathy
    Chronic polyneuropathy
      Diabetes mellitus
      Amyloidosis
      Carcinoma
      Chronic renal failure
      Alcoholism

Drug complications

Fig. 5.8. Disorders in which paralysis of baroreceptors may occur in elderly subjects, resulting in orthostatic hypotension.

ages, often, however, of young adults. It is rare in the elderly. Loss of consciousness is abrupt, and recovery rapid and complete (Lyle et al. 1961). In most cases, it occurs only occasionally, though in a few it is recurrent (Coggins et al. 1964, Lukash et al. 1964). The physiological explanation appears to be that a full bladder tends to cause peripheral vasoconstriction (Carmichael 1950), although such vasoconstriction usually does not cause arterial hypertension, since the tendency for hypertension to occur is counteracted through the baroreceptor reflexes. In micturition syncope, a full bladder is emptied quickly, the vasoconstriction gives way to dilatation, and in a few subjects the dilatation and the erect posture are enough to lower the blood pressure sufficiently to cause a faint (Lukash et al. 1964). In most subjects, however, other factors are required that also tend to lower the blood pressure. These factors include a change from the recumbent to the erect posture, as in getting out of bed; vasodilatation due to the warmth of the bed or a hot room; and alcohol (Lyle et al. 1961). Rarely, syncope may also occur during defecation (Pathy, 1975). The mechanism is probably similar to that in Valsalva's maneuver (Littler et al. 1974).

Causes of Orthostatic Hypotension

Patients with orthostatic hypotension (see Fig. 5.8) have a progressive fall of blood pressure when they sit or stand (Fig. 5.9). Many

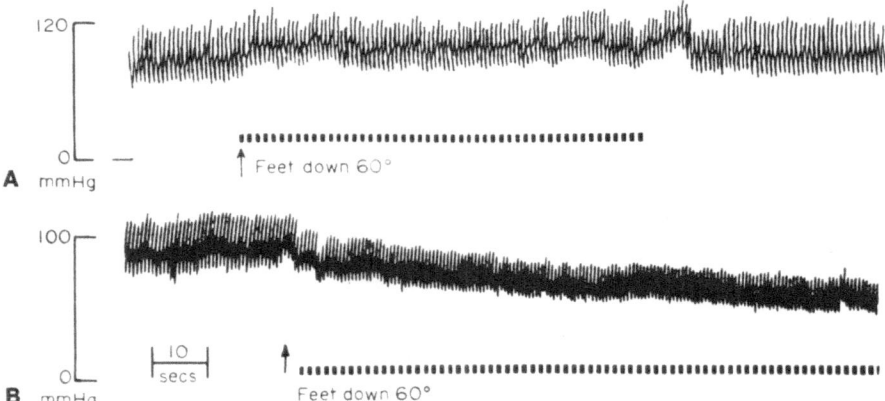

Fig. 5.9. Blood pressure with change in posture in a normal subject (A) and in a patient with orthostatic hypotension (B) from intermediolateral column degeneration (Johnson et al. 1966). The patient has a progressive fall of blood pressure when his posture is changed.

TOTAL REFLEX ARC				
Orthostatic hypotension, "blocked" blood pressure response to Valsalva's maneuver or to subatmospheric pressure to the lower part of the body				

AFFERENT LIMB OF ARC (from baroreceptors)	EFFERENT LIMB OF ARC
Abnormal tests of total reflex, arc function, but normal tests of efferent limb of arc	No blood pressure rise or vasconstriction in hand to loud noise, mental concentration, or ice pack No vasodilatation to radiant heating of trunk. Increased sensitivity of blood pressure to drug infusions (No sweating to raised central temperature)

Preganglionic pathway			Postganglionic pathway
Brain	Cervical spinal cord	Dorsal spinal cord	Peripheral fibers
Abnormal tests of efferent limb of arc, but acetylcholine axon reflex normal			Gasp reflex absent Acetylcholine axon reflex absent Failure of catecholamine release

Fig. 5.10. Indications of failure of *sympathetic* circulatory activity.

causes must be considered. These include *loss of circulating blood volume,* as may occur with hemorrhage, either external or internal, or dehydration. Failure of hydration can occur from inadequate fluid input or from excessive fluid loss, as with diarrhea, profuse sweating, diabetes insipidus, and diabetes mellitus. Orthostatic hypotension also occurs in disorders in which there is *paralysis of reflexes from baroreceptors* subserving blood pressure. This paralysis may occur in many neurological disorders and as a toxic effect of drugs. Those that are important differential diagnoses in the elderly are considered below. Unfortunately, there is no single test to determine the site of autonomic block. Localization of lesions affecting the circulatory system requires several tests to be carried out, and additional information may be gained examining other autonomic activities. The indications of failure of sympathetic circulatory activity are summarized in Fig. 5.10, those of failure of parasympathetic activity, in Fig. 5.11. The

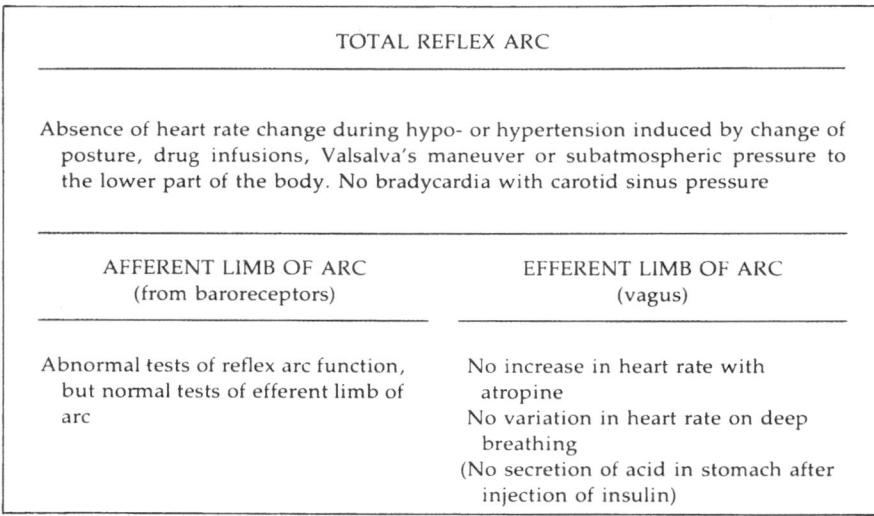

Fig. 5.11. Indications of failure of *parasympathetic* circulatory activity.

reader is referred to detailed descriptions by Johnson and Spalding (1974), who also give details of original work.

Cerebrovascular Disease. Orthostatic hypotension is more common in the elderly than in younger age groups. This section is relevant to those patients in whom it develops with evidence of cerebrovascular disease. Other diseases in which it occurs as a complication are described in subsequent sections. In one series, 11% of ambulatory residents in an old people's home had falls in systolic blood pressure of 20 mmHg or more on standing, and 4% had a systolic fall of from 40 to 62 mm Hg (Rodstein and Zeman 1957). Nevertheless, symptoms of weakness, dizziness, and headaches were not related to appreciable falls in blood pressure. In a series of 100 elderly inpatients in a geriatric hospital, 17% had falls of more than 20 mm Hg systolic blood pressure, and 5% had falls in excess of 40 mmHg (Fig. 5.12) (Johnson et al. 1965). In this series, it was found that symptoms could be related to the hypotension, as some patients developed dizziness and one had transient loss of consciousness. In 9 of these patients with orthostatic hypotension, blood pressure was measured through an intra-arterial cannula, and evidence of blocked reflex activity from baroreceptors was obtained (Fig. 5.13). Efferent sympathetic activity was present, however, and there was therefore no evidence of degeneration affecting peripheral sympathetic nerves or the spinal cord; the lesion causing the disorder was presumed to be in the brainstem.

Not all patients, however, have other evidence of neurological deficit. Some patients with a minor degree of orthostatic hypotension have hyponatremia, which responds to treatment with sodium chloride. The improvement was attributed to increased plasma volume (Fine 1969). Potassium depletion has also been found in elderly patients with orthostatic hypotension, and clinical improvement occurred with replacement therapy (Cox et al. 1973). Such changes may be related to hyperaldersteronism, but the endocrine changes in such patients remain to be clarified.

Other nonneurological disorders are frequent in elderly patients with orthostatic hypotension. Many patients with systolic falls of blood pressure in excess of 20 mm Hg have varicose veins (50%) or thrombophlebitis (18%) (Rodstein and Zeman 1957). In another series of nearly 500 people 65 years of age or more living at home, orthostatic hypotension of at least 40 mmHg systolic blood pressure was again found in 5% (Caird et al. 1973). Compared with those in whom there

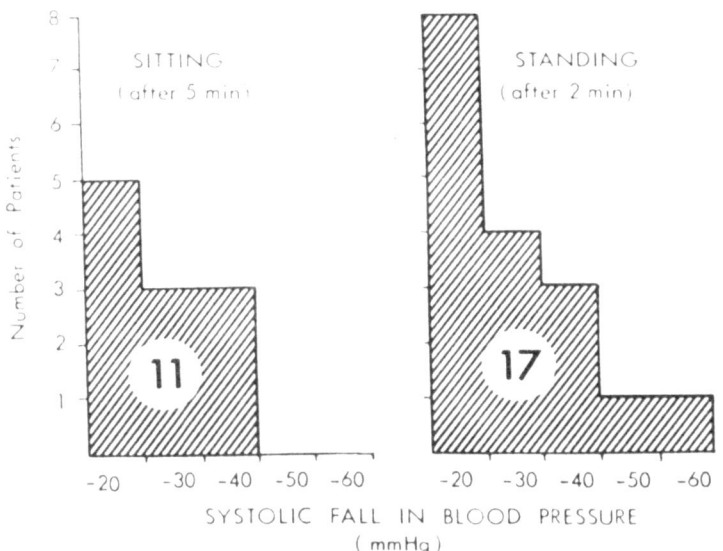

Fig. 5.12. Postural fall in systolic blood pressure in 100 elderly patients in a geriatric unit. Falls of less than 20 mm Hg are not shown (Johnson et al. 1965). Orthostatic fall in blood pressure was frequent.

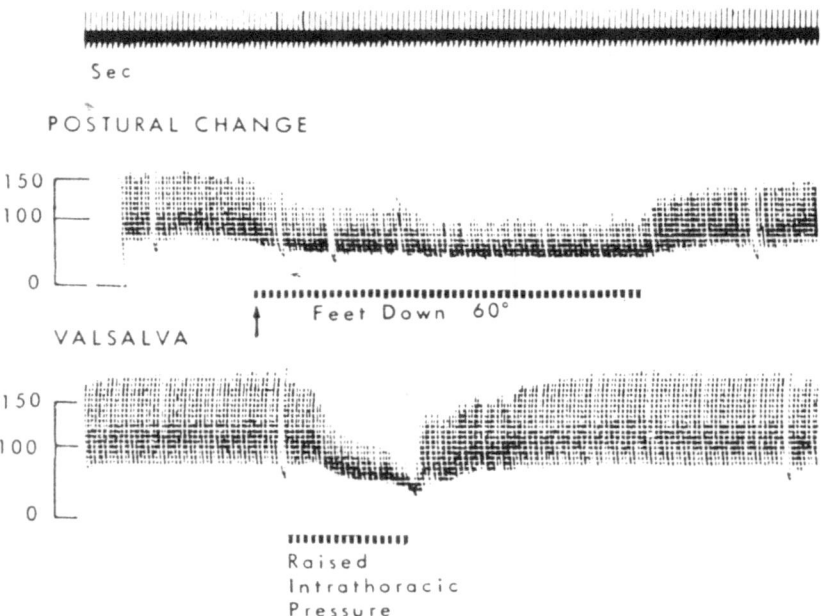

Fig. 5.13. Arterial blood pressure in a 74-year-old female with cerebrovascular disease on change of posture from supine to 60° feet down and during Valsalva's maneuver (raised intrathoracic pressure) (Johnson et al. 1965). The patient had orthostatic hypotension and a blocked response to Valsalva's maneuver.

was no fall, there was no significant difference in the frequency of various factors when taken singly (Fig. 5.14). Combinations of two or more of these factors, however, were significantly more frequent in those with orthostatic hypotension. The cause of orthostatic hypotension in elderly people is therefore likely to be multifactorial.

Idiopathic Orthostatic Hypotension and Multiple-System Disease. Some patients develop autonomic failure with no evidence of other neurological deficit. In a few of these patients, there is evidence of pure autonomic peripheral neuropathy or failure of catecholamine release (see below), but in others the lesion appears to be central. There is uncertainty about whether these patients are early cases of multiple-system disease in which degeneration occurs in other parts of the nervous system, or whether it is a separate condition (Bannister 1971). Patients with *multiple-system disease* are usually middle-aged or elderly men, and the autonomic nervous system may fail as a whole over years or decades, the symptoms progressing through loss of sweating, impotence, sphincter disturbance, and orthostatic hypotension. The orthostatic hypotension results from a defect of reflex vasoconstriction in both resistance and capacity vessels (Johnson et al. 1966, Bannister et al. 1967). Johnson et al. (1966) reported two patients with autopsy findings of marked cell loss in the intermediolateral columns of the spinal cord. They attributed the orthostatic hypotension to this cell loss, and subsequent reports have supported this view. In many cases, autonomic failure is accompanied by multiple-system degeneration elsewhere in the nervous system, notably olivo-pontocerebellar atrophy and similar syndromes (Welte 1939, Rosenhagen 1943, Greenfield 1954), and Parkinsonism (Shy and Drager 1960, Lewis 1964, Johnson et al. 1966, Nick et al. 1967, Schwarz 1967, Graham and Oppenheimer 1969, Thomas and Schirger 1970). Such patients may have degeneration of corticobulbar, corticospinal, extrapyramidal, and cerebellar tracts. A syndrome has been reported in which the condition was familial (Lewis 1964).

There is also the possibility that in multiple-system disease, lesions in structures other than the intermediolateral cell columns may be involved in causing autonomic failure. There is evidence that the afferent or the brainstem part of circulatory reflex arcs may be involved (Bannister et al. 1967). Two patients with idiopathic ortho-

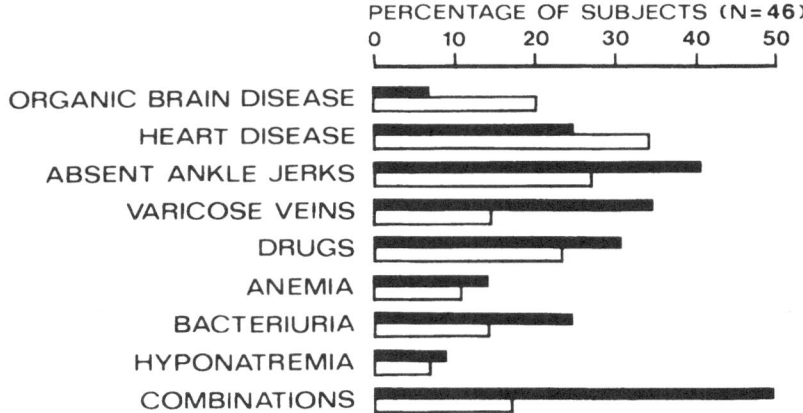

Fig. 5.14. A study of 496 patients, all 65 years old or more, living at home, in which a comparison of the frequency of a series of factors was made between (■) a group of 46 subjects with a drop in systolic pressure of 30 mm Hg or more on standing, and (□) a matched group without such a drop (Caird et al. 1973). No factor was statistically significant alone, but a combination of factors was significantly more frequent (p < 0.01) in those with orthostatic hypotension.

static hypotension have been described who had evidence of postganglionic degeneration (Love et al. 1971). In a number of subjects with severe idiopathic orthostatic hypotension, catecholamine excretion has been normal (Johnson et al. 1966, Johnson et al. 1971, Love et al. 1971). Two patients with idiopathic orthostatic hypotension have been described however, as having a deficiency in catecholamine release (Luft and von Eular 1953). Other patients with orthostatic hypotension and low excretion of cetecholamines have since been reported (Sundin 1958, Hickler et al. 1959, Goodall et al. 1967). Another possible cause of idiopathic orthostatic hypotension, therefore, is a decreased ability of sympathetic nerves to form catecholamines, due either to a failure of production by nerve endings or to absence of secretory impulses.

Parkinson's Disease. As stated above, orthostatic hypotension occurs commonly in patients with Parkinsonism associated with multiple-system disease. It may also occur in idiopathic paralysis agitans (Barbeau et al. 1969, Aminoff and Wilcox 1971, Appenzeller and Goss 1971), but its frequency is much less. Autonomic dysfunction may be related to damage of autonomic structures centrally. Peripheral involvement may also occur, as Lewy inclusion bodies have been reported in sympathetic ganglion cells (Appenzeller 1970).

Spinal Cord Lesions. After an acute lesion of the spinal cord above T6, orthostatic hypotension is the rule. It may be severe and can easily cause loss of consciousness; great care must therefore be taken to avoid raising the patient's head above the horizontal. Although evidence of autonomic dysfunction may be present in patients with chronic incomplete spinal cord lesions, e.g., signs of Horner's syndrome in cervical spondylosis, orthostatic hypotension is very rare, but may occur.

Tabes Dorsalis. Loss of circulatory reflexes and orthostatic hypotension may develop in tabes dorsalis. The loss of circulatory reflexes is attributed to interruption on the afferent side of the reflex arc from baroreceptors as part of the deep sensory loss characteristic of this disease (Sharpey-Schafer 1956).

Peripheral Neuropathy. In acute polyneuropathy (polyradiculoneuropathy, Guillain-Barré syndrome), the normal circulatory reflexes may be lost, resulting in orthostatic hypotension. The degree of autonomic failure that occurs in patients with acute polyneuropathy is variable and loosely related to the extent of muscular paralysis or sensory involvement (Johnson 1966). Some patient who are completely paralyzed and receiving artificial respiration have apparently normal blood pressure control. Others have almost complete vasomotor paralysis, while still retaining some skeletal muscle power.

Patients with chronic or recurrent polyneuropathy are also liable to autonomic disturbances, including orthostatic hypotension (Yamamoto 1967). One common disorder in which orthostatic hypotension is a complication is diabetes mellitus (Sharpey-Schafer and Taylor 1960, Bárány and Cooper 1956, Appenzeller and Richardson 1966). Primary amyloidosis may rarely present with orthostatic hypotension, 10 in a series of 138 having this dysfunction (Kyle et al. 1966), although other patients with amyloid infiltration of autonomic ganglia may be asymptomatic (Appenzeller and True 1967). Bronchial carcinoma has been reported in association with an autonomic polyneuropathy, giving profound orthostatic hypotension (Ivy 1961, Siemsen and Meister 1963). The orthostatic hypotension appears to be a nonmetastatic consequence of the carcinoma, for, in one patient, irradiation of the primary neoplasm improved chest symptoms, and orthostatic hypotension disappeared (Park et al. 1972). Autonomic failure with loss of circulatory reflexes, impotence, and inability to sweat has also been reported in association with carcinoma of the pancreas (Thomas and Shields 1970). Acute or chronic alcoholism may also disturb the circulation, and circulatory reflexes may be impaired. When alcohol is combined with dehydration, or with drugs such as barbiturates or psychotropic drugs, profound hypotension can occur, even when the patient is in the supine position (Richards 1944; Barraclough and Sharpey-Schafer 1963). The symptoms improve when alcohol is withdrawn, and may occur without peripheral neuropathy. The circulatory disturbances are therefore partly a direct toxic manifestation, though peripheral neuropathy, if it is present, may also play a part. Alcohol normally causes an increase in catecholamine excretion, but in alcoholics their excretion is significantly decreased, and this decrease may be among the causes of the hypotension (Wartburg et al. 1961, Schenker et al. 1967).

Drug Complications. A number of drugs, some of which are used frequently in the treatment of the elderly, interfere with circulatory reflexes. They include chlorpromazine, meprobamate, monoamine oxidase inhibitors, and barbiturates (Barraclough and Sharpey-Schafer 1963), and many other tranquilizers and antidepressives, as well as the drugs used to control arterial hypertension. Even when the drugs are used in therapeutic doses, severe arterial hypotension may occur if the patient's circulation is already imperfectly controlled because other conditions, such as cerebrovascular disease or peripheral neuropathy. When patients with such disorders who are receiving these drugs are first set up in bed or in a chair, postural syncope may occur, and it is important to appreciate that it may be in part iatrogenic. Severe acute poisoning with these drugs results in arterial hypotension, while the limbs remain warm and the veins dilated. The clinical picture is therefore distinguishable from that of "shock," in which the effect of a fall in cardiac output is compensated by powerful activity of resistance and capacity vessels, resulting in cold limbs with intensely constricted veins.

Management of Orthostatic Hypotension

Investigations should be directed to the cause of the orthostatic hypotension in order to determine whether it is secondary to a treatable disorder. The most convenient method of treating orthostatic hypotension is to use mechanical means to prevent pooling. These include full-length elastic stockings in combination with a firm elastic abdominal support. A more effective way is for the patient to wear a pair of trousers with inflatable compartments that compress the legs and abdomen, but still allow joint movement. These trousers, however, may be inconvenient for elderly people. The patient may also benefit by progressive adoption of a foot-down position (MacLean and Allan 1940); sleeping in a footdown position may sometimes be helpful (Stead and Ebert 1941). There is evidence that this position may be of value in elderly patients with orthostatic hypotension related to cerebrovascular disease (Johnson et al. 1965). The mechanism for the improvement may be related to increased renin release, which has been observed in patients with idiopathic orthostatic hypotension and cervical cord transection who are tipped from the supine to the vertical position several times (Love et al. 1971, Johnson and Park 1973). The value of postural training of the circulation, however, requires further study.

Two forms of drug therapy may be of value, i.e., blood-volume expanders and vasoconstrictors. Because orthostatic hypotension results from too large a proportion of the blood volume pooling in dependent capacity vessels, drugs that expand the blood volume may be of value. Fludrocortisone (Florinef), 0.5–2.0 mg/day in divided doses, has been found most effective, and has largely supplanted other drugs such as deoxycorticosterone acetate (DOCA) (Bannister et al. 1969). Drugs that cause vasoconstriction may also be tried. These drugs include ephedrine and phenylephrine, but care must be taken to avoid complications such as urinary retention in elderly men. Recently, the combination of a monoamine oxidase inhibitor with tyramine has been introduced (Lewis et al. 1972, Frewin et al. 1973, Nanda et al. 1975). It has proved successful in some patients under 70 years of age with idiopathic orthostatic hypotension. In older patients, drug therapy should be used with caution, and the mechanical means of improving the circulation described above are likely to prove of more value.

References

Aminoff, M., and Wilcox, C. S. (1971) *Br. Med. J.* **4,** 80.

Anderson, W. F., and Cowan, N. R. (1959) *Clin. Sci.* **18,** 103.

Anderson, W. F., and Cowan, N. R. (1972) *Gerontol. Clin.* **14,** 129.

Andrews, C. J. H., Andrews, W. H. H., and Orbach, J. (1971) *J. Physiol. (London)* **213,** 37P.

Appenzeller, O. (1970) *The Autonomic Nervous System,* North Holland, Amsterdam.

Appenzeller, O., and Descarries, L. (1964) *N. Engl. J. Med.* **271,** 820.

Appenzeller, O., and Goss, J. E. (1971) *Arch. Neurol.* **24,** 50.

Appenzeller, O., and Richardson, E. O. (1966) *Neurology* **16,** 1205.

Appenzeller, O., and True, C. W. (1967) *J. Neuropathol. Exp. Neurol.* **26,** 174.

Arenburg, K., Cummins, G. M., Bucy, P. C., and Oberhill, H. R. (1971) *Laryngoscope (St. Louis)* **81,** 253.

Baker, C. (1949) *Guy's Hosp. Rep.* **98,** 132.

Bannister, R. G. (1971) *Lancet* **1,** 175.

Bannister, R. G., Ardill, L., and Fentem, P. (1967) *Brain* **90,** 725.

Bannister, R. G., Ardill, L., and Fentem, P. (1969) *Q. J. Med. N.S.* **38,** 377.

Bárány, F. R., and Cooper, E. H. (1956). *Clin. Sci.* **15,** 533.

Barbeau, A., Gillo-Joffroy, L., Boucher, R., Nowacznski, W., and Genest, J. (1969) *Science* **165,** 291.

Barraclough, M. A., and Sharpey-Schafer, E. P. (1963) *Lancet* **1,** 1121.

Beacham, W. S., and Kunze, D. L. (1969). *J. Physiol. (London)* **201,** 73.

Bickelmann, A. G., Lippschutz, E. J., and Brunjes, C. F. (1961) *Am. J. Med.* **30,** 26.

Bristow, J. D., Gribbon, B., Honour, A. J., Pickering, T. G., and Sleight, P. (1969a) *J. Physiol. (London)* **202,** 45P.

Bristow, J. D., Honour, A. J., Pickering, T. G., and Sleight, P. (1969b) *Circ. Res.* **3,** 476.

Bristow, J. D., Honour, A. J., Pickering, G. W., Sleight, P., and Smyth, H. S. (1969c) *Circulation* **39,** 48.

Brody, H. (1955) *J. Comp. Neurol.* **102,** 511.

Caird, F. I. (1963) *Postgrad. Med. J.* **39,** 408.

Caird, F. I., Andrews, G. R., and Kennedy, R. D. (1973) *Br. Heart. J.* **35,** 527.

Carlsten, A., Folkow, B., Grimby, G., Hamberger, C-A., and Thulesius, O. (1958) *Acta Physiol. Scand.* **44,** 138.

Carmichael, E. A. (1950) *Br. Med. Bull.* **6,** 351.

Charcot, J. M. (1876) *Gaz. Med. Paris 4me Ser.* **5,** 588.

Coggins, C. H., Lillington, G. A., and Gray, C. P. (1964) *Arch. Intern. Med.* **113,** 14.

Corbett, J. L. (1969) D.Phil. thesis, University of Oxford.

Cox, J. R., Admani, A. K., Agarwal, M. L., and Abel, P. (1973) *Age and Ageing* **2,** 112.

Currens, J. H. (1948) *Am. Heart J.* **35,** 646.

Dastur, D. K., Lane, M. M., Hansen, D. B., Kety, S. S., Butler, R. N., and Sokoloff, L. (1963) *In: Human Aging,* U.S. Government Printing Office, p. 57.

Fazekas, J. F., Alman, R. W., and Bessman, A. N. (1952). *Am. J. Med. Sci.* **223,** 245.

Fazekas, J. F., Bessman, A. N., Cotsonas, N. J., and Alman, R. W. (1953) *J. Gerontol.* **8,** 137.

Fine, W. (1969) *Gerontol. Clin.* **11,** 206.

Folkow, B., and Neil, E. (1971) *Circulation,* University Press, Oxford.

Frewin, D. B., Robinson, S. M., and Willing, R. L. (1973) *Aust. N.Z. J. Med.* **3,** 180.

Freyham, F. A., Woodford, R. B., and Kety, S. S. (1951) *J. Nerv. Ment. Dis.* **113,** 449.

Gastaut, H., Naquet, R., and Regis, H. (1959) *Presse Méd.* **67,** 2229.

Gavey, C. J. (1949) *Lancet* **2,** 725.

Goodall, McC., Harlan, W. R., and Alton, H. (1967) *Circulation* **36,** 489.

Graham, J. G., and Oppenheimer, D. R. (1969) *J. Neurol. Neurosurg. Psychiatry* **32,** 28.

Greenfield, J. G. (1954) *The Spino-cerebellar Degenerations,* Blackwell Scientific Publications, Oxford.

Gribbon, B., Pickering, T. G., Sleight, P., and Peto, R. (1971) *Circ. Res.* **29,** 424.

Gross, M. (1970) *Clin. Sci.* **38,** 491.

Gross, M., and Marshall, J. (1970) *Clin. Sci.* **38,** 563.

Hamilton, M., Pickering, G. W., Roberts, J. A. F., and Sowry, G. S. C. (1954) *Clin. Sci.* **13,** 11.

Hauss, W. H., Kreutziger, H., and Asteroth, H. (1949) *Z. Kreislauforsh.* **38,** 128.

Hellström, R. (1961) *Acta Med. Scand.* **170,** Suppl. 371, 1.

Heron, J. R., Anderson, E. G., and Noble, I. M. (1965) *Lancet* **ii,** 214.

Heymans, C., and Neil, E. (1958) *Reflexogenic Areas of the Cardiovascular System,* Churchill, London.

Hickler, R. B., Wells, R. E., Tyler, H. R., and Hamlin, J. T. (1959) *Am. J. Med.* **26,** 410.

Humphreys, P. W., and Lind, A. R. (1963) *J. Physiol. (London)* **166,** 120.

Hutchinson, E. C., and Stock, J. P. P. (1960) *Lancet* **2,** 445.

Ivy, H. K. (1961) *Arch. Intern. Med.* **108,** 47.

James, J. E. A. (1972) *Clin. Sci.* **43,** 12P.

Johnson, R. H. (1966) M.D. thesis, University of Cambridge.

Johnson, R. H., and Park, D. M. (1973) *Clin. Sci.* **44,** 539.

Johnson, R. H., and Spalding, J. M. K. (1974) *Disorders of the Autonomic Nervous System,* Blackwell Scientific Publications, Oxford.

Johnson, R. H., and Spalding, J. M. K. (1976) *Br. J. Hosp. Med.* **15,** 266.

Johnson, R. H., Smith, A. C., Spalding, J. M. K., and Wollner, L. (1965) *Lancet* **1,** 731.

Johnson, R. H., Lee, G. de J., Oppenheimer, D. R., and Spalding, J. M. K. (1966) *Q. J. Med.* **35,** 276.

Johnson, R. H., McLellan, D. L., and Love, D. R. (1971) *J. Neurol. Neurosurg. Psychiatry* **34,** 562.

Kety, S. S. (1956) *J. Chronic Dis.* **3,** 478.

Kyle, R. A., Kottke, B. A., and Schirger, A. (1966) *Circulation* **34,** 883.

Lassen, N. A., Munck, O., and Tolley, E. R. (1957) *Arch. Neurol. Psychiatry* **77,** 126.

Lewis, P. (1964) *Brain* **87,** 719.

Lewis, R. K., Hazelrig, C. G., Fricke, F. J., and Russell, R. D. (1972) *Arch. Intern. Med.* **129,** 943.

Lind, A. R., and McNicol, G. W. (1967a) *J. Physiol. (London)* **192,** 575.

Lind, A. R., and McNicol, G. W. (1967b) *J. Physiol. (London)* **192,** 595.

Littler, W. A., Honour, A. J., and Sleight, P. (1974) *Am. Heart J.* **88,** 205.

Love, D. R., Brown, J. J., Chinn, R. H., Johnson, R. H., Lever, A. F., Park, D. M., and Robertson, J. I. S. (1971) *Clin. Sci.* **41,** 289.

Lown, B., and Levine, S. A. (1961) *Circulation* **23,** 766.

Luft, R., and von Euler, U. S. (1953) *J. Clin. Invest.* **32,** 1065.

Lukash, W. M., Sawyer, G. T., and Davis, J. E. (1964) *N. Engl. J. Med.* **270,** 341.

Lyle, C. B., Monroe, J. T., Flinn, D. E., and Lamb, L. E. (1961) *N. Engl. J. Med.* **265**, 982.
MacLean, A. R., and Allan, E. V. (1940) *J. Am. Med. Assoc.* **115**, 2162.
Mankikar, G. D., and Clark, A. N. G. (1975) *Age and Ageing* **4**, 86.
Martin, A., and Millard, P. H. (1973) *Age and Ageing* **2**, 211.
Master, A. M., Lassar, R. P., and Jaffe, H. L. (1958) *Ann. Intern. Med.* **48**, 284.
Mitchell, G. A. G. (1953) *Anatomy of the Autonomic Nervous System*, Livingstone, London.
Nanda, R. N., Johnson, R. H., and Keogh, H. J. (1975) *Clin. Sci. Mol. Med.* **49**, 13P.
Nelson, D. A., and Mahru, M. M. (1963) *Arch. Neurol.* **8**, 640.
Nick, J., Contamin, F., Escourelle, R., Guillard, A., and Marcantoni, J. P. (1967) *Rev. Neurol.* **116**, 213.
Novack, P., Shenkin, H. A., Bostin, L., Goluboff, B., and Soffe, A. M. (1953) *J. Clin. Invest.* **32**, 696.
Park, D. M., Johnson, R. H., Crean, G. P., and Robinson, J. F. (1972) *Br. Med. J.* **3**, 510.
Parry, C. H. (1799) *An Inquiry into the Symptoms and Causes of the Syncope Anginosa*, Bath, p. 102.
Pathy, M. S. (1975) Communication to British Geriatrics Society.
Pickering, G. W., Sleight, P., and Smyth, H. S. (1968) *J. Physiol. (London)* **194**, 46P.
Proudfit, W. L., and Forteza, M. E. (1959) *N. Engl. J. Med.* **260**, 328.
Purves, M. J. (1972) *Physiology of the Cerebral Circulation*, University Press, Cambridge.
Richards, D. W. (1944) *Bull. N.Y. Acad. Med.* **20**, 363.
Richardson, D. W., Honour, A. J., Fenton, C. W., Stott, F. H., and Pickering, G. W. (1964) *Clin. Sci.* **26**, 445.
Rodstein, M., and Zeman, F. D. (1957) *J. Chronic Dis.* **6**, 581.
Rosenhagen, H. (1943) *Arch. Psychiatr. Nervenkr.* **116**, 163.
Sarnoff, S. J., and Yamada, S. I. (1959) *Circ. Res.* **7**, 325.
Schenker, V. J., Kissin, B., Maynard, L. S., and Schenker, A. C. (1967) In Maickel, R. P. (ed.), *Biochemical Factors in Alcoholism*, Pergamon Press, Oxford, p. 38.
Schieve, J. F., and Wilson, W. P. (1953) *Am. J. Med.* **15**, 171.
Schwarz, G. A. (1967) *Arch. Neurol.* **16**, 123.
Sharpey-Schafer, E. P. (1953a) *Br. Med. J.* **2**, 860.
Sharpey-Schafer, E. P. (1953b) *J. Physiol. (London)* **122**, 351.
Sharpey-Schafer, E. P. (1955) *Br. Med. J.* **1**, 693.
Sharpey-Schafer, E. P. (1956) *J. Physiol. (London)* **134**, 1.
Sharpey-Schafer, E. P., and Taylor, P. J. (1960) *Lancet* **1**, 559.
Shy, G. M., and Drager, G. A. (1960) *Arch. Neurol.* **2**, 511.
Siemsen, J. K., and Meister, L. (1963) *Ann. Intern. Med.* **58**, 669.
Sleight, P. (1971) *Br. Heart J.* **33**, Suppl. 109.
Sleight, P., Gribbon, B., and Pickering, T. G. (1971) *Postgrad. Med. J.* **47**, 79.
Smyth, H. S., Sleight, P., and Pickering, G. W. (1969) *Circ. Res.* **24**, 109.
Stead, E. A. (Jr.), and Ebert, R. V. (1941) *Arch. Intern. Med.* **67**, 546.
Strandell, T. (1964) *Acta Med. Scand.* **175**, Suppl. 414, 1.
Sundin, T. (1958) *Acta Med. Scand.* **161**, Suppl. 336.
Thomas, J. E., and Schirger, A. (1970) *Arch. Neurol.* **22**, 289.
Thomas, J. P., and Shields, R. (1970) *Br. Med. J.* **4**, 32.
Ulrych, M., Tauber, J., and Shapiro, A. P. (1973) *Clin. Sci. Mol. Med.* **45**, 107.
Valsalva, A. M. (1707) *De Aure Humana Tractatus.*
Wang, H. S., and Busse, E. W. (1975) In Harper, A. M., Jennett, W. B., Miller, J. D., and Rowan, J. O. (eds.), *Blood Flow and Metabolism in the Brain*, Churchill Livingstone, Edinburgh, p. 8.17.
Wartburg, J. P. von, Berli, W., and Aebi, H. (1961) *Helv. Med. Acta* **28**, 89.

Weiss, S., and Baker, J. P. (1933) *Medicine* **12**, 297.

Welte, E. (1939) *Arch. Psychiatr. Nervenkr.* **109**, 649.

Whitty, C. W. M. (1943) *Brain* **66**, 43.

Winson, M., Heath, D., and Smith, P. (1974) *Cardiovasc. Res.* **8**, 58.

Yamamoto, K. (1967) *Brain Nerve, Tokyo* **19**, 1199.

Yoshida, S., Sawami, K., Tone, K., Fujimoto, J., and Matsabara, T. (1975) *In* Jennett, W. B., Miller, J. D., and Rowan, J. O. (eds.), *Blood Flow and Metabolism in the Brain*, Churchill Livingstone, Edinburgh, p. 7.25.

Zulch, K. J., and Hossmann, V. (1967) *Dtsch. Med. Wochenschr.* **92**, 567.

6

Clinical Examination and Investigation of the Heart

F. I. CAIRD

Introduction

It is well established that symptoms of heart disease are often modified in the elderly. Cardiac pain, both that of angina pectoris and that of cardiac infarction, may be either greatly reduced in intensity, or overshadowed by the simultaneous development of mental confusion, presumably because of reduction in cardiac output and cerebral blood flow. The dyspnea of cardiac failure is replaced as a leading symptom by fatigue, though patients in whom this occurs appear objectively to be as breathless as those who do complain of dyspnea. This frequent relative insignificance of the major symptoms of heart disease in the elderly makes proper and detailed clinical examination and investigation the more important. There are, however, numerous problems of interpretation, both of physical signs and of the results of investigations, that are particular to the cardiology of old age. Knowledge of these problems is essential in arriving at an accurate and complete cardiological diagnosis, which is often a crucial part of the overall assessment of the elderly patient.

F. I. CAIRD · University Department of Geriatric Medicine, Southern General Hospital, Glasgow, G51 4TF, Scotland.

Clinical Examination

Arterial Pulse

The principal value of examination of the arterial pulse in the elderly is to establish heart rate and rhythm. A palpable arterial wall is of no significance, since it reflects only Mönckeberg's medial sclerosis, and is totally unrelated to disease elsewhere in the cardiovascular system. The form of the pulse wave can be felt better and more easily in the brachial artery than in the radial.

The slowly rising pulse of severe aortic stenosis and the collapsing pulse of aortic incompetence can often be correctly identified. The former, however, may be masked by the age-related increase in rate of rise of the arterial upstroke, consequent on increased stiffness of the vessel wall (Wiggers 1932, Freis et al. 1966).

Blood Pressure

Recording of the arterial blood pressure in the elderly presents no particular problems. It is important to record the blood pressure, in any patient who is fit enough, in both the lying and the standing position. The demonstration of a postural drop in pressure may provide a diagnosis for symptoms such as dizziness or difficulty in standing or walking. About one-fourth of old people at home show a drop in pressure of 20 mm Hg or more (Caird et al. 1973a), but for a diagnosis of clinically significant postural hypotension, the standing systolic pressure is more important than the postural drop. The diagnosis should not usually be accepted unless the standing systolic pressure is below 110 mm Hg.

Venous Pressure and Pulse

Because the venous pressure and pulse are made more clearly visible by atrophy of the skin and subcutaneous tissue of the neck, they are often easier to observe in the elderly than in the young.

The venous pressure in the left jugular and subclavian veins may be higher than that in the right, when the left innominate vein is compressed in systole between the enlarged aorta of old age and the back of the sternum (Sleight 1962). The difference is abolished by deep inspiration, and if a disparity in venous pressures in the two sides of the neck is observed, the effects of deep inspiration should always be noted. The true central venous pressure must always be the lowest demonstrable pressure on full inspiration. Very occasionally, this pseudo-obstruction may occur on both sides of the neck, when it can obviously give rise to difficulty in the diagnosis of congestive heart failure, but it is still abolished by deep inspiration.

Examination of the venous pulse wave is of value when the large positive systolic wave of tricuspid incompetence is present, because it may then clarify the nature of a regurgitant systolic murmur, or when the cannon waves of atrioventricular dissociation can be used in the bedside diagnosis of ventricular tachycardia and of complete heart block. Less striking changes, such as an increased *a* wave due to right atrial hypertrophy, are demonstrable only in relatively rare cases.

Hepatojugular reflux is an important physical sign, unduly neglected recently because its improper performance leads to difficulties in interpretation (Matthews and Hampson 1958). The liver must be compressed during inspiration, so that the normal rise in central venous pressure during expiration is not mistaken for a positive reflux sign. A positive hepatojugular reflux is valuable confirmatory evidence of true elevation of the central venous pressure, and therefore of the presence of cardiac failure.

Cardiac Impulse

Increase in heart size is a classic indicator of the presence of heart disease, but in the elderly, kyphosis or scoliosis, or both, frequently make clinical assessment of heart size very difficult. Certainly if the spine is straight, the cardiac apex should not be palpable outside the midclavicular line, but if there is spinal deformity, it is often impossible to know where the cardiac impulse should lie.

The increased rigidity of the chest wall in the elderly may emphasize the ease with which the apical impulse can be felt, and unless obesity is gross, it is almost always possible to detect left ventricular hypertrophy or dilatation. It follows that the feel of the cardiac impulse is more important than the site of the apex beat as evidence of cardiac abnormality. The feel of the sustained impulse of a powerful hypertrophied left ventricle—or that of a dilated ventricle, which is less powerful but covers a wide area of chest wall—can be correctly identified (see Figs. 6.2 and 6.3). Presystolic outward movement of the ventricle associated with increased left atrial contraction is a further important sign of left ventricular disease (see Figs. 6.2 and 6.5).

The clinical diagnosis of right ventricular hypertrophy is much more difficult, since only relatively slight degrees of hypertrophy are

common in the elderly, and the heart is often hidden behind expanded lungs. In rheumatic mitral disease and in atrial septal defect,
however, increased pulsation at the left sternal edge can often be
detected.

Cardiac Auscultation

Heart Sounds. The problems of cardiac auscultation in the elderly
present some difficulty, but less than the necessary attention is often
paid to the correct identification of heart sounds.
  Variable intensity of the first heart sound occurs in atrioventricu-

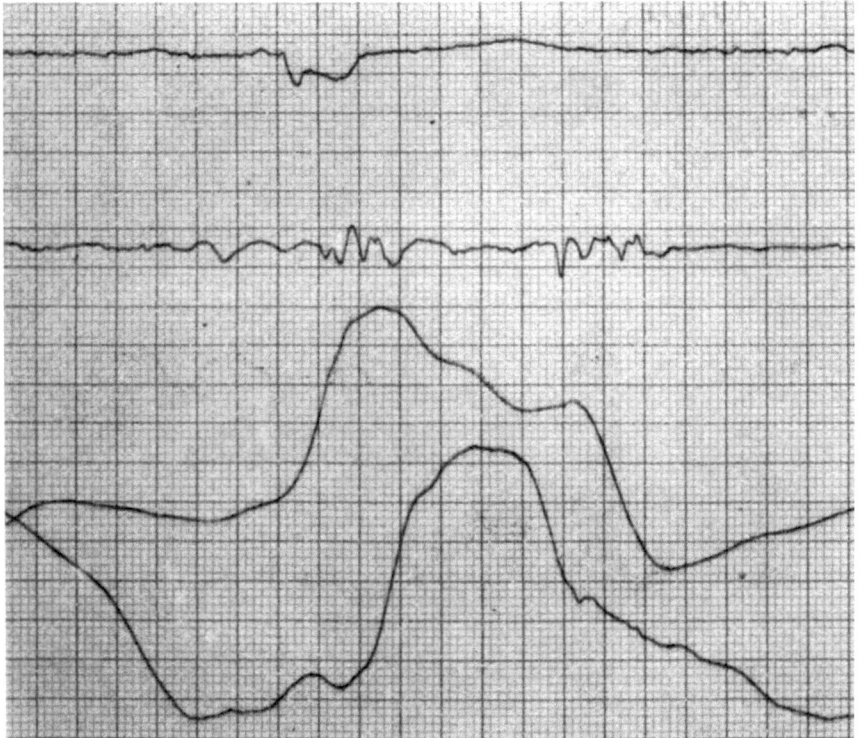

Fig. 6.1. Right bundle branch block in an 85-year-old woman. (*Top trace*) ECG Lead II;
(*2nd trace*) low-frequency phonocardiogram from left second space, showing fourth and
widely split second sound; (*3rd trace*) apexcardiogram; (*bottom trace*) external arterial
pulse trace; dicrotic notch corresponds to first (aortic) component of second sound (time,
10 and 50 msec).

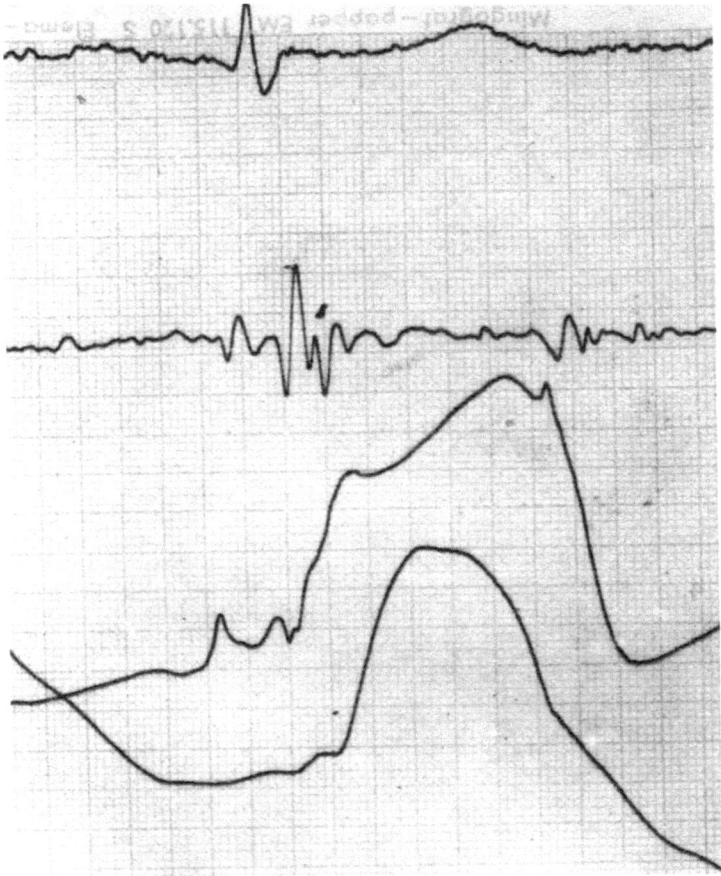

Fig. 6.2. Left ventricular hypertrophy in a 74-year-old man with high blood pressure. *(Top trace)* ECG Lead II; *(2nd trace)* low-frequency phonocardiogram from internal to apex, showing fourth sound; *(3rd trace)* apexcardiogram, showing prominent atrial component and marked late systolic outward movement of apex; *(bottom trace)* external arterial pulse trace (time, 10 and 50 msec).

lar dissociation, and also in atrial fibrillation; it cannot be used to distinguish the latter from multiple ectopic beats, because these also produce a first heart sound of widely varying intensity. Reverse splitting of the second heart sound (Gray 1956) is often difficult to demonstrate in the elderly because they cannot carry out the necessary respiratory maneuvers. When it can be clearly identified clinically, it

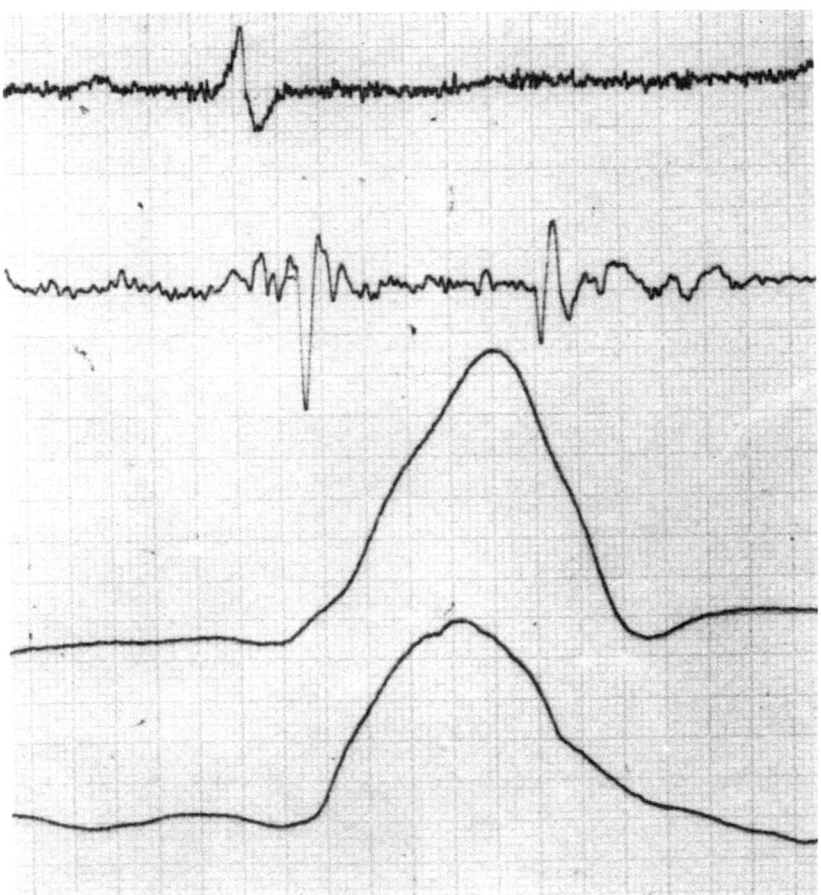

Fig. 6.3. A 78-year-old man with left heart failure. *(Top trace)* ECG Lead II; *(2nd trace)* low-frequency phonocardiogram from internal to apex, showing third heart sound, coinciding with rapid filling wave on apexcardiogram; *(3rd trace)* apexcardiogram showing late systolic outward movement of apex, and rapid filling wave; *(bottom trace)* external arterial pulse trace (time, 10 and 50 msec).

bears the same significance as in younger people, of embarrassment of the left ventricle, and delay in or prolongation of left relative to right ventricular ejection. Wide fixed splitting of the second heart sound in right bundle branch block can be more readily demonstrated at the bedside (Fig. 6.1).

   A fourth heart sound is a sign of ventricular abnormality in old age, just as it is in younger people (Fig. 6.2), and a third heart sound is a sign of ventricular failure (Fig. 6.3). Inspiratory accentuation will demonstrate the right-sided origin of third and fourth heart sounds, and can be used to support a diagnosis of pulmonary heart failure, rather than failure due to left heart disease.

Heart Murmurs. Systolic murmurs are very common in old age. Bruns and van der Hauwert (1958) and Bethel and Crow (1963) record frequencies of around 60%. Thus, there is a temptation to attribute such murmurs to aging, and not to attempt a diagnosis. In the great majority of cases, it is possible to assign the murmur to one of relatively small number of categories, and an appropriate diagnosis to each.

The initial distinction is between regurgitant and ejection murmurs (Leatham 1958), the latter being considerably more common in old age (Bethel and Crow 1963, Davison and Friedman 1968). Regurgitant murmurs may be either pansystolic with onset during the first heart sound, or late systolic, but in both cases they run with increasing or at least undiminished intensity up to the second heart sound. Ejection murmurs show midsystolic accentuation and late systolic decrescendo.

The next stage is to distinguish between left- and right-sided murmurs. Left-sided regurgitant murmurs in the elderly are heard at the customary site, the apex, and radiate around the left side of the chest. Rarely, they may also be heard at the base of the heart (Movitt and Gerstl 1953); on occasion, expiratory accentuation can be clearly demonstrated. Right-sided regurgitant murmurs are heard with maximum intensity near the left sternal edge, usually show clear inspiratory accentuation, and are accompanied by a large positive systolic wave in the venous pulse.

Virtually all ejection murmurs in the elderly are derived from the left side of the heart (Bruns and van der Hauwert 1958, Bethel and Crow 1963, Davison and Friedman 1968). The only exception is the pulmonary ejection murmur of atrial septal defect, which is heard in the left second and third spaces, does not radiate widely, and is usually accompanied by clear evidence of right ventricular hypertrophy.

Left-sided ejection murmurs arising from the aortic valve may be heard both at the base of the heart and at the apex, but their maximum intensity is usually at the base. In old people, however, the apical component of an ejection murmur may be louder than that at the base; Roberts et al. (1971) have suggested a number of reasons why this may be so. Increase in the anteroposterior diameter of the chest and systemic hypertension (with a reduction in the magnitude of the systolic gradient across the aortic valve) will both reduce the intensity of the basal murmur. Differing pathologies in the aortic valve may result in different patterns of murmur. A rigid calcified valve with commissural fusion may produce a high-velocity jet into the ascending aorta, with a more intense basal murmur. By contrast, a tricuspid stenotic aortic valve without fusion of the commissures might produce a spray rather than a jet effect, with consequent reduction in intensity of the basal component of the murmur; separate vibration of the three cusps tends to produce a pure-tone murmur, which is demonstrable in the left ventricular cavity, and so may be better transmitted to the apex. In general, soft ejection murmurs are not associated with significant stenosis of the aortic valve, but rather with aortic valvular sclerosis. Louder murmurs of grade 2/4 or 2/6 or more in intensity, on the other hand, are usually associated with evidence of significant obstruction to ejection (Davison and Friedman 1968). The diagnosis of aortic stenosis depends, however, on features other than the mur-mur—in particular, the presence of left ventricular hypertrophy and of depression and reverse splitting of the second sound at the base. As with other aspects of cardiac auscultation in the elderly, attention to detail and to the whole pattern of physical signs is the key to rational diagnosis.

By contrast with systolic murmurs, diastolic murmurs are always evidence of significant heart disease in old age. An apical middiastolic murmur indicates mitral stenosis; this is true in general, even when an Austin Flint murmur is suspected because aortic incompetence is also present (Bedford and Caird 1960). An early diastolic murmur indicates aortic incompetence; as in younger people, it is best heard at the left sternal edge, with the patient sitting up, and if possible in held expiration. Pulmonary incompetence should be diagnosed only very rarely (see Chapter 11).

Electrocardiography

The ECG is without a doubt the most valuable simple method of clinical investigation of the heart in old age. As in younger people, it provides the diagnosis of cardiac arrhythmias, ischemic heart disease, and ventricular hypertrophy, and clues to important noncardiac disorders such as potassium depletion and hypothyroidism. Many abnormalities of the ECG are so common in old age, however, that interpretation is made difficult.

Clinical experience, backed by studies of survival rates (Caird et al. 1974), suggests that it is reasonable to regard as insignificant purely positional abnormalities—such as left axis deviation without evidence of left anterior hemiblock, counterclockwise rotation, and minor degrees of clockwise rotation, insufficient to give rise to an rS complex in lead V_5. Incomplete right bundle branch block and infrequent ectopic beats, which are as often atrial as ventricular (Kennedy and Caird 1972), are also unimportant.

There is uncertainty about the significance of first degree atrioventricular block, which is found in a variable but sizable proportion of "normal" old people (see Table 1.7, page 7). The P–R interval tends to lengthen with increasing age (Harlan et al. 1967), and it may be that some instances of first degree block in old age can be regarded as normal. In many old people, however, first degree block is accompanied by evidence on His-bundle electrography of disorder in other parts of the conducting system (Narula et al. 1971).

The significance of the voltage changes of left ventricular hypertrophy when encountered alone is also uncertain, since they are not associated with any excess mortality, whereas if S-T–T changes are present in addition, mortality is increased (Caird et al. 1974). The problem may merely reflect the difficulty in establishing voltage criteria alone as firm electrocardiographic evidence of left ventricular hypertrophy (Romhilt et al. 1969).

By contrast, there is no doubt whatever that other electrocardiographic changes encountered in old age must be regarded as significant, however common they may be. These include Q/QS abnormalities, which correlate with evidence of cardiac infarction at autopsy in the elderly as well as in the young (Kurihara et al. 1967); left ventricular hypertrophy patterns with S-T–T as well as voltage changes (Caird et al. 1974); all conduction defects other than incomplete right bundle branch block and possibly first degree A-V block; all arrhythmias other than occasional ectopic beats; and all T-wave changes, including T-wave flattening. Such isolated changes in the T waves have been clearly shown to carry an excess mortality, and to be precursors of more definite evidence of cardiac ischemia (Ostrander 1966, 1970; Caird et al. 1974).

Two additional electrocardiographic techniques may have some value in special situations in old age: His bundle electrography and continuous telemetric monitoring.

His-Bundle Electrography. This technique has been used to demonstrate the nature of the abnormalities in first degree atrioventricular block (Narula et al. 1971), and the frequency of abnormal H–V intervals in right bundle branch block with left anterior hemiblock (Denes et al. 1975), when a prolonged H–V interval was found to be

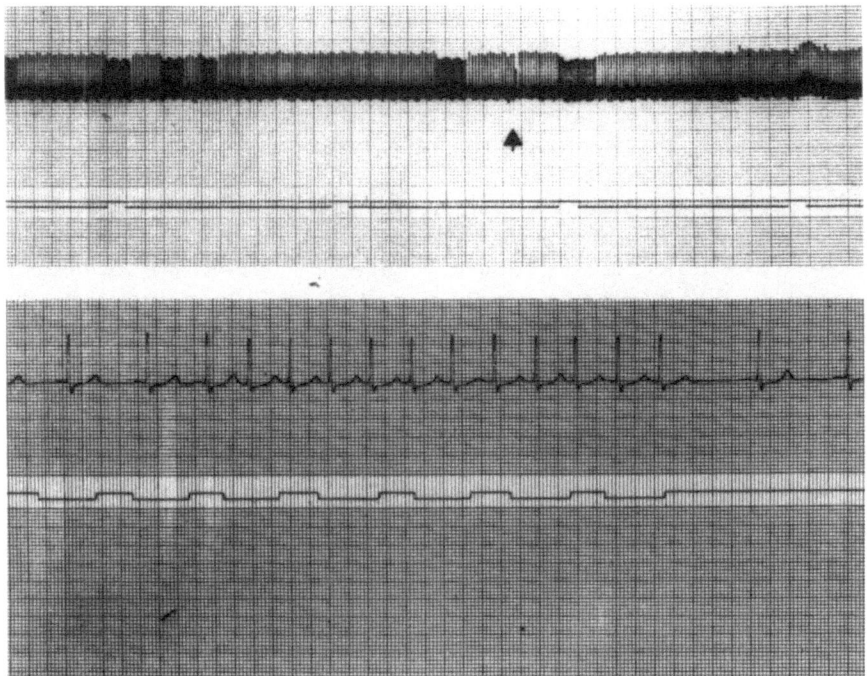

Fig. 6.4. Telemetric electrocardiogram from an 80-year-old man. (*Upper trace*) at 1 mm/ sec, showing 5 episodes of supraventricular tachycardia; *arrow* indicates ventricular ectopic beat, followed by pause (time marker, 1 min); (*lower trace*) at 25 mm/sec, showing one complete paroxysm.

associated with a worse prognosis. The practical value of this invasive procedure in the elderly has, however, not yet been established. The recent demonstration that His-bundle potentials can be recorded by a noninvasive method (Hishimoto and Sawayama 1975) may prove valuable.

Continuous Telemetric Monitoring. This technique can demonstrate paroxysmal arrhythmias (Fig. 6.4), and has been used in an attempt to demonstrate episodic digitalis toxicity in old people (Taylor et al. 1974). Again, however, the practical value of this technique in establishing that paroxysmal changes in heart rate and rhythm are a cause of an individual old person's symptoms remains to be shown (see Chapter 18).

Radiology

Radiology has an important part to play in cardiac diagnosis in the elderly, although again there are frequent difficulties in interpretation, many of which derive from the effect on the cardiac silhouette of abnormalities of the shape of the chest.

Cowan (1959, 1960, 1965) has shown that in elderly women the cardiothoracic ratio is related to the degree of thoracic kyphosis, and that values for the cardiothoracic ratio somewhat above the conventional upper limit of 50% can be found when the heart is clinically normal. Even greater difficulty results when scoliosis is also present. It may then be virtually impossible to decide what shape the cardiac silhouette should have, since scoliosis may be upper or lower dorsal in site, and to the left or to the right; there are many chest X rays in the elderly to which the term "straight" is totally inapplicable.

Despite these difficulties, enlargement of the cardiac chambers can often be correctly identified, with the help of barium in the esophagus if necessary, and the interpretation of most radiological changes, when they can be definitely identified, is essentially the same as in younger people.

The demonstration of unfolding of the aorta is of no significance in old age, and dilatation of the ascending aorta and arch is often difficult to assess. Calcification of the aortic knuckle is of no significance. It is present in about 30% ot old people, tends to increase in frequency with age, and is more common and more severe in women

TABLE 6.1. Percentage Prevalence of Calcification of the Aortic Knuckle in Old Age[a]

	65–69 Years of age		70–74 Years of age		75–79 Years of age		80+ Years of age	
	M (54)[b]	F (82)	M (41)	F (66)	M (45)	F (69)	M (29)	F (56)
Calcification[c]								
Grade 1	28	23	27	35	29	38	28	46
Grade 2	4	6	2	11	7	12	10	13
Grade 3	0	0	0	0	0	0	0	5
TOTAL:	32	29	29	46	36	50	38	64

[a] Kennedy, Caird, and Andrews (unpublished).
[b] Number of cases in parentheses.
[c] Grade 1, calcification confined to one quadrant; Grade 2, calcification in two quadrants only; Grade 3, calcification in three quadrants.

than in men (Table 6.1). There is little relationship between such calcification and any other cardiovascular phenomenon. Calcification in the ascending aorta is, however, an important sign of syphilitic aortitis which preserves its value into old age (Thorner et al. 1949). The calcification is characteristically thinner and more regular than that due to atheroma, which is no doubt the more common lesion.

Calcification in the cardiac valves is evidence of significant valvular disease, and in the aortic valve is more easily seen by image-intensification than by conventional procedures. Calcification in the mitral annulus may be of clinical significance in relationship to mitral disease and to heart block (see Chapters 2 and 3); calcification can also occasionally be identified in the myocardium (after a major infarct); in the pericardium; in the coronary arteries; and, in mitral disease, in thrombus in the left atrium. Interpretation may be rendered difficult, particularly by calcification in costal cartilages and in the tracheobronchial tree.

The radiological changes in the lungs in heart disease in the elderly are seldom marked. In particular, Kerley's lines are comparatively rare, even in patients in whom pulmonary venous hypertension is very likely. Enlargement of vessels to the upper lobes may be apparent in left heart failure and in mitral disease. Pleural effusions are common in cardiac failure.

Other Investigations

Phonocardiography

There have been several excellent studies of the phonocardiogram in old age (Aravanis and Harris 1958, Bruns and van der Hauwert 1958, Bethel and Crow 1963). The findings in 103 people over the age of 80 are summarized in Table 6.2 (Bethal and Crow 1963). Normal values for the various time intervals have been shown to be essentially the same as in younger people (Aravanis and Harris 1958).

The phonocardiogram may be of diagnostic value when a third heart sound has been queried (see Fig. 6.3), or when there is uncertainty between a fourth heart sound and splitting of the first sound (see Fig. 6.2). It is valuable in the distinction between obstructive and nonobstructive lesions of the aortic valve (Aravanis and Luisada 1957), since the length of the murmur and the time taken for it to reach its peak are related to the degree of obstruction (Fig. 6.5).

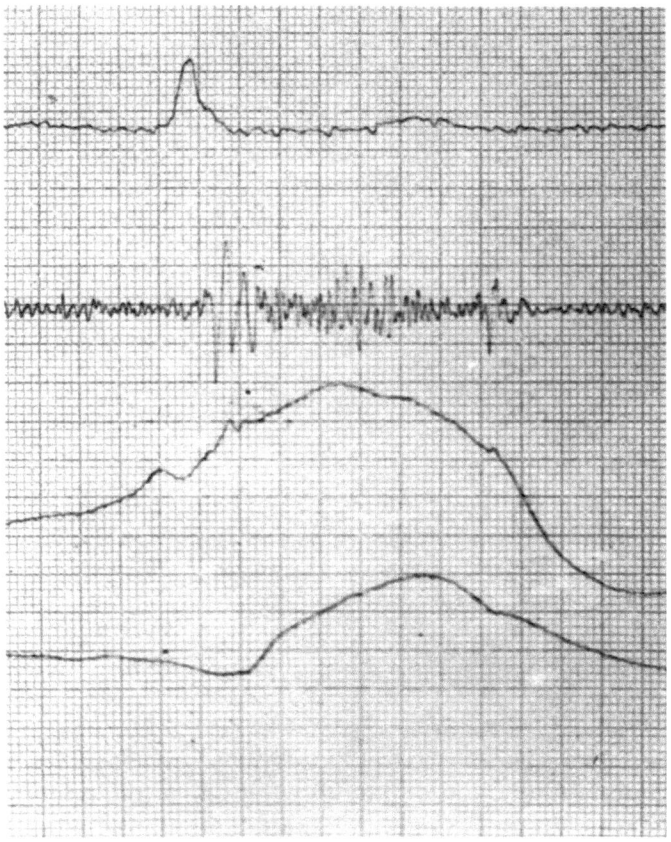

Fig. 6.5. A 74-year-old women with aortic stenosis. *(Top trace)* ECG Lead II; *(2nd trace)* phonocardiogram from right second space, showing ejection systolic murmur with late peak (250 msec after onset of QRS); *(3rd trace)* apexcardiogram, showing clear atrial component; *(bottom trace)* external arterial pulse trace (carotid), showing slow upstroke (time, 10 and 50 msec).

Combination of phonocardiography with other records such as apexcardiography and an external arterial trace greatly increases its value (Benchimol et al. 1961, Caird et al. 1973b).

Apexcardiography

This relatively simple technique has been little exploited in the elderly. An adequate apexcardiogram can be recorded only when the

TABLE 6.2. Phonocardiographic Findings in 103 People over 80 Years of Age[a]

Finding	Number shown by phono- cardiography	Comments
Fourth heart sound	59	42 heard clinically; 2 recently in cardiac failure
Third heart sound	27	12 heard clinically; 10 recently in cardiac failure
Systolic click	16	14 ejection type (10 aortic, 4 pulmonary)
Systolic murmur	60	
Grades 1 or 2		
Grade 3	48	47 ejection, 1 regurgitant
Diastolic murmur	12	All ejection
	1	Aortic diastolic

[a] From Bethel and Crow (1963).

apex is clearly clinically palpable, and the patient not unduly restless (Caird et al. 1973b). The qualitative changes that result from left atrial hypertrophy, and from left ventricular hypertrophy and dilatation, can be displayed (see Figs. 6.2 and 6.3), while the combination of apex- and phonocardiography can be used to elucidate the physical signs of mitral disease (Nixon and Wooler 1963).

Quantitative information derived from the study of time intervals in the apexcardiogram has yet to find a place in diagnosis in old age. Baragan et al. (1968) showed that four types of mechanical abnormality may underlie the single electrocardiographic pattern of left bundle branch block. This has been confirmed (Caird et al. 1973b), but the significance of the subdivision, in terms of etiology, pathology, and prognosis, is still quite uncertain.

Systolic Time Intervals

The external arterial pulse trace can be used to measure systolic time intervals. Normal values have been established for the elderly (Willens et al. 1970), and the corrections necessary for heart rate calculated. As Weissler has shown (Lewis et al. 1974), in nonvalvular heart disease, the ratio of the pre-ejection period to the left ventricular ejection time is related to the stroke volume. Although the correlation is not close enough to enable accurate prediction of stroke volume in an individual, it seems likely that this noninvasive method will be of value in demonstrating the hemodynamic consequences of heart disease in groups of elderly subjects (Caird, Roberts, and Al Badran, unpublished) and the changes in individuals that take place in changing situations, such as, for instance, in recovery from anemia.

Echocardiography

Despite its attractiveness as a noninvasive technique, echocardiography seems to have been little exploited in the elderly. Its main value would seem to lie in the diagnosis and assessment of rheumatic mitral disease (see Feigenbaum 1972, Gibson 1973, Popp and Harrison 1974), and in the diagnosis of mitral valve prolapse (Dillon et al. 1971, Popp et al. 1974). Although aortic valve movement can be visualized (Gramiak and Shah 1970), technical difficulties make the use of echocardiography in aortic valve disease of considerably less value.

The demonstration that echocardiography can be used to measure left ventricular volumes, and also, though less reliably, stroke volume and regurgitant volume (Popp and Harrison 1970, Pombo et al. 1971, Feigenbaum et al. 1972), is of great interest, and may prove to have important applications in the elderly.

Other Investigative Techniques

Cardiac catheterization and angiocardiography are justifiable in the elderly only if there is a serious consideration of cardiac surgery, and it is necessary to provide quantitative hemodynamic data or confirmation of the nature of anatomical and functional abnormalities. Other techniques such as ballistocardiography and isotope cardiography do not appear to have been exploited in the elderly.

References

Aravanis, C., and Harris R. (1958) *Dis. Chest* **33,** 214.

Aravanis, C., and Luisada, A. A. (1957) *Am. Heart J.* **54,** 32.

Baragan J., Fernandez-Carmano, F., Sozutek, Y., Coblence, B., and Lenègre, J. (1968) *Br. Heart J.* **30,** 196.

Bedford, P. D., and Caird, F. I. (1960) *Valvular Disease of the Heart in Old Age*, J. & A. Churchill, London.

Benchimol, A., Dimond, E. G., and Carson, J. C. (1961) *Am. Heart J.* **60,** 417.

Bethel, C. S., and Crow, E. W. (1963) *Am. J. Cardiol.* **11,** 763.

Bruns, D. L., and van der Hauwert, L. G. (1958) *Br. Heart J.* **20,** 370.

Caird, F. I., Andrews, G. R., and Kennedy, R. D. (1973a) *Br. Heart J.* **35,** 527.

Caird, F. I., Kennedy, R. D., and Kelly, J. C. C. (1973b) *Gerontol. Clin.* **15,** 366.

Caird, F. I., Campbell, A., and Jackson, T. F. M. (1974) *Br. Heart J.* **36,** 1012.

Cowan, N. R. (1959) *Br. Heart J.* **21**, 238.

Cowan, N. R. (1960) *Br. Heart J.* **22**, 391.

Cowan, N. R. (1965) *Br. Heart J.* **27**, 231.

Davison, E. T., and Friedman, S. A. (1968) *N. Engl. J. Med.* **279**, 225.

Denes, P., Dhingra, R. C., Wu, D., Chuqumia, R., Amat-y-Leon, F., Wyndham, C., and Rosen, K. M. (1975) *Am. J. Cardiol.* **35**, 23.

Dillon, J. C., Haine, C. L., Chang, S., and Feigenbaum, R. (1971) *Circulation* **43**, 503.

Feigenbaum, H. (1972) *Echocardiography*, Lea and Febiger, Philadelphia.

Feigenbaum, H., Popp, R. L., Wolfe, S. B., Troy, B. L., Pombo, J. F., Haine, C. L., and Dodge, H. T. (1972) *Arch. Intern. Med.* **129**, 461.

Freis, E. D., Heath, W. C., Luchsinger, P. C., and Snell, R. E. (1966) *Am. Heart J.* **71**, 757.

Gramiak, R., and Shah, P. M. (1970) *Radiology* **96**, 1.

Gray, I. R. (1956) *Br. Heart J.* **18**, 21.

Gibson, D. (1973) *In* Hamer, J. (ed.), *Recent Advances in Cardiology*, 6th edition, Churchill Livingstone, London and Edinburgh, p. 266.

Harlan, W. R., Graybiel, A., Mitchell, R. E., Oberman, A., and Osborne, R. K. (1967) *J. Chronic Dis.* **20**, 853.

Hishimoto, Y., and Sawayama, T. (1975) *Br. Heart J.* **37**, 635.

Kennedy, R. D., and Caird, F. I. (1972) *Gerontol. Clin.* **14**, 5.

Kurihara, H., Kuramoto, K., Terasawa, F., Matsushita, S., Seki, M., and Ikeda, M. (1967) *Jpn. Heart J.* **8**, 514.

Leatham, A. (1958) *Circulation* **17**, 601.

Lewis, R. P., Leighton, R. F., Forester, W. F., and Weissler, A. M. (1974) *In* Weissler, A. M. (ed.), *Non-Invasive Cardiology*, Grune and Stratton, New York and London, p. 301.

Matthews, M. B., and Hampson, J. (1958) *Lancet* **1**, 873.

Movitt, E. R., and Gerstl, R. W. (1953) *Ann. Intern. Med.* **38**, 981.

Narula, O. S., Schering, B. J., Samet, P., and Javier, R. P. (1971) *Am. J. Med.* **50**, 146.

Nixon, P. G. F., and Wooler, G. H. (1963) *Br. Heart J.* **25**, 246.

Ostrander, L. D. (1966) *Circulation* **34**, 1069.

Ostrander, L. D. (1970) *Am. J. Cardiol.* **25**, 325.

Pombo, J. F., Troy, B. L., and Russell, R. O. (1971) *Circulation* **43**, 480.

Popp, R. L., and Harrison, D. C. (1970) *Circulation* **41**, 493.

Popp, R. L., and Harrison, D. C. (1974) *In* Weissler, A. M. (ed.), *Non-Invasive Cardiology*, Grune and Stratton, New York and London, p. 149.

Popp, R. L., Brown, O. R., Silverman, J. F., and Harrison, D. C. (1974) *Circulation* **49**, 428.

Roberts, W. C., Perloff, J. K., and Costantino, T. (1971) *Am. J. Cardiol.* **27**, 497.

Romhilt, D. W., Bove, K. E., Norris, R. J., Conyers, E., Conradi, S., Rowlands, D. T., and Scott, R. C. (1969) *Circulation* **40**, 185.

Sleight, P. (1962) *Br. Heart J.* **24**, 726.

Taylor, B. B., Kennedy, R. D., and Caird, F. I. (1974) *Age and Ageing* **3**, 79.

Thorner, M. C., Carter, R. A., and Griffith, G. C. (1949) *Am. Heart J.* **38**, 641.

Wiggers, C. J. (1932) *Ann. Intern. Med.* **6**, 72.

Willens, J. L., Roelandt, J., De Geest, H. Kesteloot, H., and Joossens, J. V. (1970) *Circulation* **42**, 37.

7

Blood Pressure and the Development of Cardiovascular Disease in the Aged

WILLIAM B. KANNEL

Introduction

Prospective epidemiological investigations of population samples at Framingham and elsewhere have produced a body of data that emphasize the importance of hypertension as a contributor to the high incidence of cardiovascular morbidity and mortality in affluent parts of the world (Kannel et al. 1969, Paul 1970, Page and Sidd 1972, Intersociety Commission for Heart Disease Resources 1970, Tibblin 1967, A.H.A.–N.H.I. 1965). In particular, the impact of each component of the blood pressure and its net and joint contribution to cardiovascular disease as an ingredient of a cardiovascular risk profile have been ascertained (Kannel 1974).

   At all ages, in each sex, hypertension is among the most readily and objectively detected risk factors promoting cardiovascular disease. Theoretically, it is an easily controllable contributor to cardiovascular disease. It can be detected early in its course, and there are available a

---

WILLIAM B. KANNEL · National Institutes of Health, National Heart and Lung Institute, Heart Disease Epidemiology Study, 123 Lincoln Street, Framingham, Massachusetts 01701.

variety of antihypertensive pharmaceuticals with tolerable side effects that, if skillfully used, can normalize most elevated blood pressures. There is now convincing evidence that when this is done, even in persons of middle age and beyond with fixed diastolic hypertension and target organ involvement, a considerable reduction in cardiovascular morbidity and mortality ensues, and within a relatively short period of time (Freis 1971).

Because cardiovascular disease is an even more prominent cause of death and disability in the aged, a detailed examination of the role of blood pressure in cardiovascular disease in relation to age and the factors that affect its impact and the indications and need for treatment is warranted.

The Framingham Study

This chapter will rely heavily on data from the Framingham Study, in which a cohort of 5,209 men and women originally 30–62 years of age has been followed biennially for the development of cardiovascular disease in relation to their antecedent blood pressure status determined every two years. The net and joint effects of hypertension

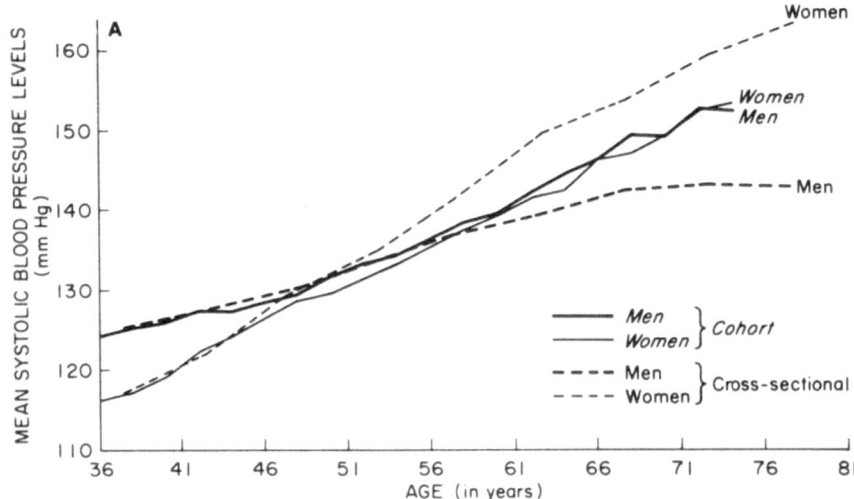

Fig. 7.1a. Average age trends in systolic blood pressure levels for cross-sectional and cohort data (Framingham Study, Exams 3–10).

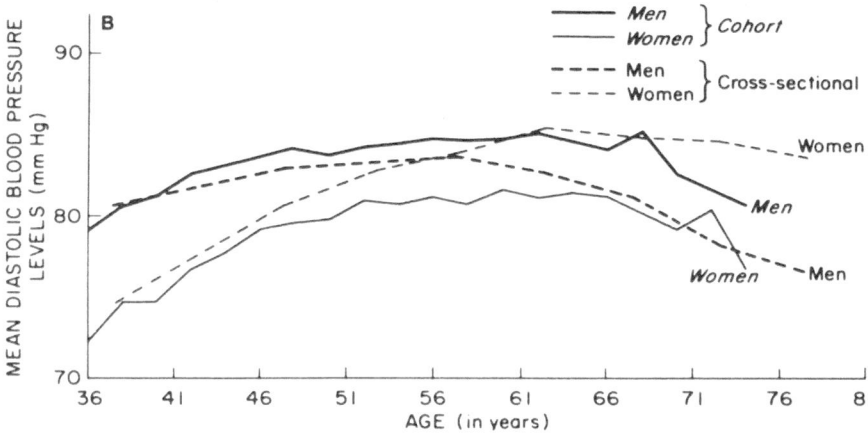

Fig. 7.1b. Average age trends in diastolic blood presssure levels for cross-sectional and cohort data (Framingham Study, Exams 3–10).

are examined, taking other contributors to the incidence of cardiovascular disease into account by comparing univariate with multivariate regression coefficients, using the method of Walker and Duncan (Walker and Duncan 1967, Shurtleff 1974). The criteria and methods employed in the Framingham Study have been published in detail elsewhere (Shurtleff 1974).

Because of the focus on the impact of hypertension in older persons, the effect is examined in the 65–74 age group in particular, as well as in younger age groups. During the 18 years of follow-up, there were enough people who reached this age range to provide 2,872 person–years of experience in men and 4,382 in women. In the period of follow-up, they developed 190 cardiovascular events, 86 in the men and 104 in the women. The cardiovascular sequelae examined include: coronary heart disease, atherothrombotic brain infarction, congestive heart failure, and intermittent claudication. There were also 132 deaths in men and 103 in women, of which 72 in men and 66 in women were from cardiovascular causes.

Age Trends in Blood Pressure

Prevalence data make it clear that blood pressure increases with age in most population samples, except possibly in primitive, isolated cultures (Page and Sidd 1972, Gordon and Devine 1966, P.H.S. 1964,

Lovell 1967, Feinleib et al. 1969, Miall 1969, Maddocks 1961). Longitudinal data are required, however, if a clear picture of age trends is to be obtained (Gordon and Shurtleff 1973, Dawber et al. 1973). In crosssectional data, both systolic and diastolic pressures increase with age in adult life, with systolic pressures continuing to rise into the 80's in women and into the 70's in men (Figs. 7.1a,b). Diastolic pressures tend to level off sooner and, in men, to decline precipitously beyond age 56. The pressures start lower in women and rise more steeply with age until they equal those of men at about 50 and then increasingly exceed those in men. This crossover in pressures is observed for both the systolic and the diastolic component.

Longitudinal data, which reflect pressures in the cohort as they actually age, reveal diastolic pressures that are essentially parallel in the sexes, with women's pressures persistently lower than men's. These cohort data show systolic pressures of women initially lower

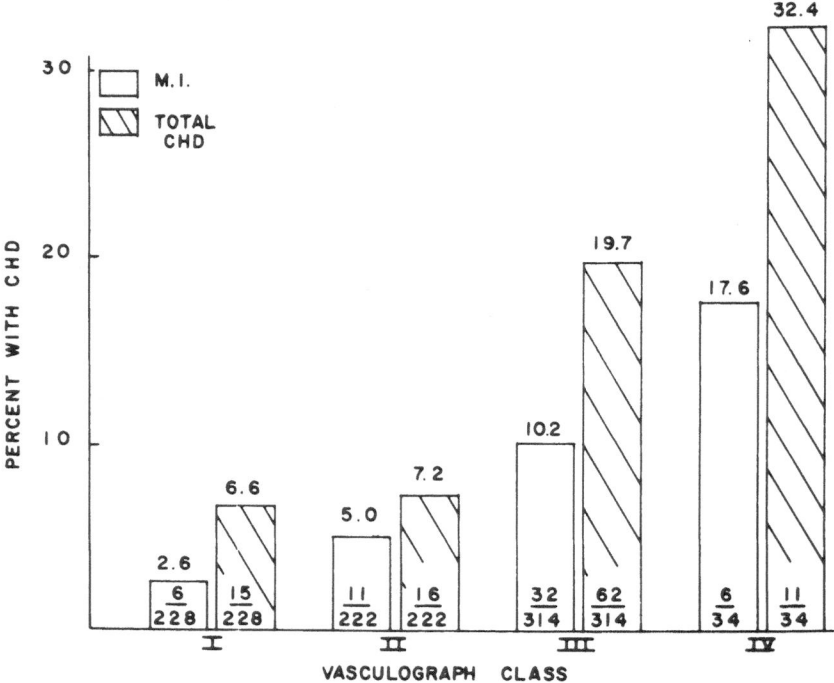

Fig. 7.2. Prevalence of coronary heart disease in men 45–77 years old according to vasculograph class (Framingham Study).

than those of men, converging on those of men by age 60, but never exceeding them. The data indicate that there is a disproportionate rise in systolic pressure in advanced age (relative to diastolic pressure), presumably due to progressive loss of arterial elasticity.

The reason for the difference in the picture of age trends obtained cross-sectionally and longitudinally is not entirely clear, but could well be due to differential mortality in the two sexes in relation to hypertension.

Age, Blood Pressure, and Cardiovascular Risk

Although it is clear that blood pressure (particularly systolic) tends to rise with age, and continues to do so into advanced age, it is not clear that this rise is inevitable. It is certainly detrimental to cardiovascular health. It is sometimes implied that because blood pressure commonly increases with age, the increase is physiologic and may even be necessary to compensate for progressive stenosis of the arterial circulation by maintaining adequate flow to vital organs. Those who hold this point of view would argue that the excess cardiovascular risk associated with high pressures in the aged is really a product of the underlying vascular stenosis, of which hypertension is more a sign than a cause.

Rigidity of vessels, as determined from the depth of the dicrotic notch in pulse wave recordings in the Framingham cohort increases precipitously with age (Dawber et al. 1973). In males, the proportion with normal prominent dicrotic notches has dropped to less than 50% by age 45–54, and by age 65–74, less than 10% are normal. Since the prevalence and incidence of cardiovascular disease is proportional to the degree of rigidity of the arterial circulation so assessed (Fig. 7.2), and because this rigidity is independent of the associated blood pressure level (Dawber et al. 1973), it is suggested that loss of elasticity per se is associated with increased risk.

This association does not mean, however, that the disproportionate rise in systolic pressure with age is merely an innocuous accompaniment of aging inelastic vessels. If this were so, the risk gradients associated with systolic pressure should become progressively attenuated with advancing age. Instead, they are observed actually to increase (Fig. 7.3), even in persons otherwise at low risk of cardiovascular disease. Although higher pressures are characteristic of older persons, an examination of cardiovascular disease incidence reveals

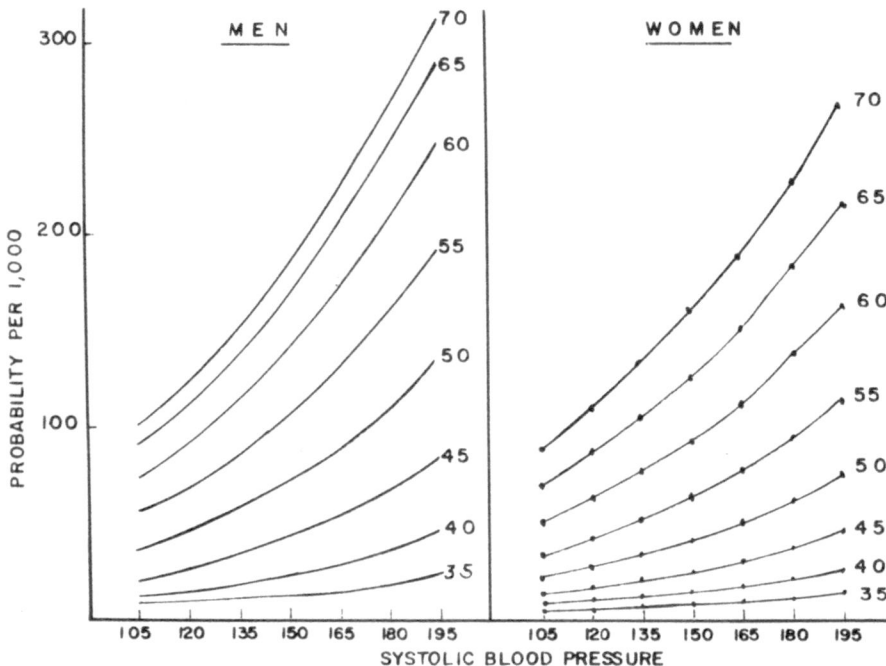

Fig. 7.3. Probability of cardiovascular disease in 8 years according to systolic blood pressure at specified ages in each sex (Framingham Study: 18 year follow-up, low-risk subjects).

prominent gradients of risk proportional to blood pressure at all ages (Fig. 7.3). Thus, hypertension is a distinct threat to life in the old as well as in the young, in terms of both relative and absolute risk.

The impact of blood pressure on cardiovascular disease incidence could be to some extent an intrinsic aging phenomenon. It is clear from age-specific analysis, however, that at any age those who have higher pressures are at considerably greater risk than those in the cohort with lower pressures. In the age range 45–74, less than 10% of the risk gradient according to blood pressure is accounted for by age, as can be judged from a comparison of univariate coefficients, including age as well as blood pressure. This comparison reveals, only a modest reduction of the coefficients in the bivariate case (Table 7.1).

Comparison of mortality in hypertensives versus normotensives reveals that it is more than doubled, and that the difference increases with age for overall mortality (Table 7.2), for cardiovascular mortality

TABLE 7.1. Regression of Systolic Blood Pressure on Cardiovascular Disease Incidence, Taking Age into Account in Men and Women 45–74 (Framingham Study: 18-Year Follow-Up)

	Regression coefficients[a]					
	Total C-V disease		Congestive heart failure		Atherothrombotic brain infarction	
	Men	Women	Men	Women	Men	Women
Univariate	0.0208	0.0221	0.0278	0.0262	0.0324	0.0288
Bivariate	0.0182	0.0180	0.0247	0.0225	0.0290	0.0262
	Coronary heart disease		Intermittent claudication		Cardiovascular mortality	
	Men	Women	Men	Women	Men	Women
Univariate	0.0174	0.0219	0.0137	0.0229	0.0198	0.0216
Bivariate	0.0151	0.0183	0.0101	0.0187	0.0156	0.0163

[a] Univariate, systolic blood pressure. Bivariate, age and systolic blood pressure.

TABLE 7.2. Overall Mortality According to Hypertensive Status by Age and Sex in Men and Women 45–74 (Framingham Study: 18-Year Follow-Up)

	Men			Women		
Age in years:	45–54	55–64	65–74	45–54	55–64	65–74
Blood pressure status	Five-year incidence per 100 at risk					
Normotensive	3.55	7.05	12.15	1.95	3.50	5.35
Borderline	3.55	8.10	18.45	2.30	4.20	9.35
Hypertensive	7.65	14.40	23.75	4.00	4.55	12.40
Regression coefficient	0.369	0.371	0.359	0.351	0.131	0.401
HBP vs. Normotensive						
Risk ratio	2.15	2.04	1.95	2.05	1.30	2.32
Difference in risk	4.10	7.35	11.60	2.05	1.05	7.05
Attributable risk (%)	53.6	51.0	48.8	51.3	23.1	56.9
t Value	3.22	4.08	3.10	2.53	1.10	2.85

TABLE 7.3. Cardiovascular Mortality According to Hypertensive Status by Age and Sex in Men and Women 45–74 (Framingham Study: 18-Year Follow-Up)

	Men			Women		
Age in years:	45–54	55–64	65–74	45–54	55–64	65–74
Blood pressure status	Five-year incidence per 100 at risk					
Normotensive	1.45	3.90	3.90	0.45	1.20	1.25
Borderline	2.00	5.30	11.30	0.50	2.25	5.35
Hypertensive	4.75	10.80	13.00	1.90	2.75	9.95
Regression coefficient	0.608	0.534	0.527	0.725	0.390	0.851
HBP vs. Normotensive						
Risk ratio	3.28	2.77	2.41	4.22	2.29	7.96
Difference in risk	3.30	6.90	7.60	1.45	1.55	8.70
Attributable risk (%)	69.5	63.9	58.5	76.3	56.4	87.4
t Value	3.85	4.74	2.81	2.90	2.27	4.28

(Table 7.3), and for cardiovascular morbidity (Table 7.4). These findings suggest that the yield in lives saved and in cardiovascular illness avoided by treating hypertension could be, if anything, greater in older hypertensives. Examination of the attributable risk (hypertensive mortality minus normotensive mortality divided by hypertensive mortality) reveals that for morbidity and mortality alike, a sizable proportion of each age group's death and illness is attributable to hypertension (Tables 7.2–7.4). About 69–75% of the morbidity and more than half the mortality in the elderly is attributable to their hypertension. The absolute risk of cardiovascular disease conveyed by hypertension increases with age. Proportionally, even considering other causes of death that might increase more rapidly with age, hypertension still accounts for almost as many deaths in the old as in the young (Table 7.3). In women, the relative risk for cardiovascular disease and for cardiovascular mortality (as well as for overall mortality) does not decrease with age (Tables 7.2–7.4). In men, it appears to do so for mortality, but not for morbidity.

The etiology of essential hypertension is as obscure in the aged as in the young. In both the aged and younger members of a cohort, what is regarded as normal and "hypertensive" is actually part of a continuum of pressures without any discernible critical value demarcating the hypertensive from the normotensive. Except on *a priori* statistical grounds, there is no logical basis for choosing normal limits of pressure for each decade of age. Some other basis for determining the acceptable or optimal values is required, rather than the usual values found in each age group. An examination of the cardiovascular morbidity and mortality in relation to blood pressure in persons 65–74 years old should provide the best guide to the ideal pressure in this age group. This examination reveals that the risk varies linearly in proportion to the blood pressure, so that, in general, the lower the pressure the better (Fig. 7.3.) Computations reveal that, on the average, there is a 30% change in risk for each 10% change in pressure (Kannel and Sorlie 1974). Pressures average higher in the elderly than in the young, but at any level of pressure, both the absolute and the relative risk is greater in the elderly.

Impact in the Sexes

Since the risk of cardiovascular sequelae is proportional to the height of the blood pressure in the "hypertensive," the aforementioned regression coefficients based categorically on "hypertensive status" could be misleading. The average "hypertensive" 65–74 years

TABLE 7.4. Incidence of Cardiovascular Disease According to Hypertensive Status by Age and Sex in Men and Women 45–74 (Framingham Study: 18-Year Follow-Up)

	Men			Women		
Age in years:	45–54	55–64	65–74	45–54	55–64	65–74
	Five-year incidence per 100 at risk					
Blood Pressure Status						
Normotensive	4.15	7.75	8.20	1.20	3.10	4.15
Borderline	7.33	14.65	15.95	2.50	7.10	12.45
Hypertensive	11.70	22.20	26.15	4.45	11.35	16.60
Regression coefficient	0.534	0.554	0.613	0.662	0.639	0.579
HBP vs. Normotensive						
Risk ratio	2.82	2.86	3.19	3.71	3.66	4.00
Difference in risk	7.55	14.45	17.95	3.25	8.25	12.45
Attributable risk (%)	64.5	65.1	68.6	73.0	72.7	75.0

old could have higher pressures than those 45–54 years old. An examination of the regression of cardiovascular disease incidence on blood pressure per se, however, yields similar information; the impact of high blood pressure, systolic or diastolic, is about the same at all ages. In men, the relative impact may be less pronounced in the oldest age group, although there is no clear trend.

The *relative* impact in women is just as great as in men; for older women, it may be even greater than for older men. The *absolute* risk for men is about double that of women at all ages, but this is true even for normotensives (Table 7.4). There is a clinical impression that postmenopausal women tolerate hypertension well, but prospectively obtained data do not support this contention. Compared to normotensive women the same age, the liability incurred by women who develop hypertension is just as great as the disadvantage incurred by men (Tables 7.1–7.5). True enough, the *absolute* risk for women is lower at any level of blood pressure, but it is far from negligible. The attributable risk, however, is even higher in women than in men. The *relative* risk (risk ratio) for cardiovascular morbidity (Table 7.4), for cardiovascular mortality (Table 7.3), and for mortality in general is, if anything, larger for women than for men. Thus, there is no justification for withholding treatment from elderly hypertensive women.

Systolic vs. Diastolic Pressures

Because the disproportionate rise in systolic pressure in the elderly (see Fig. 7.1a) is often considered inevitable and an innocuous accompaniment of aged, inelastic vessels, only diastolic hypertension is considered worthy of treatment. An examination of the risk of each of the major cardiovascular sequelae of hypertension in persons followed over 18 years in relation to their systolic and diastolic pressures, however, reveals little to suggest that diastolic pressures are more closely linked to cardiovascular incidence, particularly in the aged (Table 7.5). There is no consistent pattern in the regression coefficients favoring one over the other. To judge from the t values (which have the effect of adjusting for the different range of values for the two components of the pressure), systolic pressure appears to be, if anything, uniformly more closely related to cardiovascular disease incidence of any variety than diastolic pressure (Table 7.5).

Other studies of isolated systolic hypertension (Colandrea et al. 1970) have shown that even in the elderly, such hypertension is associated with an increased morbidity. In addition, life insurance

TABLE 7.5. Regression of Incidence of Cardiovascular Sequelae on Blood Pressure According to Age and Sex in Men and Women 45–74 (Framingham Study: 18-Year Follow-Up)

Age	CHD[a]		ABI[a]		IC[a]		CHF[a]	
	Men	Women	Men	Women	Men	Women	Men	Women
				Regression coefficients				
Systolic Blood Pressure								
45–54	0.016	0.018	0.027	0.026	0.008	0.032	0.040	0.023
55–64	0.017	0.019	0.035	0.029	0.015	0.018	0.022	0.023
65–74	0.009	0.018	0.021	0.023	−0.000	0.010	0.018	0.023
Diastolic Blood Pressure								
45–54	0.026	0.033	0.028	0.057	0.007	0.048	0.048	0.033
55–64	0.024	0.028	0.073	0.058	0.003	0.033	0.027	0.048
65–74	0.020	0.024	0.014	0.049	−0.027	0.010	0.028	0.012
				t Values				
Systolic Blood Pressure								
45–54	4.04	4.23	2.49	3.38	0.83	4.72	6.16	2.96
55–64	6.67	7.16	5.91	5.67	3.09	3.18	4.41	5.40
65–74	1.92	4.22	2.48	3.49	−0.04	1.36	2.86	4.11
Diastolic Blood Pressure								
45–54	3.78	3.69	1.25	3.36	0.41	2.60	3.63	1.71
55–64	4.47	4.53	5.92	4.78	0.30	2.61	2.56	5.05
65–74	2.25	2.72	0.74	3.70	−1.50	0.64	2.10	0.91

[a] CHD, coronary heart disease; ABI, atherothrombotic brain infarction; IC, intermittent claudication; CHF, congestive heart failure.

TABLE 7.6. Correlation of Systolic Blood Pressure
Between Biennial Examinations in Men and
Women (Framingham Study: 18-Year Follow-Up)

Exams	Men	Women
1,2	0.750	0.802
1,3	0.695	0.767
1,4	0.677	0.742
1,5	0.602	0.704
1,6	0.583	0.684
1,7	0.568	0.643
1,8	0.521	0.609
1,9	0.482	0.588
1,10	0.466	0.554

data have shown that mortality is proportional to systolic pressure at either high or low diastolic pressures (Gubner 1962).

The emphasis on diastolic over systolic pressure appears to stem from three misconceptions: (1) that the diastolic component better reflects the increased peripheral resistance, (2) that the evil consequences of hypertension derive entirely from the diastolic component of the pressure (Page and Sidd 1972), and (3) that the benefits of treatment necessarily derive entirely from lowering the diastolic pressure. There is little evidence to support any of these contentions.

Casual Blood Pressures

Most physicians are reluctant to commit patients to prolonged antihypertensive therapy on the basis of casual office blood pressures. Such pressures are often regarded as unreliable and hence misleading, so that treatment based on them is ill-advised. Since about 40% of the elderly have some degree of hypertension, however, it is not feasible to obtain basal pressures in the hospital or even with prolonged monitoring.

Examination of casual office blood pressures as a predictor of cardiovascular sequelae reveals nothing to suggest that they are often misleading. The pressure is fairly reproducible from one office visit to the next, and such office pressures correlate highly with each other even after extended periods of observation (Table 7.6), so that they are fairly characteristic of persons. More important, the risk of cardiovascular events is decidedly and strikingly related to these casual values

(Tables 7.1–7.6). It is evidently not even prudent to ignore casual elevations that subside under basal conditions. Even excluding those whose basal pressures are closer than 20 mm Hg to the casual pressures, risk is still strikingly related to the casual office blood pressure. With reasonable care, a series of casual office pressures can be used to select patients who are in jeopardy of a cardiovascular catastrophe because of elevated blood pressure. The risk gradients associated with the highest of three office pressures are surprisingly similar to those obtained using the lowest (Fig. 7.4).

In taking casual office blood pressures, the question often arises as to how many pressures are needed to arrive at a reasonable assessment of the pressure status. The data are based on single casual pressures, and it is clear that even such a single casual pressure is

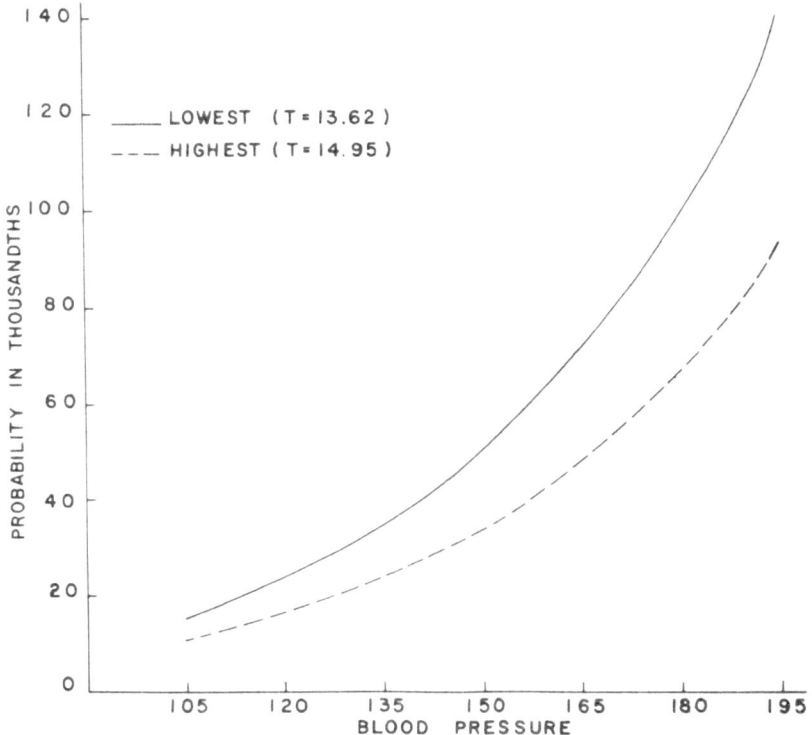

Fig. 7.4. Risk of cardiovascular disease for the lowest vs. the highest systolic blood pressure (mm Hg) at each exam (Framingham study: 18-year follow-up).

TABLE 7.7. Association of Trends in Systolic Blood
Pressure and Incidence of Cardiovascular Disease
(Framingham Study: 18-Year Follow-Up)

| Sex | Age | Regression[a] | |
		Value	χ^2 (1 D.F.)
Men	35–44	0.436	3.48
	45–54	0.750	11.45
	55–62	1.246	12.29
Women	35–44	0.262	0.50
	45–54	−0.071	0.07
	55–62	0.418	1.00

[a] Analyzed by the method of Truett and Sorlie (1971).

highly related to subsequent morbidity and mortality (Tables 7.1–7.5). It is not unreasonable, however, to expect that multiple observations of pressure over a period of time would more accurately select those likely to get into trouble. Analysis of blood pressure data at Framingham has indicated that not much is gained by remeasuring pressures over a prolonged period of time. Multiple measurements during one or more office visits are all that is required if further refinement of the casual pressure is desired.

Changes in Blood Pressure

Analysis of data from the Framingham cohort indicates that the *change* in pressure observed over a long period of observations is another matter.

Blood pressure information from 10 biennial examinations showed that in men, but not in women, a pressure rising more rapidly than average is associated with a greater than average risk. This risk is more pronounced at older ages. Thus, not only is an established high pressure ominous in older people, but a rapidly rising pressure in men augurs ill as well (Table 7.7).

Direct Sequelae

Hypertension directly affects cardiac performance, renal function, and cerebral blood flow, and also directly precipitates rupture and dissection of aortic aneurysms and cerebral vascular bleeding.

The rate of development of cardiac enlargement or hypertrophy, as judged from X-ray and ECG, was distinctly and strikingly related to the blood pressure level in the Framingham cohort in both sexes, especially at advanced ages (Fig. 7.5). Congestive failure was a common and lethal sequela of this sequence of events (Table 7.8).

Aortic Dissection. Although aortic dissection is a highly lethal consequence of hypertension, it is relatively uncommon. There is little prospective population-based data, but clinical studies reveal that hypertension accompanies 52–78% of dissecting hematomas of the aorta, and that an enlarged heart or electrocardiographic left ventricular hypertrophy (ECG–LVH), presumably reflecting hypertensive heart

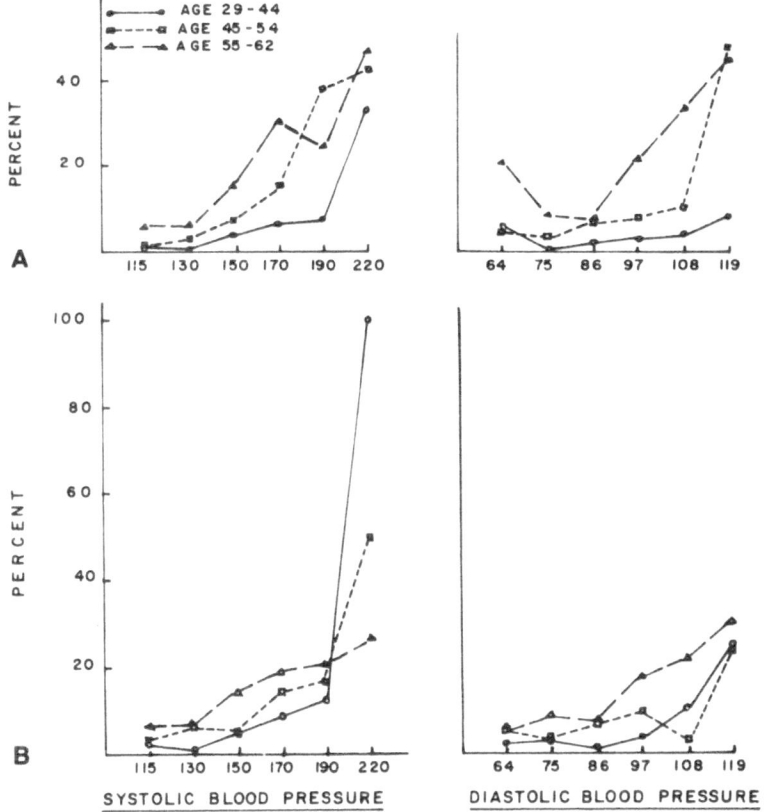

Fig. 7.5. Prevalence of LVH by ECG (A) or cardiac enlargement by X ray (B) according to initial systolic and diastolic blood pressure in men 30–62 years of age at entry (Framingham study).

TABLE 7.8. Incidence of Congestive Heart Failure According to X-Ray and ECG Finding of Heart Enlargement in Men and Women 65–74 (Framingham Study: 18-Year Follow-Up)[a]

Degree of abnormality at biennial exam	Five-year incidence per 100 at risk			
	Cardiac enlargement by X-ray		ECG–LVH	
	Men	Women	Men	Women
Negative	1.25	1.45	2.80	2.60
Possible	3.60	3.05	4.30	4.65
Definite	10.45	5.85	17.85	17.70
t Value	4.54	3.35	3.88	4.38

[a] Framingham monograph No. 30.

disease, is present in 64% (Levinson et al. 1950, Hume and Porter 1963). Dissecting aneurysm in the aged is most frequently associated with atherosclerosis, as well as hypertension, and may result either from an intimal tear or from hemorrhage from the vasa vasorum with expanding interluminal hematoma. Untreated, it is associated with an 83% mortality by one month from onset, and prognosis is especially poor in the aged, particularly where it is accompanied by severe hypertension and lesions in the ascending aorta. It seems likely that treatment of hypertension will reduce the incidence of this hypertensive catastrophe.

Intracerebral Hemorrhage. This is another highly lethal direct sequela of hypertension that can very likely be avoided by sustained control of hypertension. Subarachnoid hemorrhage, which is also more frequent in hypertensives, should likewise be reduced in frequency by antihypertensive treatment. It is important to recognize, however, that the predominant kind of stroke in the hypertensive, as in the nonhypertensive, is an atherothrombotic brain infarction. In the elderly, 55% of strokes are of this variety.

Nephrosclerosis. This is a frequent finding at necropsy in either mild or severe hypertensives (Smith et al. 1950). Usually, the pathology encountered is incidental, the patient having succumbed to the more lethal hypertensive cardiovascular sequelae. Renal insufficiency culminating in a uremic death is usually encountered in accelerated hypertension, accompanied by severe grades of hypertensive retinopathy. In common with the other sequelae of hypertension, the severity of postmortem nephrosclerosis is better correlated with systolic than with diastolic blood pressure (Goss et al. 1969). Even in those who exhibit azotemia, it has been found that further deterioration of renal function can be retarded by lowering blood pressure (Page and Sidd 1972).

Accelerated Atherogenesis

The direct sequelae of hypertension are undoubtedly lethal, but an even greater toll is exacted by the accelerated atherogenesis promoted by hypertension. It is likely that the atherogenic effect prevails in moderate hypertension, while the more direct effects, which acutely damage vessels and overwork the heart, predominate in severe grades of hypertension.

Hypertension is a powerful member of an atherogenic triad of risk

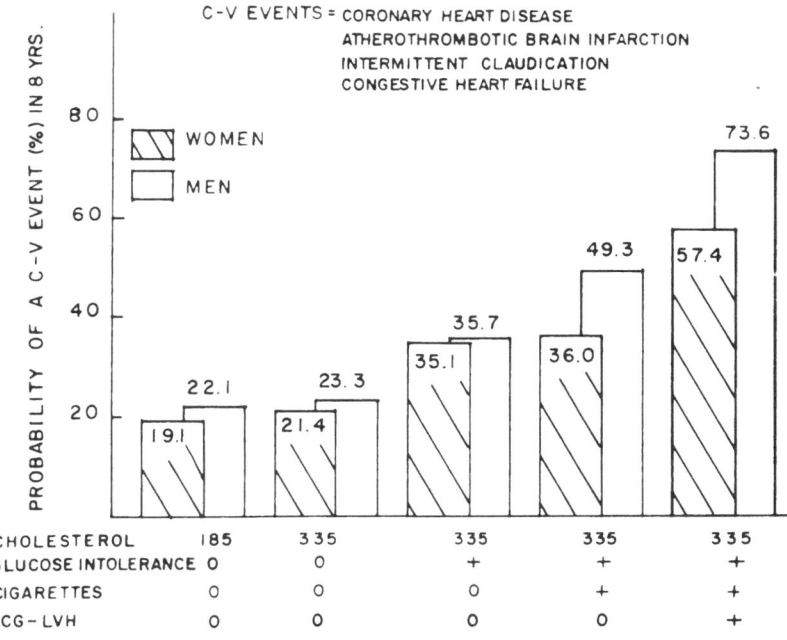

Fig. 7.6. Probability in men and women 70 years of age of cardiovascular disease at systolic blood pressure of 165 mm Hg according to dose of other risk factors (Framingham study: 18-year follow-up. Source, Monograph No. 28).

factors that also includes hyperlipidemia and impaired glucose tolerance. Risk of major atherosclerotic diseases, such as brain infarction,
and coronary disease mounts in proportion to the number of these
traits persons exhibit (Fig. 7.6).

Only in intermittent claudication is there no clear-cut relationship. Blood pressure must play a critical role in atherogenesis. Atheromata almost never develop in the low-pressure segments of the
circulation, such as the pulmonary arteries or veins, even though they
are bathed by the same lipid-laden blood as the systemic arterial
circulation, where atherosclerosis simultaneously abounds. This absence of atheromata is not a consequence of a different vascular
anatomy, since atheromata will appear when veins are grafted to
bypass coronary arteries, or when pathology produces pulmonary
hypertension. Although atheromata do occur in "normotensive" persons, there are evidently pressures below which they are exceedingly
rare. Whether hypertension accelerates atherogenesis primarily by
damaging the vessel wall or by enhancing filtration of lipid into the
vessel is a matter of some controversy. It seems likely that both
processes are involved. Whatever the mechanism, and whether hypertension is only a contributor or a direct cause, elderly hypertensives
are at increased risk of brain infarction, coronary heart disease, and
possibly peripheral arterial disease (Table 7.9)—diseases that are
unequivocally atherosclerotic in nature.

In addition to promoting occlusive atherosclerotic disease, hypertension promotes saccular aneurysms of the aorta, also believed to be
on an atherosclerotic basis. This condition is particularly likely to
affect the elderly hypertensive.

Variable Impact on Cardiovascular End Points

Blood pressure is a major risk factor for cardiovascular disease in
the elderly. It is distinctly more important as a precursor of brain
infarction and of congestive failure, on a relative scale, than it is for
coronary heart disease and intermittent claudication (Table 7.9). Because coronary heart disease is much more common on an absolute
scale, however, it is still the most frequently encountered vascular
complication in the hypertensive elderly (as it is in the normotensive
in this age group).

Hypertensives 65–74 years of age develop a clear excess of myocardial infarctions, in particular (Table 7.10). The impact on other clinical
manifestations of coronary heart disease is less consistent in the

Table 7.9. Incidence of Cardiovascular Disease According to Hypertensive Status in Men and Women 65–74 (Framingham Study: 18-Year Follow-Up)

	Coronary heart disease		Brain infarction		Congestive heart failure		Intermittent claudication	
	Men	Women	Men	Women	Men	Women	Men	Women
				Five-year incidence per 100 at Risk				
Blood pressure status								
Normotensive	5.35	2.20	0.70	—	1.05	1.25	3.60	1.70
Borderline	11.55	6.55	2.15	2.15	2.85	2.65	1.85	1.45
Hypertensive	14.85	11.30	3.50	3.95	8.90	5.15	3.80	2.85
Regression Coefficient	0.508	0.728	0.751	1.044	1.113	0.708	−0.034	0.341
t Value	2.98	3.92	2.10	2.98	3.84	2.69	−0.12	1.13
Hypertensive vs. normotensive								
Difference in risk	9.50	9.10	2.80	3.95	7.85	3.90	0.20	1.15
Attributable risk (%)	64	81	80	100	88	76	5	40
Risk ratio	2.8	5.1	5.0	—	8.5	4.1	1.1	1.7

William B. Kannel

TABLE 7.10. Incidence of Clinical Manifestations of Coronary Heart Disease According to Hypertensive Status at Each Biennial Examination in Men and Women 65–74 (Framingham Study: 18-Year Follow-Up)

	Myocardial infarction		Angina pectoris		Coronary insufficiency		Sudden death	
	Men	Women	Men	Women	Men	Women	Men	Women
	Five-year incidence per 100 at Risk							
Blood pressure status								
Normotensive	1.65	0.90	2.90	0.45	0.40	0.45	0.40	
Borderline	7.00	1.55	2.05	3.65	1.25	0.50	1.25	0.50
Hypertensive	7.40	4.15	2.95	4.75	1.50	0.60	2.25	1.20
Regression coefficient	0.636	0.858	-0.023	0.713	0.578	0.147	0.791	1.194
t Value	2.65	2.54	-0.07	2.62	1.08	0.25	1.54	1.63
Hypertensive vs. normotensive								
Difference in risk	5.75	3.25	0.05	4.30	1.10	0.15	1.85	1.20
Attributable risk (%)	78	78	2	1	73	25	82	100
Risk ratio	4.5	4.6	1.0	10.6	3.8	1.3	5.6	

TABLE 7.11. Regression of Incidence of Cardiovascular Disease on Hypertensive Status in Men and Women 45–74 (Framingham Study: 18-Year Follow-Up)[a]

Status	Total cardiovascular disease				Congestive heart failure			
	Regression coefficient		t Value		Regression coefficient		t Value	
	Men	Women	Men	Women	Men	Women	Men	Women
Univariate	0.588	0.789	10.21	11.23	1.012	0.992	7.47	6.72
Bivariate	0.552	0.609	9.49	8.30	0.963	0.764	7.04	4.97
Multivariate	0.482	0.487	7.83	6.29	0.738	0.635	5.12	3.91

Status	Intermittent claudication				Atherothrombotic brain infarction			
	Regression coefficient		t Value		Regression coefficient		t Value	
	Men	Women	Men	Women	Men	Women	Men	Women
Univariate	0.422	0.865	3.38	4.90	1.118	1.217	5.71	6.19
Bivariate	0.364	0.644	2.89	3.49	1.060	1.028	5.37	5.05
Multivariate	0.277	0.565	2.10	2.84	0.982	0.818	4.82	3.88

Status	Coronary heart disease				Cardiovascular mortality			
	Regression coefficient		t Value		Regression coefficient		t Value	
	Men	Women	Men	Women	Men	Women	Men	Women
Univariate	0.497	0.784	7.73	9.45	0.584	0.838	7.47	7.66
Bivariate	0.462	0.617	7.12	7.12	0.519	0.585	6.54	5.09
Multivariate	0.391	0.505	5.66	5.51	0.265	0.337	3.09	2.77

[a] Bivariate: High blood pressure and age. Multivariate: High blood pressure and age, plus serum cholesterol, glucose tolerance, cigarettes per day, and ECG-LVH.

Framingham cohort, probably owing to a paucity of data in this elderly age group.

Multivariate analysis designed to assess the net effect of hypertension on the cardiovascular sequelae of hypertension indicates that its contribution is unique and not mediated to any great extent through, or dependent on, the existence of other risk factors. This finding can be demonstrated by a comparison of the size of bivariate coefficients, adjusting only for age, with multivariate coefficients, adjusting for all the major risk factors as well (Table 7.11). For men, there is an 87% net effect; for women, 80%. Thus, hypertension is a potent *independent* contributor to the incidence of cardiovascular disease.

Cardiovascular Risk Profiles

Although the risk of cardiovascular sequelae in the elderly hypertensive is high, it is far from uniform and depends to some extent on the dose of other risk factors (Fig. 7.6). If any one factor were to be chosen to identify high-risk candidates for cardiovascular disease in the elderly, it would be hypertension. Using blood pressure alone to detect persons at high risk of a stroke would be reasonably effective. Some 57% of the incidence of brain infarction arises in the 19% of the population having systolic pressures exceeding 160 mm Hg. The statistics for congestive heart failure are quite similar.

The screening efficacy for candidates for cardiovascular disease in the aged hypertensive can be further improved, however, by considering other risk factors and treating blood pressure as one ingredient of a cardiovascular risk profile. Major contributors to cardiovascular disease incidence can be synthesized quantitatively into a composite risk score, using a multiple logistic formulation. This synthesis provides an estimate of the conditional probability of any of the major cardiovascular diseases for any set of risk factors (McGee 1973). An efficient set of variables for this purpose, in addition to blood pressure, is a glucose and cholesterol determination, an ECG, and a cigarette history. The risk associated with any combination of these can be displayed in handbooks (McGee 1973).

These variables have a varying impact on the incidence of particular cardiovascular events in the elderly. The impact of cholesterol and cigarettes wanes markedly with advancing age, particularly for coronary heart disease (Shurtleff 1974). The combined risk factors will, however, appreciably enhance risk assessments in the hypertensive for intermittent claudication (Table 7.12), for brain infarction (Table 7.13), and for congestive heart failure (Table 7.14). For coronary heart disease in this age group, risk-profile handbook tabulations can only estimate risk over a 6-fold range, compared to the 40-fold range for the other cardiovascular endpoints.

Organ Damage

While it is apparently not common knowledge that the risk in the hypertensive varies depending on the associated cardiovascular risk profile, it is well recognized that hypertension is more dangerous when accompanied by evidence of organ damage. This increased danger is present even if the patient is asymptomatic. The rate of development of cardiac impairments such as ECG–LVH, intraventricular conduction disturbances, nonspecific ST–T wave abnormalities, and cardiac enlargement on X-ray is strikingly related to blood pressure level. The excess risk associated with each of these blood pressure–related findings is substantial (Table 7.15), and at any level of hypertension, those with such impairments are substantially worse off (Shurtleff 1974).

Awaiting organ damage before instituting treatment would seem, however, most imprudent. Fully half the cardiovascular morbidity and mortality in hypertensives in the Framingham cohort occurred prior to evidence of organ damage. Thus, more often than not, a stroke or coronary attack is the first evidence of organ damage in the hypertensive.

In the elderly hypertensive, ECG–LVH, in particular, is an extremely ominous finding. Within 5 years, 50% will develop a cardiovascular event, and from 40 to 60% will be dead (Table 7.16). The bulk of the cardiovascular mortality is not from coronary heart disease, but from stroke and congestive failure.

Albuminuria is associated with hypertension. Its occurrence even in asymptomatic patients is associated with a distinct increase in cardiovascular as well as renal disease incidence (Shurtleff 1974). In those 65–74 years of age, there is almost a 3-fold increase in cardiovascular as well as overall mortality (Table 7.17).

Thus, in addition to the height of the blood pressure—systolic or diastolic, at all ages, in either sex—there is a greater penalty for the

TABLE 7.12. Probability (per 1,000) in 70-Year-Old Men of Developing Intermittent Claudication in 8 Years According to Specified Characteristics (Framingham Study: 18-Year Follow-Up)

ECG–LVH Negative

Nonsmokers

Chol	105	120	135	SBP 150	165	180	195
Glucose intolerance absent							
185	8	9	11	12	14	16	19
210	9	10	12	13	16	18	21
235	10	11	13	15	17	20	23
260	11	12	14	16	19	22	25
285	12	13	15	18	21	24	28
310	13	15	17	20	23	26	30
335	14	16	19	22	25	29	33
Glucose intolerance present							
185	21	24	28	33	38	43	50
210	23	27	31	36	41	47	55
235	26	29	34	39	45	52	60
260	28	32	37	43	50	57	66
285	31	36	41	47	54	62	72
310	34	39	45	52	59	68	78
335	37	43	49	57	65	75	86

Smokers

Chol	105	120	135	SBP 150	165	180	195
Glucose intolerance absent							
185	27	31	36	41	47	54	62
210	29	34	39	45	52	59	68
235	32	37	43	49	57	65	75
260	35	41	47	54	62	71	82
285	39	45	51	59	68	78	89
310	42	49	56	65	74	85	97
335	47	54	62	71	81	93	106
Glucose intolerance present							
185	69	79	91	104	119	135	153
210	76	87	99	113	129	147	166
235	83	95	108	123	140	159	180
260	90	103	118	134	152	172	195
285	99	113	128	146	165	187	210
310	107	123	139	158	179	202	227
335	117	133	151	171	193	218	244

ECG-LVH Positive

Glucose intolerance absent

Chol	SBP 105	120	135	150	165	180	195
185	19	22	25	29	34	39	45
210	21	24	28	32	37	43	49
235	23	26	30	35	41	47	54
260	25	29	33	39	44	51	59
285	28	32	37	42	49	56	65
310	30	35	40	46	53	61	71
335	33	38	44	51	59	67	77

Chol	SBP 105	120	135	150	165	180	195
185	62	72	82	94	107	122	139
210	68	78	90	102	117	133	151
235	75	85	98	112	127	145	164
260	81	93	107	122	138	157	177
285	89	102	116	132	150	170	192
310	97	111	126	144	163	184	207
335	106	121	137	156	176	199	224

Glucose intolerance present

Chol	SBP 105	120	135	150	165	180	195
185	50	57	66	76	87	99	113
210	55	63	72	83	94	108	123
235	60	69	79	90	103	118	134
260	65	75	86	98	112	128	145
285	72	82	94	107	122	139	158
310	78	90	102	117	133	151	171
335	85	98	112	127	144	164	185

Chol	SBP 105	120	135	150	165	180	195
185	153	173	195	220	246	275	305
210	166	187	211	237	264	294	326
235	180	202	227	254	284	315	347
260	194	218	245	273	303	336	369
285	210	235	263	293	324	358	392
310	226	253	282	313	346	380	415
335	243	272	302	334	368	403	439

Framingham men 70 years of age have an average SBP of 145 mm Hg and an average serum cholesterol of 231 mg%; 37% smoke cigarettes, 4.0% have definite LVH by ECG, and 15.2% have glucose intolerance. At these average values, the probability of developing intermittent claudication in 8 years is 26/1,000.

TABLE 7.13. Probability (per 1,000) in 65-Year-Old Men of Developing Atherothrombotic Brain Infarction in 8 Years According to Specified Characteristics (Framingham Study: 18-Year Follow-Up)

ECG–LVH Negative

Nonsmokers

Chol	SBP						
	105	120	135	150	165	180	195
Glucose intolerance absent							
185	4	7	10	15	23	35	52
210	4	6	10	15	23	34	52
235	4	6	10	15	22	34	51
260	4	6	10	15	22	33	50
285	4	6	9	14	22	33	49
310	4	6	9	14	21	32	49
335	4	6	9	14	21	32	48
Glucose intolerance present							
185	9	13	20	31	46	69	102
210	9	13	20	30	45	68	100
235	9	13	20	30	45	67	99
260	8	13	19	29	44	66	97
285	8	13	19	29	43	65	96
310	8	12	19	28	43	64	95
335	8	12	19	28	42	63	93

Smokers

Chol	SBP						
	105	120	135	150	165	180	195
Glucose intolerance absent							
185	8	13	19	29	44	66	98
210	8	13	19	29	44	65	96
235	8	12	19	29	43	64	95
260	8	12	19	28	42	63	94
285	8	12	18	28	42	62	92
310	8	12	18	27	41	61	91
335	8	12	18	27	40	61	90
Glucose intolerance present							
185	17	26	39	58	86	126	181
210	17	25	38	57	85	125	179
235	17	25	38	57	84	123	176
260	16	25	37	56	83	121	174
285	16	24	37	55	82	120	172
310	16	24	36	54	80	118	170
335	16	24	36	53	79	116	167

ECG–LVH Positive

Glucose intolerance absent

Chol	105	120	135	150	165	180	195
185	5	8	12	18	27	41	62
210	5	8	12	18	27	41	61
235	5	8	12	18	27	40	60
260	5	7	11	17	26	39	59
285	5	7	11	17	26	39	58
310	5	7	11	17	25	38	57
335	5	7	11	16	25	38	56

Chol	105	120	135	150	165	180	195
185	10	15	23	35	52	78	114
210	10	15	23	34	51	76	112
235	10	15	22	34	51	75	111
260	10	14	22	33	50	74	109
285	9	14	22	33	49	73	108
310	9	14	21	32	48	72	106
335	9	14	21	32	48	71	105

Glucose intolerance present

Chol	105	120	135	150	165	180	195
185	10	16	24	36	54	81	118
210	10	16	24	36	54	80	117
235	10	15	23	35	53	78	115
260	10	15	23	35	52	77	114
285	10	15	23	34	51	76	112
310	10	15	22	34	50	75	110
335	9	14	22	33	50	74	109

Chol	105	120	135	150	165	180	195
185	20	30	46	68	101	146	208
210	20	30	45	67	100	144	205
235	20	30	44	66	98	143	203
260	19	29	44	65	97	141	200
285	19	29	43	65	95	139	198
310	19	28	43	64	94	137	195
335	18	28	42	63	93	135	193

Framingham men 65 years of age have an average SBP of 141 mm Hg and an average serum cholesterol of 239 mg%; 44% smoke cigarettes, 1.4% have definite LVH by ECG, and 8.1% have glucose intolerance. At these average values, the probability of developing atherothrombotic brain infarction in 8 years is 16/1,000.

TABLE 7.14. Probability (per 1,000) in 70-Year-Old Men of Developing Hypertensive Heart Failure in 8 Years According to Specified Characteristics (Framingham Study: 18-Year Follow-Up)

ECG-LVH Negative

Nonsmokers

				SBP			
Chol	105	120	135	150	165	180	195
Glucose intolerance absent							
185	4	5	8	11	17	25	36
210	4	6	8	12	18	26	38
235	4	6	9	13	19	28	40
260	4	6	9	14	20	29	43
285	4	7	10	14	21	31	45
310	5	7	10	15	22	33	48
335	5	7	11	16	24	35	50

				SBP			
Chol	105	120	135	150	165	180	195
Glucose intolerance present							
185	13	19	28	41	59	85	120
210	14	20	29	43	62	89	127
235	14	21	31	45	66	94	133
260	15	22	33	48	69	99	140
285	16	24	35	51	73	105	148
310	17	25	37	54	77	110	155
335	18	27	39	57	82	116	163

Smokers

				SBP			
Chol	105	120	135	150	165	180	195
Glucose intolerance absent							
185	5	8	12	17	25	37	54
210	6	8	12	18	27	39	57
235	6	9	13	19	28	41	60
260	6	9	14	20	30	44	63
285	7	10	15	22	32	46	67
310	7	11	16	23	34	49	71
335	8	11	17	24	36	52	75

				SBP			
Chol	105	120	135	150	165	180	195
Glucose intolerance present							
185	19	29	42	60	87	123	172
210	21	30	44	64	92	130	181
235	22	32	47	67	97	137	190
260	23	34	49	71	102	144	199
285	24	36	52	75	107	151	208
310	26	38	55	79	113	159	218
335	27	40	58	84	119	167	228

ECG–LVH Positive

Glucose intolerance absent

Chol	SBP						
	105	120	135	150	165	180	195
185	12	18	26	39	56	81	115
210	13	19	28	41	59	85	121
235	14	20	30	43	62	90	127
260	15	21	31	46	66	95	134
285	15	23	33	48	70	100	141
310	16	24	35	51	74	105	148
335	17	25	37	54	78	111	156

Chol	SBP						
	105	120	135	150	165	180	195
185	18	27	40	57	83	118	165
210	20	29	42	61	87	124	173
235	21	30	44	64	92	130	182
260	22	32	47	68	97	137	190
285	23	34	49	71	102	144	200
310	25	36	52	75	108	152	209
335	26	38	55	80	114	159	219

Glucose intolerance present

Chol	SBP						
	105	120	135	150	165	180	195
185	43	63	90	128	179	243	323
210	46	66	95	135	187	254	335
235	49	70	100	142	196	266	349
260	51	74	106	149	206	277	362
285	54	78	111	157	216	289	376
310	57	82	117	164	226	301	389
335	61	87	124	173	236	314	403

Chol	SBP						
	105	120	135	150	165	180	195
185	65	93	131	183	249	329	420
210	68	98	138	192	260	342	434
235	72	103	145	201	271	355	449
260	76	109	153	210	283	369	463
285	80	114	160	220	295	382	478
310	85	120	168	231	307	396	493
335	89	127	177	241	320	410	507

Framingham men 70 years of age have an average SBP of 145 mm Hg and an average serum cholesterol of 231 mg%; 37% smoke cigarettes, 4.0% have definite LVH by ECG, and 15.2% have glucose intolerance. At these average values, the probability of developing hypertensive heart failure in 8 years is 17/1,000.

TABLE 7.15. Incidence of Cardiovascular Disease According to Evidence of Cardiac Impairments in Men and Women 65–74 (Framingham Study: 18-Year Follow-Up)

	Five-year incidence per 100 at risk							
	Electrocardiographic left ventricular hypertrophy		Nonspecific ST-T abnormality		Intraventricular conduction defect		X-ray cardiac enlargement	
Cardiac abnormality	Men	Women	Men	Women	Men	Women	Men	Women
Normal	14.0	10.4	13.6	11.5	14.7	11.7	14.2	10.7
Abnormal	44.9	51.0	29.6	16.3	20.9	24.2	21.6	16.4
Risk ratio	3.2	4.9	2.2	1.4	1.4	2.2	1.5	1.5
t Value	2.93	5.31	2.82	1.18	0.86	1.27	1.37	2.00

TABLE 7.16. Mortality According to ECG–LVH Status at Biennial
Examination, in Men and Women 65–74 (Framingham Study:
18-Year Follow-Up)[a]

	Five-year mortality per 100 at risk					
	CHD death		C-V death		Overall mortality	
ECG–LVH	Men	Women	Men	Women	Men	Women
Negative	1.9	1.5	6.9	4.3	14.1	7.6
Doubtful	18.3	5.8	23.1	14.9	34.6	19.1
Definite	16.4	6.3	47.4	34.6	63.2	40.7
t Value for trend	4.32	2.36	7.30	7.53	6.99	6.97

[a] Source: Framingham monograph No. 30.

hypertensive who is allowed to progress to the stage where he exhibits
evidence of even presymptomatic involvement (Shurtleff 1974).

Preventive Implications

Perhaps as insidious as hypertension itself is the confusion and
the misconceptions that have retarded its treatment and control.

TABLE 7.17. Risk of Mortality According to Albuminuria Status at
Biennial Examination in Men and Women 65–74 (Framingham Study:
18-Year Follow-Up)

	Five-year mortality per 100 at risk			
	Overall mortality		Cardiovascular mortality	
Albuminuria	Men	Women	Men	Women
Absent	16.1	9.1	8.8	5.9
Present	39.5	27.1	21.1	15.1
Factor of increased risk	2.5	3.0	2.4	2.6
t Value	3.37	3.19	2.36	2.05

TABLE 7.18. Percent on Antihypertensive Therapy
According to Systolic Blood Pressure in Men
and Women 65–74 (Framingham Study:
18-Year Follow-Up)

Systolic blood pressure	Percent on treatment	
	Men	Women
140–149	1.7	6.0
150–159	7.0	8.0
160–169	7.0	9.5
170–179	14.8	16.1
180–189	14.3	20.3
190–199	17.4	26.9
200+	20.8	32.3

Effective drug treatment has been shown to control hypertension and
to substantially reduce the amount of illness and death it causes (Page
and Sidd 1972, Freis 1971). Even so, hypertension remains the greatest
contributor to cardiovascular disease, the greatest killer of persons
over 65.

Hypertension is easy to detect, even in its asymptomatic stage,
yet it is permitted to exact its toll in cardiovascular morbidity and
mortality, undetected and uncontrolled more often than not. Even in
the Framingham cohort, no more than 21% of men and 32% of women
receive treatment in the age group 65–74, despite systolic blood
pressures of 200 mm Hg or greater (Table 7.18). As a result, treatment
often begins too late, after the occurrence of organ damage or a
cardiovascular catastrophe that could have been delayed or prevented
by prudent treatment.

Reduction of this unnecessary toll of death and disability would
appear to require increased professional understanding of recent
developments in hypertension control and better public awareness, to
ensure compliance in long-term detection and treatment programs.
Until recently, hypertension was not considered a public health
problem, since it is not a contagious disease. It must now be so
considered, because it has been demonstrated to be the most powerful
contributor to cardiovascular disease (Shurtleff 1974) and a condition
that afflicts 27% of men and 48% of women 65–74 years of age.
Furthermore, this common and serious disease process is one for
which effective treatment is available; yet, for some reason, treatment

is not helping more than a fraction of those who need it. In hypertension, as in communicable disease, we are confronted with a problem of bringing care to people who do not know they are at risk and cannot act in their behalf to protect themselves. Also, particularly in the elderly, the cardiovascular sequelae of hypertension impose an enormous economic and social burden on the family and the community, and a huge drain on the medical resources available to cope with the problem.

References

A. H. A.–N. H. I. (1965) *Cardiovascular Disease in the U.S.*, American Heart Association and National Heart Institute.

Colandrea, M. A., Friedman, G. D., Nichaman, M. Z., and Lynd, C. N. (1970) *Circulation* **41**, 239.

Dawber, T. R., Thomas H. E., Jr., and McNamara, P. M. (1973) *Angiology* **24**, 244.

Feinleib, M., Gordon, T., and Kannel, W. B. (1969) 2nd Ann. Meeting, Soc. Epid. Res.

Freis, E. D., (1971) *Med. Conc. Cardiovasc. Dis.* **40**, 17.

Gordon, T., and Devine, B. (1966) *Vital and Health Stas.*, Series 11, No. 13.

Gordon, T., and Shurtleff, D. (1973) *In* Kannel, W. B., and Gordon, T. (eds.), DHEW Publ. No. (NIH) 74–478, U.S. Govt. Printing Office, Washington, D.C.

Goss, L. Z., Rosa, R. M., O'Brien, W. M., Ayers, C. R., and Wood, J. E. (1969) *Arch. Intern. Med.* **124**, 160.

Gubner, R. S. (1962) *Am. J. Cardiol.* **9**, 773.

Hume, D. M., and Porter, R. R. (1963) *Surgery* **53**, 122.

Intersociety Commission for Heart Disease Resources (1970) Report.

Kannel, W. B. (1974) *Prog. Cardiovasc. Dis.* **17**, 5.

Kannel, W. B., Castelli, W. P., McNamara, P. M., and Sorlie, P. (1969) *Millbank Mem. Fund Q.* **27**, 116.

Kannel, W. B., and Sorlie, P. (1974) *Proceedings of the Second International Symposium on the Epidemiology of Hypertension*, Chicago Symposia Specialists.

Levinson, D. C., Edmeades, D. J., and Griffith, G. C. (1950) *Circulation* **1**, 360.

Lovell, R. R. H. (1967) *In* Stamler, J., Stamler, R., and Pullman, T. R. (eds.), *The Epidemiology of Hypertension*, Grune and Stratton, New York, p. 122.

Maddocks, I. (1961) *Lancet* **2**, 396.

McGee, D. (1973) *In* Kannel, W. B., and Gordon, T. (eds.), DHEW Publ. No. 74-618, U.S. Govt. Printing Office, Washington, D.C.

Miall, W. E. (1969) *Millbank Mem. Fund Q.* **47**, 107.

P.H.S. (1964) Public Health Service Publ. No. 1,000, Series 11, No. 4.

Page, L. B., and Sidd, J. J. (1972) *N. Engl. J. Med.* **287**, 960.

Paul, O. (1970) *Br. Heart J. (Suppl.)* **33**, 116.

Shurtleff, D., (1974) *In* Kannel, W. B., and Gordon, T. (eds.), DHEW Publ. No. (NIH) 74-599, U.S. Govt. Printing Office, Washington, D.C.

Smith, D. E., Odel, H. M., and Kernohan, J. W. (1950) *Am. J. Med.* **9**, 516.

Tibblin, G. (1967) *Acta. Med. Scand. Suppl.* **470**, 1.

Truett, J., and Sorlie, P. (1971) *J. Chronic Dis.* **24**, 349.

Walker, S. H., and Duncan, D. B. (1967) *Biometrics* **54**, 167.

8

High Blood Pressure and Its Management

R. D. KENNEDY

Introduction

For the clinician, the definition of hypertension in older people presents some problems. If WHO guidelines are used, a high proportion of the elderly can be regarded as being hypertensive, with blood pressures in excess of 160/95 mm Hg.

Master et al. (1958) collected information from 5,000 physicians regarding blood pressure of those 65 years old and over. Their data demonstrated that while there is relatively little increase over the age of 65, the range of values is wide, and that the middle 80% of the range includes diastolic pressures up to 100 mm Hg in both sexes, and systolic pressures up to 185 mm Hg in men and 190 mm Hg in women (Table 8.1). Anderson and Cowan (1959) assessed the blood pressure in 546 men and women 60–89 years old selected as healthy by strict criteria, excluding those with gross adiposity. They showed that both mean systolic and diastolic blood pressures increase gradually with age, the increase being greater for the systolic values. At all ages, females showed a higher mean value than men. They confirmed the wide range of blood pressure, particularly systolic, with advancing years (Table 8.2).

Anderson and Cowan (1972) attempted to correlate the levels of

R. D. KENNEDY · University Department of Geriatric Medicine, Stobhill, Hospital, Glasgow, G21 3UW, Scotland.

TABLE 8.1. Range of Blood Pressure in People over 65 Years of Age without Heart Disease[a]

Age	Number examined	Systolic blood pressure (mm Hg)			Diastolic blood presure (mm Hg)		
		Mean ± SD	Upper 80% limit	Upper 95% limit	Mean ± SD	Upper 80% limit	Upper 95% limit
Men							
65–69	911	143 ± 26	191	195	83 ± 10	101	103
70–74	694	145 ± 26	193	198	92 ± 15	110	113
75–79	534	146 ± 22	186	190	81 ± 13	105	107
80–84	385	145 ± 26	192	196	82 ± 10	100	102
85–89	325	145 ± 24	190	193	79 ± 15	106	109
90–94	124	145 ± 23	188	192	78 ± 12	100	102
95–106	25	145 ± 28	196	198	78 ± 13	101	103
Women							
65–69	856	154 ± 29	207	212	85 ± 14	110	113
70–74	682	159 ± 26	207	211	85 ± 15	113	116
75–79	464	158 ± 26	206	210	84 ± 13	108	110
80–84	344	157 ± 28	208	213	83 ± 17	115	109
85–89	263	154 ± 28	205	210	82 ± 12	104	107
90–94	122	150 ± 24	197	198	79 ± 13	102	103
95–106	28	149 ± 24	192	197	81 ± 15	108	110

[a] Master et al. (1958).

TABLE 8.2. Range of Blood Pressure in Clinically Healthy Old People[a]

Age	Number		Systolic (mm Hg)[b]		Diastolic (mm Hg)[b]	
	Male	Female	Male	Female	Male	Female
60–64	44	48	151 ± 2.8	158 ± 2.7	85 ± 1.2	86 ± 1.2
65–69	63	42	154 ± 2.8	163 ± 3.3	85 ± 0.94	86 ± 1.2
70–74	69	54	164 ± 2.4	168 ± 2.6	86 ± 0.97	87 ± 1.1
75–79	59	35	168 ± 2.7	179 ± 4.2	86 ± 1.2	88 ± 1.9
80–84	50	35	171 ± 2.9	187 ± 4.1	88 ± 1.2	89 ± 2.1
85–89	21	26	173 ± 5.6	189 ± 5.0	87 ± 2.9	92 ± 2.0

[a] Anderson and Cowan (1959).
[b] Mean ± SE.

arterial pressure with detectable vascular abnormalities in an elderly population; they chose the presence or absence of abnormal findings on ophthalmoscopy, palpation of the radial artery, and palpation of the foot pulses. The population surveyed was otherwise considered to be healthy. When all three criteria examined were normal, the upper limits of systolic blood pressure were found to be 185 mm Hg at 60 years and 200 mm Hg at 85 years of age for both sexes. When all three were abnormal, the upper limits of systolic blood pressure were 204 mm Hg for men and 211 mm Hg for women at 60 years, and 218 mm Hg for men and 225 mm Hg for women at 85 years. The diastolic blood pressure was uninfluenced by age for either sex, and only in women were the vascular abnormalities related significantly to the diastolic pressure level.

The effects of hypertension in the elderly population were further studied by Bechgaard (1946), who followed up 1,000 hypertensive patients attending a general outpatient department in Copenhagen. All these patients had blood pressures in excess of 160/100 mm Hg at their first attendance. Reexamination was carried out at 10 and 20 years after admission to the survey, and if possible, a third examination was carried out. Of those who survived to this third examination, 80% had lived beyond the age of 60. The mortality in elderly women was not increased unless the systolic blood pressure was in excess of 200 mm Hg. Further evidence suggesting that the elderly female can sustain increased levels of blood pressure without any great increase in mortality can be found in the study of Miall and Chinn (1974). In this study, raised systolic or diastolic pressures were not associated with any increase in deaths due to cardiovascular causes among women 65–74 years old. The same did not hold true for men in the same age group.

There is considerable evidence, however, to suggest that the elderly person with either systolic or diastolic hypertension has an increasing risk of cardiovascular or cerebrovascular complications (Chapter 7), though possibly to a lesser degree than his younger counterpart. The findings of the Chicago Stroke Study suggest that 28% of the total incidence of strokes in persons 65–74 years old may be attributable to hypertension (Shekelle et al. 1974). The increasing risk of cardiovascular disease and congestive cardiac failure in association with raised pressure levels has been demonstrated by Kannel and his colleagues (Chapter 7, Kannel et al. 1971, Shurtleff 1970), suggesting that the absence of symptoms or signs of target organ involvement is no guarantee against a sudden vascular catastrophe when hypertension is present. While there is evidence to suggest that asymptomatic hypertension is of adverse influence with regard to atherothrombotic brain infarction, congestive cardiac failure, and possibly coronary artery disease in later years, it seems less so with regard to peripheral vascular disease, in the absence of other pathology. The systolic blood pressure in the elderly is frequently labile, which in itself may be of adverse significance. Colandrea et al. (1970) investigated a retired "leisure" community in the United States and showed that in this elderly population, isolated systolic hypertension was a relatively infrequent and labile condition; it was associated, however, with an increased risk of developing cardiovascular complications.

The effect of raised blood pressure on the cardiovascular systems of elderly people has been demonstrated in a population survey of the ambulant elderly (Kennedy 1974). Of this population, 65 years of age and over, 21% had pressures in excess of 180/110 mm Hg. Hypertensive heart disease was diagnosed in the presence of left ventricular hypertrophy, left bundle branch block, an arrhythmia noted in the absence of valvular or ischemic heart disease, or an increase in the cardiothoracic ratio. Of those with elevated blood pressures, 62% of men and 55% of women showed evidence of direct cardiac involvement, though symptoms in relation to this involvement were infrequent.

While these statistics point to the influence of high blood pressure as a risk factor in cardiovascular conditions in old age, the circumstances of the affected patient must be borne in mind. It has been shown that in some instances, untreated hypertensives with no evidence of target organ involvement will fare well in comparison with those treated (Stewart 1971). The difficulty lies in the identification of such groups, especially with regard to the elderly.

Etiology

The cause of hypertension in the elderly, as in the younger person, is frequently elusive. Malignant hypertension with papilledema is rare in those over 70 (Kincaid-Smith et al. 1958). Hypertension of renal origin does occur in older patients, but with no greater frequency than in younger subjects. When the blood pressure of an elderly person on no relevant drug therapy has risen rapidly over a period of several months, hypertension of renal origin may be implicated. This hypertension can be due to structural damage such as renal artery occlusion, but is more likely to result from chronic pyelonephritis.

Bacteriuria is a not infrequent finding in the elderly. It is more common in women than in men, and has an incidence of upward of 10% in the total elderly population (Sourander 1966, Brocklehurst et al. 1968). Only one-third of these with bacteriuria also have pyuria (Akhtar et al. 1972), and when the blood pressures of those elderly people in the community with a urinary tract infection are compared with those who are infection-free, no significant elevation is noted in either group.

Occult or reactivated pyelonephritis is probably the most common renal cause of hypertension in later years. There may also be endocrine causes, but they are infrequent. Primary aldosteronism, Cushing's syndrome, or pheochromocytoma occur as rarities. Most instances of raised blood pressure in the elderly are classified as essential or primary, a diagnosis reached by exclusion of known causes. Many factors have been suggested as contributing to this situation. Salt intake has been suspected for a considerable time of having some influence on blood pressure levels. The evidence for this influence remains conflicting, but the renal handling of sodium is abnormal in hypertension, and patients with high blood pressure may have a higher taste threshold and appetite for salt (Wotman et al. 1967).

Emotion and stressful situations can result in the elevation of blood pressure. This elevation may occur as a result of increased catecholamine secretion in susceptible individuals, leading eventually to sustained hypertension (Nestel 1969).

Interaction between renal and nervous effects on the circulation has demonstrated the important role of the kidney in arterial pressure control. The role of renin in patients with either primary or secondary hypertension continues to provoke interest and controversy. About one-third of patients found to have essential hypertension have subnormal renin levels; a small percentage have raised values; in most, plasma renin is normal. Low plasma renin levels in association with essential hypertension, however, appear in some to be related to increasing age. It has been postulated that plasma renin has fallen in these circumstances as a result of the long-term effect of raised blood pressure on the kidney (Padfield et al. 1975).

Pathology

With age, structural changes occur in the kidneys, affecting renal function. The changes include a reduction of renal mass corresponding to the general decrease in the size and weight of most organs with advancing years. Microscopically, there is reduction in the number of nephrons and in the size of each nephron. Vascular changes initially involve smaller arteries and arterioles, with a consequent diminution in the renal arterial tree. This diminution has been demonstrated by angiography, which shows changes in the intrarenal arterial pattern in the normotensive elderly similar to that found in the hypertensive younger patient (Davidson et al. 1969). Pathological lesions attributed to hypertension in young and middle-aged patients are not necessarily due to the same cause in the elderly. The degree and incidence of renovascular damage in elderly subjects with moderate hypertension has been noted to be approximately the same as that in comparable age groups who are normotensive (McKeown 1965). Decreasing renal glomerular and tubular function occurs with advancing years as a result of these structural changes in the kidney (Davies and Shock 1950, Shock 1968). These functional, age-related changes may be confused with hypertensive effects where arterial pressure is only moderately raised.

Renal lesions caused by the vascular changes of aging may coexist with chronic infective scarring in kidneys that have been the seat of chronic pyelonephritis. Care must be taken that such changes are not wholly ascribed to the pyelonephritic process.

The influence of hypertension on cardiac pathology has been mentioned in Chapter 2. While myocardial hypertrophy is the usual cardiac result of sustained hypertension, several studies have shown that such hypertension in the elderly is not necessarily associated with an increase in heart weight (Pomerance 1968, McKeown 1965).

Hypertension as a causative factor in major-vessel atherosclerosis has been dealt with in Chapter 7. It is unusual for arteriolar wall damage of a severe nature, such as fibrinoid necrosis, to be found in the elderly, who rarely suffer from malignant hypertension (Kincaid-Smith et al. 1958). It is often difficult at autopsy to determine whether the arteriosclerotic cerebral vessel changes are related to age or to hypertension (McKeown 1965). Microaneurysms of the cerebral perforating arteries—the *état lacunaire* and *état criblé* described by Marie and Vogt—are common in elderly and hypertensive patients (Cole and Yates 1968), and are not necessarily implicated in the occurrence of clinical strokes (Dayan 1973).

Intracerebral cellular degeneration occurs commonly in later years. This degeneration may be associated with small-vessel disease, causing cystic softening in brain tissue in association with arteriosclerosis, which itself may be related to hypertension or may occur in normotensive individuals as an aging process. McKeown (1965) has described medial fibrosis in large and smaller cerebral vessels, and capillary fibrosis that can possibly be attributed to hypertension in later years. It has been suggested by some that this fibrosis forms the basis for vascular dementia, by an association with the clinical picture of gradual and progressive impairment of mental function, though obviously factors other than hypertension may well be involved. Older people with severe diastolic hypertension show significant intellectual decline over a set span of time when validated intelligence ratings are used. In the setting of moderate diastolic hypertension (i.e., 96–105 mm Hg), however, no such impairment was found, and some individuals even showed an increase in rating scales (Wilkie and Eisdorfer 1971).

Clinical Manifestations

Minor complaints such as headaches, dizziness, poor memory, and impairment of concentration are often attributed incorrectly in the elderly to raised blood pressure. Such symptoms are often present in old people with normal blood pressure.

Secondary hypertension may give rise to characteristic clinical pictures. Cushing's syndrome, extremely rare in old age, causes weight increase and redistribution of body fat with striae, hirsutism, and carbohydrate intolerance. Polyuria, thirst, fatigue, and muscle weakness may be present with Conn's syndrome. Sweating, glycosuria, and paroxysmal hypertension occur in the presence of a pheochromocytoma. Renal causes may be associated with hematuria, dysuria and pyuria, and rapidly accelerating hypertension. In contrast, essential hypertension is usually symptomless until organ involvement is marked, the patient's well-being then being compromised.

Hypertensive heart disease may cause left heart failure with pulmonary edema, signs of cardiac stress, and cerebral anoxia. Myocardial ischemia, with or without cardiac pain, may be present. At all ages, cerebral infarction and, particularly, cerebral hemorrhage are associated with increased blood pressure, though this risk may diminish in later years (Miall and Chinn 1974, Cole and Yates 1968).

Management

Where a remediable lesion has been detected, treatment should be directed to it, provided the current state of health of the patient is fully considered. Where a renovascular cause has been found, conservative management may often be in the patient's best interests. The diagnosis of chronic pyelonephritis requires prolonged treatment in its own right with sulfonamides or antibiotics. In the rare instances where an endocrine cause has been discovered, appropriate drug therapy or surgical intervention should be considered, depending on the state of the patient's health.

The management of high blood pressure in the elderly, however, is basically the management of essential hypertension. Antihypertensive therapy is indicated where there is definite evidence of target organ involvement. Thus, appropriate drug therapy should be employed where congestive cardiac failure has occurred, either solely or partly as a result of hypertensive heart disease. The situation with regard to patients over the age of 65 with stroke is different from that for younger subjects, for there is no good evidence yet that antihypertensive therapy prolongs life or reduces the recurrence rate in the elderly (Adams and Merritt 1961, Barham Carter 1970). Hypertensive cerebrovascular disease with diffuse cerebral signs of dementia is generally regarded as a contraindication to therapy, because further deterioration in intellectual capacity frequently results when drugs are employed (Hughes et al. 1954, Caird 1963).

Many physicians with experience in treating elderly patients find difficulty in determining whether the symptom-free but hypertensive old person merits antihypertensive treatment and, if so, at what pressure levels. Possible reasons for this uncertainty are that epidemiological surveys have included very few elderly subjects; that clinical trials of antihypertensive therapy have concentrated on the young and middle-aged; and that in the elderly, the risks of such therapy are increased in the presence of multiple pathology, and of mental changes, which are frequently unrecognized. The older person may be at risk from enhanced drug activity or unwanted side effects as a result of alterations in the body's capacity to metabolize and excrete the prescribed agent or its metabolites.

In the absence of definite contraindications, antihypertensive therapy should be considered in the setting of symptomless hypertension when the diastolic pressure is persistently in excess of 110 or possibly 105 mm Hg, especially where there is documented evidence of previous left ventricular failure. It is more difficult to decide at what systolic level such therapy should be employed in older subjects, and the decision must await the results of further controlled clinical trials.

Certain considerations with regard to the elderly must be stressed. If there is an element of mental confusion, the question of antihypertensive therapy requires very full appraisal. The frequently encountered situation of a patient with diminished renal function requires careful monitoring of drug dosage. The ability of the patient and his relatives to cope with the complex drug regime required for several conditions may modify the therapeutic approach. Treatment of the raised pressure may be of less relevance in the light of the patient's other conditions. Furthermore, many elderly people suffer a considerable drop of blood pressure on standing (Caird et al. 1973), which may be potentiated by hypotensive agents.

General measures include weight reduction to not more than 25% in excess of standard weight for height and age, and a complete review of the subject's current therapy. Salt restriction has little part to play in the control of blood pressure in elderly subjects, on several grounds: the degree of salt restriction required to lower blood pressure satisfactorily is such that patient cooperation is unlikely, and more suitable measures are currently available. For an elderly person, the ideal drug is one that has a mild and consistent action, and no postural side effects, and needs to be taken only once daily. There are few hypotensive agents that meet these requirements. There are certain drugs, however, that seem more applicable to the treatment of hypertension in the elderly (Kennedy 1975). The thiazide diuretics are widely employed, and probably act by decreasing both peripheral arteriolar resistance and plasma volume. Other diuretics have a hypotensive action, but that of the thiazide group is more prolonged

than that of the "loop" diuretics, such as frusemide (Lasix) or
ethacrynic acid (Edecrin). Bendrofluazide (Neonaclex), given in a dose
of 5–10 mg daily, is suitable. The hypotensive effect is not dose-
dependent, so that further increase in dosage does not provide further
benefit.

Diuretics may cause hypokalemia, which is much more likely to
occur in older than in younger patients (Judge and Macleod 1968).
Supplementation with a suitably palatable oral potassium preparation
in appropriate dosage is often necessary. Combined thiazide and
potassium preparations may be inadequate to maintain satisfactory
potassium balance in some elderly patients who may already be
potassium-depleted before starting therapy (Dall et al. 1971). Alternatively, a potassium-sparing agent such as triamterene (Dytac) or
amiloride, alone or in combination with a thiazide (e.g., Dyazide or
Moduretic), may be effective (Kennedy and MacFarlane 1973). Spironolactone (Aldactone) conserves potassium due to its action on the
distal tubule, but is a relatively weak hypotensive agent. It can be
given in combination with a thiazide, such as Aldactide. Long-term
treatment with thiazides may increase 5-fold the chance of developing
diabetes mellitus (Caird 1967); it is less commonly associated with
hyperuricemia, giving rise to acute gout only infrequently.

β-Adrenergic blocking agents cause a sustained and moderate fall
in blood pressure that is little influenced by postural changes. In the
United Kingdom and elsewhere, these drugs are frequently employed
in this role. They are all chemically related, but often differ in
pharmacological activity and in metabolism. Their hypotensive action
may be due to a reduction in cardiac output (Frohlich et al. 1968), to a
lowering of plasma renin levels (Ganong 1972), and to a possible
central depressant effect on general sympathetic activity (Dollery et al.
1973). Not all β-adrenergic blocking agents act by similar pathways.
The absence of any postural effect increases the value of these drugs in
elderly subjects. The action of β-adrenergic blocking compounds on
myocardial function, however, may precipitate cardiac failure in
patients so predisposed, and also induce bradycardia. As the drugs
can also increase airway resistance, care must be shown where there is
chronic bronchitis or a history of bronchial asthma.

A satisfactory response is obtained in upward of 50% of old
people with 40–120 mg propanolol (Inderal) t.i.d. or q.i.d.; pindolol
(Visken), 5–15 mg t.i.d.; oxprenolol (Trasicor), 80–160 mg b.i.d.; or
other allied agents. Apart from the contraindications already mentioned, side effects are slight, consisting mainly of gastrointestinal
intolerance. An exception is practolol (Eraldin), which has recently

been associated with the development of keratitis, retroperitoneal fibrosis, sclerosing peritonitis, and a psoriasiform skin condition in a few instances. When these drugs alone prove inadequate, the addition of a thiazide diuretic may allow satisfactory control of blood pressure.

Of the more potent antihypertensive agents, methyldopa (Aldomet) is widely used in elderly people. This drug was originally thought to compete in the normal synthetic pathways with pressor amines. Further work (Coupar and Turner 1970) has cast doubt on this sole mode of action, however, and it may be that the drug has a significant effect on the central nervous system (Finch and Haeusler 1973). It is rapidly absorbed from the gut, and about 50% is excreted in the urine within 24 h. Maximum hypotensive effect is achieved 6–8 h after ingestion.

Although methyldopa is widely used, it is not free from disadvantages. Elderly subjects require very careful dose adjustment, particularly if renal function is impaired. The dose should start at no more than 250 mg daily in divided doses, and increase gradually every 3 or 4 days by 125 mg until control is achieved, or a maximum of 2 g daily is reached. Amounts in excess of this maximum are infrequently required; if they are, the addition of a thiazide diuretic or β-blocking agent may produce the required effect. The literature on unwanted side effects of this drug is extensive. The most common is drowsiness, which may merge into stupor, particularly in the old. This side effect renders the subject liable to other illnesses, such as infections, or to home accidents. The most disturbing in the older patient is the precipitation or deepening of a depressive state that may be unrecognized. Other effects include drug rashes, autoimmune hemolytic anemia, and a hepatitis-like syndrome. Various forms of eczema may occur or worsen due to methyldopa (Church 1973).

The rauwolfia alkaloids and, in particular, reserpine (Serpasil) have a moderate hypotensive effect and appear to act by depleting peripheral adrenergic nerve endings, as well as by reducing the amines in the adrenal medulla and central nervous system. The usual dose of reserpine is 0.20–1 mg daily in two or three divided doses, and the lowest dose compatible with satisfactory blood pressure control should be sought. This action is not usually evident for 3–6 days after starting the drug; also, since the drug has a cumulative effect, care must be taken when the dosage is being increased. Postural hypotension is unlikely, but side effects often seen with therapeutic doses include depression and fluid retention; Parkinsonism may occur with very high dosage.

Hydrallazine (Apresoline), a vasodilator, was formerly used extensively in the treatment of hypertension, but fell into disrepute when a lupus erythmatosus–like syndrome was ascribed to it (Morrow et al. 1953). It is well absorbed, however, and metabolism is rapid, but high plasma levels are found in the presence of renal failure, indicating the need for caution. Side effects of hydrallazine include tachycardia, headache, and flushing, which may be abolished by β-adrenergic blockers.

Other vasodilators currently of value in treating hypertension include minoxidil, which has a prolonged duration of action despite rapid metabolism, and also requires β-adrenergic blocking agents to counteract some of the changes consequent on vasodilation. It may also cause fluid retention, requiring diuretic therapy. Diazoxide is also thought to act by vasodilatation. It also causes fluid retention and may induce hyperglycemia, thus severely limiting its role in the elderly.

Postganglionic sympathetic blocking agents and related compounds have little place in the treatment of the elderly hypertensive. They generally have a short half-life, and therefore require administration two or more times daily. All produce postural hypotension, which can be enhanced in the elderly with dangerous results. Other side effects include alimentary upsets such as diarrhea. Impaired renal function may result in unexpected and severe hypotension as a result of drug accumulation. Such powerful agents should be reserved for the severely hypertensive elderly subject with evidence of target organ involvement who does not respond to more gentle medication. Because such elderly patients are rare, the need for such drugs is correspondingly rare.

The aim of therapy should be to reduce the diastolic pressure to a level below 110 mm Hg without producing unpleasant side effects. Blood pressure should be estimated with the patient in the standing position, and preferably after gentle exercise. Iatrogenic disease in the elderly due to overzealous administration or haphazard ingestion of antihypertensive therapy is not infrequent. Many elderly patients will be rendered housebound or chairfast if drug therapy is directed toward achieving the statistically ideal pressure, rather than the therapeutically feasible.

Drug interactions with antihypertensive therapy are frequent, for many elderly people are taking several drugs. Such a situation demands extra vigilance (Table 8.3). Postural hypotension is a frequent occurrence in the elderly; 24% of the ambulant elderly show a systolic drop of 20 mm Hg or more, 5% a drop of 40 mm Hg or more (Caird et al. 1973). Misapplied antihypertensive therapy can dangerously enhance this decrease in an old person, with the consequent possibility

TABLE 8.3. Some Possible Drug Interactions with Antihypertensive Agents

Antihypertensive agent	Potentiate	Inhibit	Potentially serious interactions
Thiazides	Antihypertensive drugs β-Adrenergic blockers	Allopurinol Sulfonylureas	Phenothiazines MAO inhibitors
Ethacrynic acid	Antihypertensive drugs β-Adrenergic blockers	Allopurinol	Sulfonylureas Aminoglycoside antibiotics
Frusemide	Antihypertensive drugs β-Adrenergic blockers Aspirin	Sulfonylureas	MAO inhibitors Aminoglycoside antibiotics
Methyldopa	Coumarin anticoagulants β-Adrenergic blockers	—	Alcohol
Guanethidine	Coumarin anticoagulants	Tricyclic antidepressants (Oral contraceptives) Phenothiazines	Alcohol
Debrisoquine	MAO inhibitors β-Adrenergic blockers	Tricyclic antidepressants	—
Clonidine	—	Tricyclic antidepressants	—

**TABLE 8.4. Commonly Used Drugs Likely
to Cause Postural Hypotension**

Antihypertensive agents
  Methyldopa
  Reserpine
  Ganglion-blocking agents
Thiazides and other diuretics
Phenothiazines
Tricyclic antidepressants
Tranquilizers, especially Diazepam
Chlormethiazole
Anticholinergic drugs for Parkinsonism
Levodopa
Barbiturates
Antihistamines

of incapacity, or indeed injury. Hypotensive drugs are not alone in causing postural hypotension; other drugs that may have this effect are listed in Table 8.4.

Every therapeutic regime should be accompanied by explanation and reassurance about the patient's future mode of life. Time is well spent explaining to the patient and his relatives the value of regular drug therapy, and the need to prevent unnecessary "risk" situations, with particular reference to abrupt postural changes. Antihypertensive therapy is not justified if the patient is less well after the institution of therapy than before. Even so, the often erroneous fear of the complications of hypertension in the minds of many older people often ensures that antihypertensive drugs are the last rather than the first to be discontinued when harmful side effects occur.

Apparent resistance to antihypertensive therapy is occasionally postulated, but in the elderly, this "resistance" usually means failure to take the prescribed drugs. Where patient compliance is doubtful, potent antihypertensive therapy should not be prescribed without adequate supervision. The need to treat the patient, not just the blood pressure, is even more important in the older person than in his younger colleagues.

References

Adams, G. F., and Merritt, J. D. (1961) *Br. Med. J.* **1**, 309.
Akhtar, A. J., Andrews, G. R., Caird, F. I., and Fallon, R. J. (1972) *Age and Ageing* **1**, 48.
Anderson, W. F., and Cowan, N. R. (1959) *Clin. Sci.* **18**, 103.

Anderson, W. F., and Cowan, N. R. (1972) *Gerontol. Clin.* **14,** 129.

Barham Carter, A. (1970) *Lancet* **1,** 485.

Bechgaard, P. (1946) *Acta Med. Scand. Suppl.* **172.**

Brocklehurst, J. C., Dillane, J. B., Griffiths, L., and Fry, J. (1968) *Gerontol. Clin.* **10,** 242.

Caird, F. I. (1963) *Postgrad. Med. J.* **39,** 408.

Caird, F. I. (1967) Communication to Medical and Scientific Section, British Diabetic Association.

Caird, F. I., Andrews, G. R., and Kennedy, R. D. (1973) *Br. Heart J.* **35,** 527.

Church, R. E. (1973) *Br. J. Dermatol.* **89,** Suppl. **9,** 10.

Colandrea, M. A., Friedman, G. D., Nichaman, M. A., and Lynd, C. M. (1970) *Circulation* **41,** 239.

Cole, F. M., and Yates, P. O. (1968) *Neurology (Minn.)* **18,** 255.

Coupar, I. M., and Turner, P. (1970) *Br. J. Pharmacol. Chemother.* **38,** 463.

Dall, J. L. C., Paulose, S., and Ferguson, J. A. (1971) *Gerontol. Clin.* **13,** 114.

Davidson, A. J., Talner, L. B., and Downs, W. M. (1969) *Radiology* **92,** 975.

Davies, D. R., and Shock, N. W. (1950) *J. Clin. Invest.* **29,** 496.

Dayan, A. D. (1973) *In* Brocklehurst, J. C. (ed.), *Textbook of Geriatric Medicine and Gerontology,* Churchill Livingstone, Edinburgh, p. 183.

Dollery, C. T., Lewis, P. J., Myers, M. G., and Reid, J. L. (1973) *Br. J. Pharmacol. Chemother.* **48,** 343.

Finch, L., and Haeusler, G. (1973) *Br. J. Pharmacol. Chemother.* **47,** 217.

Frohlich, E. D., Tarazi, R. C., Dustan, H. P., and Page, I. H. (1968) *Circulation* **37,** 417.

Ganong, W. F. (1972) *In* Assayheen, T. (ed.), *Control of Renin Secretion,* Plenum Press, New York and London, p. 17.

Hughes, W., Dodgson, M. C. H., and MacLennan, D. C. (1954) *Lancet* **2,** 770.

Judge, T. G., and Macleod, C. C. (1968) *Proceedings of the Fifth European Meeting of Clinical Gerontology,* Brussels, p. 295.

Kannel, W. B., Gordon, T., and Schwartz, M. J. (1971) *Am. J. Cardiol.* **27,** 335.

Kennedy, R. D. (1974) *Mod. Geriatrics* **4,** N9, 360.

Kennedy, R. D. (1975) *J. Am. Geriatr. Soc.* **23,** 113.

Kennedy, R. D., and MacFarlane, J. P. R. (1973) *Mod. Geriatrics* **3,** 266.

Kincaid-Smith, P., McMichael, J., and Murphy, E. A. (1958) *Q. J. Med. N.S.* **27,** 117.

Master, A. M., Lasser, R. P., and Jaffe, H. L. (1958) *Ann. Intern. Med.* **48,** 284.

McKeown, F. (1965) *Pathology of the Aged,* Butterworth, London.

Miall, W. E., and Chinn, S. (1974) *Br. Med. J.* **3,** 595.

Morrow, J. D., Schroeder, H. A., and Perry, H. N. (1953) *Circulation* **8,** 829.

Nestel, P. J. (1969) *Lancet* **1,** 692.

Padfield, P. L., Beevers, D. G., Brown, J. J., Davies, D. L., Lever, A. F., Robertson, J. I. S., Schlekamp, M. A. D., and Tree, M. (1975) *Lancet* **1,** 548.

Pomerance, A. (1968) *Geriatrics* **23,** 4, 101.

Shekelle, R. B., Ostfeld, A. M., and Klawans, H. L. (1974) *Stroke* **5,** 71.

Shock, N. W. (1968) *In* Powers, J. H. (ed.), *Surgery of the Aged and Debilitated Patient,* Saunders, London, p. 10.

Shurtleff, D. (1970) Framingham Study, 16-year follow-up. Section 26. National Heart and Lung Institute, National Institutes of Health. U.S. Govt. Printing Office.

Sourander, L. B. (1966) *Ann. Med. Intern. Fenn.* **55,** Suppl. 45.

Stewart, I. McD. G. (1971) *Lancet* **1,** 671.

Wilkie, F., and Eisdorfer, C. (1971) *Science* **172,** 959.

Wotman, S., Mandel, I. D., Thompson, R. H., and Laragh, J. H. (1967) *J. Chronic Dis.* **20,** 833.

9

Clinical Features of Ischemic Heart Disease

M. S. PATHY

Introduction

Coronary heart disease is essentially due to coronary atherosclerosis, though at times the rare exceptions of syphilitic involvement of the coronary ostia, polyarteritis nodosa, giant cell arteritis, coronary embolism, and coronary aneurysm may demand critical attention. Although the term ischemic heart disease is reasonably used as synonymous with coronary heart disease, it would logically also cover the clinical situation of angina pectoris due to aortic valve disease or severe anemia.

Pathologically, the degree of coronary atherosclerosis increases progressively until the age of 60 in men (White et al. 1950) and 80 in women (Ackerman et al. 1950). The Registrar General's figures for deaths from ischemic heart disease in England and Wales (Registrar General 1969) showed a fall in the male preponderance from 67.4% in the quinquennium 65–69 to 40.6% in those 80–84 years of age. The incidence of myocardial infarction is difficult to determine, particularly in the elderly, in whom the condition may produce few or no symptoms and be discovered only at autopsy.

Assessment of the clinical features of disease in old age is meaningful only if it is viewed as part of an overall assessment of the

M. S. PATHY · Department of Geriatric Medicine, University Hospital of Wales, Heath Park, Cardiff, CF4 4XW, Wales.

sick person. More than one etiological factor may be operative before a diseased heart produces symptoms. Hypertension or severe anemia may precipitate or exacerbate cardiovascular symptoms in the presence of coronary heart disease of modest severity. Anemia can induce subendocardial ischemia (Master et al. 1950) and infarction (Elliott 1934), even in the absence of significant coronary artery disease, and is of more serious import in the presence of coronary atheroma (Hoffman and Buckberg 1975).

Symptoms of Chronic Coronary Heart Disease

Symptoms of coronary heart disease are often insidious in onset and ill-defined in character. Multiple small myocardial infarcts are surprisingly common in old age, and often result in diffuse myocardial damage. Historical evidence—fallible as this can be in old age—of focal cardiac lesions is commonly absent. Ultimately, the residual functional myocardium is inadequate to sustain the restricted physiological demand of later life, and signs of heart failure supervene, frequently insidiously, but sometimes accelerated acutely by a superimposed infection, often respiratory. Thus, gradually developing congestive heart failure most frequently characterizes coronary ischemia. The failure is often mild in degree and responds readily to treatment. Increasing exertional dyspnea may be initially accepted as an expected symptom of aging by the elderly. If associated disease severely limits mobility, dyspnea may not be obvious until heart failure has reached an advanced stage. Left ventricular failure may herald myocardial infarction; as a recurrent phenomenon, it is a common feature of coronary heart disease in the absence of infarction. Left heart failure may disturb sleep for minutes due to short-lived dyspnea or for most of the night because of persistent cough or acute and frightening attacks of intense breathlessness, which leave the victim fearful for future nights; they may persuade him to spend each night in a chair. The combination of left and right heart failure with gross evidence of systemic venous engorgement, hepatic enlargement, peripheral edema, and left or bilateral pleural effusions is common experience.

Angina Pectoris

This clinical syndrome may be the only manifestation of ischemic heart disease in the history. It is a symptom complex that diminishes progressively in frequency after the age of 80. Using the Rose questionnaire (Rose 1962, Rose and Blackburn 1968), Kitchin et al. (1973) noted that a history of angina was admitted by 10% of a random sample of subjects 62–90 years old in a defined area of Edinburgh. Severe anemia, tachyarrhythmias, hypoglycemia, and the overenthusiastic use of L-thyroxin in the treatment of hypothyroidism may precipitate pain in asymptomatic coronary heart disease. Aortic valve disease and syphilitic aortitis can give rise to intractable angina in the absence of coronary heart disease.

Pain, frequently accompanied by apprehension, is the hallmark of angina, but the picture varies from a sense of substernal oppression to severe, dull, constant gripping or choking pain behind the sternum. Pain may extend more widely across the chest, up to the neck and jaw, or radiate a variable distance down the left arm or both arms. Occasionally, pain is limited to the wrists, with a denial of chest discomfort. Chest pain may be accompanied by a sensation of giddiness or followed by a syncopal episode, possibly due to transient arrhythmias. Typically, pain is induced by a known amount of exertion, and is rapidly relieved by rest and glyceryl trinitrate (Trinitrin) tablets, but in cold, frosty, or windy weather, minimal activity can produce angina.

Angina precipitated by exercise rarely persists for more than a few minutes after resting. If rest pain continues for more than 30 min, it is strongly suggestive of a myocardial infarction. A small group of patients with acute myocardial infarction give a clearly defined history of recurrent attacks of chest pain of progressive severity and duration over the two or three weeks preceding the major ischemic insult. Prolonged rest pain in the absence of infarction may result from uncontrolled tachyarrhythmia, bradyarrhythmia, or persistent emotional stress, or may follow severe blood loss.

Cardiac Arrhythmias

Cardiac arrhythmias are commonly associated with coronary heart disease, though they are not specific to the condition. Left bundle branch block, or right bundle branch block with or without left anterior hemiblock, may draw attention to possible coronary heart disease in an asymptomatic patient, but Lewis et al. (1970) and Haft et al. (1971) consider that coronary heart disease accounted for only 50% of cases of left bundle branch block. Atrial fibrillation is common, particularly in the presence of heart failure, but rarely gives rise to symptoms of palpitation. Ventricular ectopic beats are common, but if present in coupled form in the absence of digitalis administration, are suggestive of coronary heart disease. Multiple ventricular ectopic beats is the arrhythmia most prone to produce a sensation of palpitation in old age. Heart block may announce itself by symptoms of weakness, unsteadiness of gait, confusion, or recurrent syncope, but it is an infrequent manifestation of coronary heart disease. Bilateral branch fibrosis affecting both bundles and of unknown etiology is the most common cause of heart block (Chapter 3).

General Symptoms

Diminished cardiac output associated with arrhythmias or with mild unsuspected heart failure may express itself by complaints of ill-defined fatigue, loss of energy, or undue tiredness and weakness by the early afternoon. Preexisting renal impairment is sometimes aggravated. Anorexia, weight loss, and postprandial gaseous abdominal distension with frequent eructations may subside following treatment of marginal heart failure. Episodic confusion or a history of faints and falls may be associated with the transient arrhythmias of coronary heart disease.

Coronary heart disease produces few physical signs, and in a typical case, none is found. Left ventricular hypertrophy is occasionally noted: A third heart sound is audible relatively frequently, and signs of mitral regurgitation are to be found if dysfunction of the papillary muscles occurs.

Coronary Artery Occlusion and Myocardial Infarction

The pathological and clinical sequelae of sudden coronary artery occlusion depend on several factors. In general, acute, complete occlusion of the proximal segment of one of the main coronary arteries results in major cardiac infarction or sudden death. Obstruction of a small distal branch may be associated with little or no necrosis of cardiac muscle. The gradual atherosclerotic narrowing of coronary arteries seen in later life may enable anastomotic vessels to enlarge sufficiently to obviate the effect of final arterial occlusion. Though functional anastomoses may develop, the results of coronary artery occlusion must depend on the integrity of the remaining vessels. If coronary artery perfusion is already critical due to gross generalized atherosclerotic narrowing or to previous arterial occlusions, sudden or even gradual obstruction of a small artery may precipitate infarction.

In a meticulous histopathological study, Roberts (1974) found that 80% of thrombi were totally occlusive in patients with fatal transmural infarctions, and the remainder were partially occlusive. In contradistinction, coronary artery thrombi were absent in 9 fatal cases of subendocardial infarction. Roberts maintains that coronary artery thrombosis is consequential to myocardial infarction, and not causal.

In old age, coronary atherosclerosis is widespread, and areas of myocardial fibrosis are often irregularly disposed throughout the myocardium, particularly in the subendocardial region. At this age, infarction of the myocardium is to be seen as but a phase in the course of coronary heart disease. The area of necrosis may be small and subintimal or massive and transmural. It is therefore understandable that the accompanying symptoms may range from the insignificant to the catastrophic.

The presence of cardiac hypertrophy from long-standing coronary heart disease or hypertension often magnifies the effect of acute coronary occlusion.

Symptoms

Myocardial infarction may produce few or no symptoms and be discovered only at necropsy. Barnes and Ball (1932) found necropsy evidence of myocardial infarction in 4.9% of hearts; Gould and Cawley (1958) noted one or more healed cardiac infarcts in 3.5% of 5,000 consecutive autopsy examinations. In clinicopathological studies, Lee et al. (1957) and Johnson et al. (1959) estimated, respectively, that 10% and 50% of anatomically proved myocardial infarctions gave rise to no diagnostic clinical symptoms in life. The collation of pathological findings with retrospective documentary clinical data, frequently culled from notes of other observers, may be inaccurate with respect to the incidence or disease symptoms, and should be interpreted with caution.

Since Hammer (1878) clinically diagnosed myocardial infarction, *substernal pain* with characteristic qualities and radiation of variable extent has for long been accepted as a cardinal symptom of acute infarction of cardiac muscle. Chest pain is indeed a major presenting symptom in the very old, as in younger persons, but the frequency with which pain marks the occurrence of infarction decreases with advancing age. Pain may be mild and brief in duration, lasting for about an hour, or agonizing and persisting for several hours to one or two days. Prolonged pain may be intermittent over one to three or more days. The pain is dull and compressing in quality, and the patient sometimes graphically likens it to being constricted in a vise or compressed by a heavy weight. At times, the complaint is one of substernal discomfort or a sense of choking or oppression. The pain or discomfort may be limited to the retrosternal region, but frequently spreads across both sides or the anterior chest: It may radiate to the neck, jaw, or down one or both arms. If limited to one side, the pain is usually on the left. Occasionally, the pain is epigastric and ascribed to indigestion.

Symptoms associated with the pain of infarction are common and include breathlessness, nausea or vomiting, faintness, sweating, palpitation, and a sense of marked weakness. The dominance of these symptoms in the clinical picture of myocardial infarction in the elderly has not always received due emphasis. In old age, myocardial infarction, in common with many diseases, may give rise to vague, ill-defined, or multiple symptoms of a general character that cannot be profitably classified.

The presenting clinical features in a group of patients 65 years of age and over with a myocardial infarction confirmed by defined electrocardiographic and, in fatal cases, histopathological criteria are shown in Table 9.1 (Pathy 1967). Due to the strict serial electrocardiographic criteria laid down for accepting a diagnosis of recent myocardial infarction, patients with localized subintimal infarction had to be excluded with unavoidable selectivity. Within the limits of any study conforming to specified criteria, the data in the table make it clear that the presenting symptoms of infarction of the myocardium in the elderly are protean.

The frequency with which symptom complexes present are often biased in hospital-orientated data due to admission policy and selectivity. Nevertheless, the frequent *absence of pain* in reliable elderly witnesses with unequivocal infarction and the cardinal importance of the many other presenting features is undeniable. The factors that determine absence of the pain of infarction have been the subject of considerable speculation. In his original classic paper, Herrick (1912) considered gradual atherosclerotic narrowing of the coronary arteries to be significant, though later (1931) he postulated that involvement of "silent areas" of myocardium might give rise to painless infarction. Libman (1919), Keefer and Resnik (1928), and Carr (1935) proposed hyposensitivity to pain as a possible explanation. Wearn (1923) and Hamman (1934) noted that pain might be absent if infarction supervenes on preexisting heart failure; Hay (1933) similarly considered pain to be less common if a previous infarction had been experienced. A degree of coronary ischemia insufficient to induce pain, but of

TABLE 9.1. Clinical Presentation of Myocardial Infarction and Acute Coronary Occlusion in 597 Patients 65 Years of Age and Over[a]

Group	Mode of presentation	Number of cases	%
1	Sudden dyspnea or exacerbation of heart failure	119	19.9
2	Onset with chest pain	115	19.3
3	Acute confusion	69	11.6
4	Sudden death	42	7.0
5	Syncopal attacks	39	6.6
6	Strokes	38	6.4
7	Limb ischemia	28	4.7
8	Giddiness or vertigo	27	4.5
9	Palpitation	26	4.4
10	Weakness	19	3.2
11	Renal failure	18	3.0
12	Recurrent vomiting	16	2.7
13	Pulmonary embolus	12	2.0
14	Uncontrolled diabetes	11	1.8
15	Restlessness	9	1.5
16	Cough	5	0.8
17	Sweating	4	0.7

[a] Pathy (1967).

adequate duration to cause infarction, was proposed by Snow et al. (1956). Evans and Sutton (1956) stressed the importance of dyspnea, hypertension, and arrhythmias as factors influencing absence of pain.

The sudden onset of *intense dyspnea* often dominates the clinical scene of acute infarction of the myocardium in old age. Pulmonary edema may result from a rise of pulmonary venous pressure consequential on the elevation of ventricular end-diastolic pressure. The pressure rise responsible for hypoxia and metabolic acidosis need not be great enough to induce sufficient engorgement of the pulmonary veins to cause dyspnea at rest, nor flood the lungs with fluid. Evidence of left ventricular failure with breathlessness, cough, apprehension, and variable cyanosis is common. If wheezing is marked, the symptoms may be mistaken for true asthma, though this rarely occurs for the first time in the elderly. The sputum is often frothy, copious, and white, though exceptionally it may have the classic pink appearance. Fine crepitations are audible over the chest, or in mild cases at the lung bases, but may be obscured by loud respiratory wheezes. With less intense symptoms, recurrent episodes of dyspnea on recumbency or with activity or a disturbing nocturnal cough may denote otherwise symptomless infarction. Right heart failure may follow left heart failure at a variable interval. Rapid intensification of signs of preexisting mild congestive heart failure may mark the supervention of myocardial infarction. Boyd and Werblow (1937) noted that the syndrome of painless myocardial infarction was represented most commonly by the occurrence of unexplained dyspnea during the course of congestive cardiac failure. Parkinson and Bedford (1928), Bedford and Simpson (1939), Lewis (1946), Gilchrist (1951), Herrman (1952), Papp (1952), Roseman (1954), Friedberg (1956), Evans and Sutton (1956), and Ebert (1965) commented that pain may be overshadowed by intense dyspnea. In an autopsy examination of the hearts of 370 patients 75 years of age and over, Pomerance (1965) found evidence of ischemic heart disease in 48% of subjects with a record of heart failure, and in 18% of the nonfailure group. Much of the difference was due to recent infarction, which was present in 23% of those in failure, but in only 0.5% of others.

It is common for infection, metabolic disorders, and traumatic interludes to be overtly announced in old age by *acute confusion*. The unexpected development of noisy, restless agitation with disorientation in a previously fit old person may be the only symptomatic expression of myocardial infarction. An infraction is readily overlooked if it exacerbates preexisting confusion. Rodstein (1956) attributed the confusion to cerebral anoxia, but it is common experience that an acute ischemic change in a lower-limb digit in later life is at times symptomatically ushered in by confusion, which often intensifies as the tissue necrosis increases.

Sudden death is reportedly the first clinical manifestation of acute myocardial infarction in 20–25% of all cases. A joint committee of the American Heart Association and the International Society of Cardiology has defined sudden death as death occurring within 24 h of the onset of acute symptoms and signs. In our study, the term was used only for abrupt death occurring within seconds and without preceding symptoms. Paul and Schatz (1971) recorded that 49% of coronary deaths in their study occurred within 15 min of an acute ischemic episode in middle-aged men. The 7% of patients recorded in Table 9.1 as dying suddenly were without electrocardiographic or clinical evidence of a myocardial infarction during the previous month. The incidence of sudden death among hospital patients with known recent infarction is considerably higher. The histochemical method used to indicate and date infarction (Mallory et al. 1939) in our survey does not show diagnostic histological changes for at least 10 h. Electron microscopy and more recent histochemical techniques provide much earlier characterization of cellular ischemic changes (Jennings et al. 1965, Shnitka and Nachlas 1963). Thrombi were frequently absent, but severe and widespread atherosclerosis with gross luminal narrowing was a major feature. The presence of histological evidence of infarction between 10 and 48 h old in a few subjects suggests that silent infarction may at times occur, with sudden death coming many hours later. It is probable that most sudden coronary deaths are due to an acute dysrhythmia, probably ventricular fibrillation. Cardiac rupture may cause sudden death, but was noted in only 3 of our 42 cases.

Syncope is frequent in older people with cardiac infarction. Frequently, it is accompanied by more diagnostic symptoms, especially severe chest pain (Garland and Phillips 1953). At times, syncope may be the presenting symptom (Pollard and Harvil 1940, Cookson 1942, Gilchrist 1951, Pathy 1967). Characteristically, sudden loss of consciousness lasting 5–30 min is noted, and pain is absent before and after the syncopal episode. Transient heart block, or bradycardia, tachyarrhythmias, or hypotension, are possible factors. With marked postinfarction hypotension, attempts to sit up in bed may result in repeated transient faints, but these are to be distinguished from isolated syncopal attacks.

Distal Embolization

Thromboembolism varies in incidence from 6% (Doscher and Poindexter 1950) to 60% (Garvin 1942) and is a significant cause of death from cardiac infarction, though embolic episodes are not always fatal. Distal emboli occur most frequently from the second to third week and involve, in order of frequency, lungs, kidney, spleen, brain, extremities, mesentery, carotids, and aorta (Bean 1938). Hellerstein and Martin (1947) suggested that distal embolization was the cause of death in 12% and a contributory cause in 15% of subjects examined at autopsy.

Parkinson and Bedford (1928) drew attention to the coexistence of *cerebrovascular accidents* and silent myocardial infarction. Levine considered that sudden hemiplegia may be due, in some instances, to a cerebral embolus secondary to a symptomless myocardial infarction. Subsequent studies have confirmed that the symptoms and signs of a stroke may overshadow the coexisting myocardial infarction (Bean and Read 1942, Race and Lisa 1945, Fisher and Zuckerman 1946, Bean et al. 1949, Rogers 1955, Gupta et al. 1965, Heron and Anderson 1965). In a study of the relationships between coronary thrombosis and cerebral lesions, Dozzi (1937) reviewed 1,000 consecutive autopsies; 41 had a myocardial infarction, and 12 (29%) of these were associated with a cerebral embolus or thrombosis. We noted a stroke to be the sole presenting feature in 38 patients with confirmed infarction of the myocardium. Carter (1964) suggested that cardiac infarction was responsible for embolic strokes as frequently as mitral stenosis. Wright et al. (1954) found that 64% of all arterial emboli from cardiac infarction involved arteries of the brain.

Strokes subsequent to cardiac infarction are by no means always due to cerebral embolic incidents. In our experience, the cerebrovascular episodes commonly occur either within the first 24 h or between 8 and 14 days following the myocardial infarction. If cerebrovascular disease is present, a marked fall in blood pressure might impair cerebral artery perfusion, with resulting cerebral infarction (Stürup 1952, Rogers 1955). Conversely, the possibility must be entertained that in the presence of extensive coronary artery disease, infarction of the myocardium could be subsequent to hypotension due to the stroke (Bean and Read 1942, Wilson et al. 1951). Hypertensive subjects are particularly prone to cerebral infraction following abrupt falls of blood pressure (Low-Beer and Phear 1961).

Where the only clinical manifestation of myocardial infarction is the complicating stroke, electrocardiographic changes must be critically appraised. Byer et al. (1947) described T-wave abnormalities in the ECG in intracranial hemorrhage. In a valuable study, Burch et al. (1954) described the electrocardiographic pattern in cases of cerebrovascular accidents without heart disease. Fentz and Gormsen (1962) found 16% of subjects with cerebrovascular accidents to have abnormal ECGs in the absence of heart disease. Abnormal electrocardiographic patterns in subarachnoid hemorrhage are well documented (Levine 1953, Shuster 1960, Cropp and Manning 1960, Koskelo et al. 1964, Shrivastava and Robson 1964). Careful scrutiny of serial ECGs will distinguish these T-wave and S–T segment changes from those of myocardial infarction, though exceptionally this distinction is impossible to make (Menon 1964).

Embolic occlusion of arteries of the limbs may mask other evidence of the causal cardiac infarction, or may present as a unique feature of a heart attack. Severe pain and ischemic changes progressing to gangrene of digits or limb are usually indicative of embolic arterial occlusion. Where the ischemic change is less severe, spontaneous resolution may occur.

Acute limb ischemia complicating myocardial infarction is not always due, however, to embolic phenomena. A fall in cardiac output in the presence of extensive peripheral arterial disease may reduce perfusion in the extremities of the lower limbs sufficiently to precipitate severe ischemic changes in the feet or legs. In our survey, 39 patients had ischemic limb complications following a myocardial infarction, but in 28 cases, the limb symptoms formed the cardinal presenting features. Two cases with extensive transmural infarcts presented with rapidly progressive gangrene, in the distal third of both lower limbs in one case, and in approximately the distal half of both upper and lower limbs in the other. No evidence of peripheral embolism was obtained following detailed autopsy examination. Jacobs (1959) found that a myocardial infarction was responsible for 9 of 122 embolic incidents involving the limbs. Reviewing 100 cases of sudden arterial occlusion of a limb artery, Allen et al. (1962) recorded coronary artery disease in 21 cases, of whom 20 had symptoms of peripheral arterial disease. Of Bean's (1937) 300 cases of myocardial infarction, 4 presented with arteriosclerotic gangrene.

Massive *pulmonary embolism* complicates myocardial infarction less frequently than when prolonged immobolity was the cornerstone of management of the disease. Pulmonary embolism may present with acute breathlessness or with sudden death. Rapid circulatory failure with peripheral cyanosis, syncope, or the development of right heart failure may characterize pulmonary infarction. When infarction is less extensive, cough with pleuritic pain or hemoptysis, tachycardia, and mild dyspnea are more frequent.

The reported incidence of pulmonary embolus complicating myocardial infarction varies widely. Evans (1964) recorded an incidence of 15%; Eppinger and Kennedy (1938), of 23%. The clinical features of pulmonary infarction may be the only overt picture of a recent myocardial infarction.

The interpretation of both symptoms and serial ECGs is often equivocal. In our survey, 12 patients with confirmed myocardial infarction presented with features of a pulmonary infarction.

Arrhythmias and disorders of conduction and rate are almost invariable following acute myocardial infarction. Often evanescent, and occurring most frequently within the first 2 or 3 h following the ischemic insult, disorders of rate and rhythm may be overlooked. Sinus tachycardia, sinus bradycardia, and nodal arrhythmias are frequent, early, and usually transient findings. Atrial fibrillation and flutter may be more persistent and increase the likelihood of heart failure and subsequent embolic phenomena. Ventricular ectopic beats are common and normally benign, but if they are frequent or multifocal, they may be associated with unstable ventricular rhythm, and ventricular tachycardia or fibrillation may supervene. The aging heart is unable to tolerate ventricular tachycardia, and signs of heart failure appear readily if the rapid heart rate is protracted. Ventricular fibrillation is probably the cause of most sudden deaths, but response to immediate DC shock is surprisingly good in older subjects, except for those currently in heart failure or cardiogenic shock. Bradycardia due to second degree heart block, nodal block, or complete heart block may emerge as an early and transient symptom, or as a later and often more persistent feature of infarction. Heart block may manifest itself as weakness, giddiness, syncope, or confusion. Cardiac arrhythmias following myocardial infarction may give rise to palpitation, but this symptom is frequently submerged by more dominant features. Evans and Sutton (1956) found palpitation to be a significant symptom in 30% of cases with an average age of 59 years. Palpitation was the cardinal presenting symptom in 4.4% of our patients.

Progressive *renal failure* marked by the rapid onset of increasing lethargy, lassitude, and anorexia associated with a rising blood urea was the overt clinical expression of acute infarction of the myocardium in 18 of our elderly subjects. In a study of 142 patients, Kennedy (1937) records that 5 had uremia. Reduced glomerular perfusion due to prolonged hypotension or a fall in cardiac output may be significant. Studies of renal function in old age show a decrease in glomerular filtration (Shock 1946, 1952; Olbrich et al. 1950) and tubular activity (Miller et al. 1952). The interplay of diminished renal function, increased metabolic stress, and decreased cardiac output may induce postinfarction uremia.

Vomiting has long been recognized as a frequent accompaniment of myocardial infarction. Where it is the dominant feature, diagnostic difficulties arise. Vomiting or nausea may be induced by administration of opiates for pain or by digitalis therapy. Pollard and Harvill (1940) and Evans and Sutton (1956) observed that sudden vomiting might be the cardinal symptom of myocardial infarction.

Herrick (1912) observed marked *weakness* to be a symptom of coronary occlusion. General weakness is particularly seen in elderly patients (White 1951), may be a presenting feature (Boyd and Werblow 1937), and is often very striking, even when there are but few other symptoms (Levine 1958). A complaint of weakness, often profound, was the outstanding feature in 19 patients with myocardial infarction. The sense of weakness, limpness, and exhaustion may last for up to 6 weeks and tends to fluctuate in intensity. The complaint of weakness may seem at times to overwhelm the patient, who may respond by marked depressive symptoms. Muscle hypotonia may be present, and in some cases is so striking as to give rise to a "rag doll" state.

Giddiness or unsteadiness is among the most frequent symptoms expressed by the elderly. It is a common associated feature of myocardial infarction, but may at times occur acutely as a distressing and disturbing presentation of underlying infarction. It is readily explicable where there is marked hypotension or a dysrhythmia, but intense giddiness or true vertigo is frequently present in the apparent absence of these features. Continuous monitoring indicates that some cases are indeed due to transient dysrhythmias or conduction defects. A reduction of previous hypertension to normotensive levels in the presence of widespread cerebrovascular or vertebral artery atherosclerosis may be causal, particularly if cardiac output also falls.

An uneasy *restlessness* in which the subject feels compelled to flex, extend, and rotate his arm, his leg, and his neck, and to shrug or retract one or the other shoulder at irregular intervals throughout the day or night, forms a peculiar and uncommon manifestation of myocardial infarction. Leydon (1884) recorded restlessness as a symptom of coronary occlusion. Bean (1938) noted that restlessness was present in 44% of his patients, though in none was it noted as the sole or even the predominant symptom.

Troublesome *cough* may be an early symptom of left ventricular failure; we have seen it as the presenting feature of 5 patients with acute myocardial infarction. In each instance, cough represented an early sign of left heart failure consequent on the acute ischemic incident.

Sweating is common in cardiac infarction. Bean (1938) found it to be present in 60% of his series. It may be one of the predominant complaints (Logue and Hurst 1956).

The reported incidence of *cardiogenic shock* has varied from 8% (Heyer 1961) to 52% (Friedberg 1961), the difference being due largely to differing criteria for assessing shock. Of our elderly patients with acute myocardial infarction reviewed over a period of 15 years, 9% had the syndrome of cardiogenic shock. Characteristically, the blood pressure is below 90 mm Hg, and is associated with cold, clammy face and extremities and a rapid, thready, regular or irregular pulse. Respiration is shallow and rapid, but sometimes irregular or interspersed with frequent sighing. Attempts to momentarily sit the patient up in bed for examination or administration of oral fluids may promptly precipitate a faint. A variable picture of gentle restlessness and quiet disorientation or intense apprehension or apathetic resignation is sometimes noticeable. Where shock is less intense, weakness, faintness, nausea or vomiting, gaseous abdominal distention and discomfort, and thirst are noted. Oliguria is an important feature.

Physical Signs

The physical signs of acute myocardial infarction are often those of arrhythmias or conduction defects, left or right heart failure, or cardiogenic shock. A rise of temperature is common after the first 24 h. Where previous infarctions or prolonged hypertension have been features, a degree of left ventricular hypertrophy is common. In the absence of hypertension, a fourth heart sound is of considerable diagnostic value: Gallop rhythm may indicate developing or established left ventricular failure. A transient pericardial rub may be detected in about 10% of patients within 3 days of the infarction.

Conclusion

Coronary heart disease in the elderly graphically illustrates many aspects of the medicine of old age. The pathogenesis is measured over most of a lifetime. Concurrent disease may precipitate or magnify symptoms. The historical aspect of coronary heart disease may be at best uncertain and on occasions misleading; it is subject to the vagaries of memory. Clinical features often differ from the classic presentation in younger people, and may simulate other diseases or be dismissed as merely the inevitable consequences of aging. The disease may introduce itself so quietly as to be barely audible or explosively with a plethora of signs and symptoms. The protean manifestations of the various phases of atherosclerotic disease of the coronary arteries have chastened each and every one of us who practice the medicine of old age.

References

Ackerman, R. F., Dry, T. J., and Edwards, J. E. (1950) *Circulation* **1**, 1345.
Allen, E. V., Barker, N. W., and Hines, E. A. (1962) *In: Peripheral Vascular Disease*, 3rd edition, W. B. Saunders, Philadelphia and London.
Barnes, A. R., and Ball, R. G. (1932) *Am. J. Med. Sci.* **183**, 215.
Bean, W. B. (1937) *Am. Heart J.* **14**, 684.
Bean, W. B. (1938) *Ann. Intern. Med.* **12**, 71.
Bean, W. B., and Read, C. T. (1942) *Am. Heart J.* **23**, 362.

Bean, W. B., Flamm, G. W., and Sapadin, A. (1949) *Am. J. Med.* **7**, 765.
Bedford, D. E., and Simpson, K. (1939) *Trans. Med. Soc. London* **62**, 165, 177.
Boyd, L. J., and Werblow, S. C. (1937) *Am. J. Med. Sci.* **194**, 814.
Burch, G. E., Meyers, R., and Abildskov, J. A. (1954) *Circulation* **9**, 719.
Byer, E., Ashman, R., and Toth, L. A. (1947) *Am. Heart J.* **33**, 796.
Carr, J. G. (1935) *Illinois Med. J.* **68**, 155.
Carter, A. B. (1964) *Cerebral Infarction*, Pergamon Press, Oxford.
Cookson, H. (1942) *Br. Heart J.* **4**, 163.
Cropp, G. J., and Manning, G. W. (1960) *Circulation* **22**,25.
Doscher, N., and Poindexter, C. A. (1950) *Am. J. Med.* **8**, 623.
Dozzi, D. L. (1937) *Am. J. Med. Sci.* **194**, 824.
Ebert, R. B. (1965) *Modern Treatment*, Vol. 2, Harper and Row, New York, p. 233.
Elliott, A. H. (1934) *Am. J. Med. Sci.* **187**, 185.
Eppinger, E. C., and Kennedy, J. A. (1938) *Amer. J. Med. Sci.* **195**, 104.
Evans, W. (1964) *In: Disease of the Heart and Arteries*, E. and S. Livingstone, Edinburgh and London.
Evans, W., and Sutton, G. C. (1956) *Br. Heart J.* **18**, 259.
Fentz, V., and Gormsen, J. (1962) *Circulation* **25**, 22.
Fisher, R. L., and Zuckerman, M. (1946): *J. Am. Med. Assoc.* **131**, 385.
Friedberg, C. K. (1956) *In: Disease of the Heart*, 2nd edition, W. B. Saunders, Philadelphia and London.
Friedberg, C. K. (1961) *Circulation* **23**, 325.
Garland, H. G., and Phillips, W. (1953) *In: Medicine*, Macmillan, London.
Garvin, C. F. (1942) *Am. J. Med. Sci.* **203**, 473.
Gilchrist, A. R. (1951) *Br. Med. J.* **1**, 874, 937.
Gould, S. E., and Cawley, L. P. (1958) *Arch. Intern. Med.* **103**, 524.
Gupta, P. D., Bawa, Y. S., and Wahi, P. L. (1965) *Indian Heart J.* **17**, 57.
Haft, J. I., Herman, M. V., and Gorlin, R. (1971) *Circulation* **43**, 279.
Hamman, L. (1934) *Ann. Intern. Med.* **8**, 417.
Hammer, A. (1878) *Wien. Med. Wochenschr.* **28**, 97.
Hay, J. (1933) *Lancet* **2**, 787.
Hellerstein, H. K., and Martin, J. W. (1947) *Am. Heart J.* **33**, 443.
Heron, J. R., and Anderson, E. G. (1965) *Lancet* **2**, 405.
Herrick, J. B. (1912) *J. Am. Med. Assoc.* **59**, 2015.
Herrick, J. B. (1931) *Am. Heart J.* **6**, 589.
Herrman, G. R. (1952) *Diseases of the Heart and Arteries*, 4th edition, Henry Kimpton, London.
Heyer, H. E. (1961) *Am. Heart J.* **62**, 436.
Hoffman, J. I. E., and Buckberg, G. C. (1975) *Brit. Med. J.* **1**, 76.
Jacobs, A. L. (1959) *In: Arterial Embolism in the Limbs*, E. and S. Livingstone, Edinburgh and London.
Jennings, R. B., Baum, J. H., and Herdson, P. B. (1965) *Arch. Pathol.* **79**, 135.
Johnson, W. J., Achor, R. W. P., Burchell, H. B., and Edwards, J. E. (1959) *Arch. Intern. Med.* **103**, 253.
Keefer, C. S., and Resnik, W. H. (1928) *Arch. Intern. Med.* **41**, 769.
Kennedy, J. A. (1937) *Am. Heart J.* **14**, 703.
Kitchin, A. H., Lowther, C. P., and Milne, J. S. (1973) *Br. Heart J.* **35**, 946.
Koskelo, P., Punsar, S., and Sipilä, W. (1964) *Br. Med. J.* **1**, 1479.
Lee, K. T., Thomas, W. A., Rabin, E. R., and O'Neal, R. M. (1957) *Circulation* **15**, 197.
Levine, H. D. (1953) *Am. J. Med.* **15**, 344.

Levine, S. A. (1958) *In: Clinical Heart Disease*, 5th edition, W. B. Saunders, Philadelphia and London.

Lewis, C. M., Dagenais, G. R., Friesinger, G. C., and Ross, R. S. (1970) *Circulation* **41,** 299.

Lewis, T. (1946) *In: Disease of the Heart*, 4th edition, Macmillan, London.

Leydon, E. (1884) *Z. Klin. Med.* **7,** 459.

Libman, E. (1919) *Trans. Assoc. Am. Physicians* **34,** 138.

Logue, R. B., and Hurst, J. W. (1956) *In* Meakins, J. C. (ed.), *Practice of Medicine*, 6th edition, Mosby, St. Louis.

Low-Beer, T., and Phear, D. (1961) *Lancet* **1,** 1303.

Mallory, G. K., White, P. D., Salcedo-Salgar, J. (1939) *Am. Heart J.* **18,**647.

Master, A. M., Dack, S., Horn, H., Freedman, B. I., and Field, L. E. (1950) *Circulation* **1,** 1302.

Menon, I. S. (1964) *Lancet* **2,** 433.

Miller, J.H., McDonald, R.K., Shock, N.W. (1952) *J. Geront.* **7,** 196.

Olbrich, O., Ferguson, M. H., Robson, J. S., and Stewart, C. P. (1950) *Edinburgh Med. J.* **57,** 117.

Papp, C. (1952) *Br. Heart J.* **14,** 250.

Parkinson, J., and Bedford, D. E. (1928) *Lancet* **1,** 4.

Pathy, M. S. (1967) *Br. Heart J.* **29,** 190.

Paul, C., and Schatz, M. (1971) *Circulation* **43,** 7.

Pollard, H. M., and Harvil, T. H. (1940) *Am. J. Med. Sci.* **199,** 628.

Pomerance, A. (1965) *Br. Heart J.* **27,** 697.

Race, G. A., and Lisa, J. R. (1945) *Am. J. Med. Sci.* **210,** 732.

Registrar General Statistical Review of England and Wales (1969) Her Majesty's Stationary Office, London.

Roberts, W. C. (1974) *In:* Braunwald, E. (ed.), *The Myocardium: Failure and Infarction*, H. P. Publishing Ent. Inc., New York, p. 192.

Rodstein, M. (1956) *Arch. Intern. Med.* **98,** 84.

Rogers, F. B. (1955) *J. Am. Geriatr. Soc.* **3,** 714.

Rose, G. A. (1962) *Bull. W.H.O.* **27,** 645.

Rose, G. A., and Blackburn, M. (1968) *Cardiovascular Survey Methods*, WHO, Geneva.

Roseman, M. D. (1954) *Ann. Intern. Med.* **41,** 1.

Shnitka, T. K., and Nachlas, M. M. (1963) *Am. J. Pathol.* **42,** 507.

Shock, N. W. (1946) *Geriatrics* **1,** 232.

Shock, N. W. (1952) *In* Cowdraeys (ed.), *Problems of Ageing*, 3rd edition, Williams and Wilkins, Baltimore, p. 614.

Shrivastava, S. C., and Robson, A. O. (1964) *Lancet* **2,** 431.

Shuster, S. (1960) *Br. Heart J.* **22,** 316.

Snow, P. J. D., Jones, A., Morgan, J., and Daber, K. S. (1956) *Br. Heart J.* **18,** 435.

Stürup, H. (1952) *Acta Med. Scand.* **144,** 189.

Wearn, J. T. (1923) *Am. J. Med. Sci.* **165,** 250.

White, N. K., Edwards, J. E., and Dry, T. J. (1950) *Circulation* **1,** 645.

White, P. D. (1951) *In: Heart Disease*, 4th edition, Macmillan, New York.

Wilson, G., Rupp, D., Riggs, H. E., and Wilson, W. W. (1951) *J. Am. Med. Assoc.* **145,** 1227.

Wright, I. S., Marple, C. D., and Beck, D. F. (1954) *In: Myocardial Infarction: Its Clinical Manifestations and Treatment with Anticoagulants*, Grune and Stratton, New York.

10

Pulmonary Heart Disease

T. HANLEY

Introduction

The term "pulmonary heart disease" (PHD) is often used as synonymous with the World Health Organization's (1961) definition of cor pulmonale:

> Hypertrophy of the right ventricle resulting from disease affecting the function and/or the structure of the lung, except when these alterations are the result of diseases that primarily affect the left side of the heart, or of congenital heart disease.

This definition excludes cases of chest disease with intermittent changes in the pulmonary circulation, but no material right ventricular hypertrophy. The term pulmonary heart disease as it is used here also embraces these patients.

Causes

There are many possible causes of chronic pulmonary heart disease (WHO 1961), but advancing age prunes the list radically, as many of the underlying lung lesions have already run their natural course before old age is reached. Four basically different kinds of lung

T. HANLEY · Harrogate District Hospital, Lancaster Park Road, Harrogate, HG2 7SX, England.

lesion give rise to pulmonary heart disease in old age:

1) Obstructive airway disease
2) Diffuse infiltration of the lungs by fibrous tissue or granulomata—
   the "stiff lungs syndrome"
3) Obliterative disease of the pulmonary vessels
4) Kyphoscoliosis

The underlying pathology, clinical picture, and disturbances of pulmonary function of these lesions are quite distinct, so they will be described separately, though it must be said at once that obstructive airway disease is far and away the most common.

Special Aspects of Pulmonary Heart Disease in the Elderly

Two factors influence the evolution and clinical picture of pulmonary heart disease in old people:

1) The frequent coexistence of other forms of heart disease, especially ischemic or hypertensive. The clinical and electrocardiographic findings can be dominated by such intrinsic cardiac disease.
2) Age-dependent changes in lung function and in the pulmonary circulation. Many aspects of lung function change steadily as age advances; maximum breathing capacity, vital capacity, and FEV decline, and residual volume increases (see Bates et al. 1971). The alveoloarterial PO_2 difference increases (Tenney and Miller 1956), probably because of impaired ventilation/perfusion relationships resulting from a relative increase in ventilation of the upper lobes (Holland et al. 1968). These changes do not cause disability in ordinary quiet daily activities, but limit the maximum capacity for physical effort and may set the stage for more rapid progression of disability if lung disease supervenes.

Prevalence

Heart disease is very common in old age. Kennedy et al. (1972) found a cardiac lesion in 40% of old people 65–74 years of age living at home, and in 50% of those over 75. Only a small proportion of these cardiac patients, however, had pulmonary heart disease: 6% of the men 65–74 years of age and 7% of those over 75. Not a single case of

TABLE 10.1. Age at Onset and at Death in 110 Patients with Pulmonary Heart Disease with Failure[a]

Age (yr):	15–24	25–34	35–44	45–54	55–64	65–74
Onset (%)	0.9	5.4	10.9	34.5	34.5	13.6
Death (%)	0	4.5	10.4	28.4	34.3	22.4

[a] Data of Stuart-Harris and Hanley (1957).

pulmonary heart disease was encountered in the 320 women in the survey.

The age incidence of PHD (with congestive heart failure) at onset and at death in 110 patients seen in a general medical department is shown in Table 10.1. The incidence reached a peak at 45–64 years, then declined sharply at 65–74. There were no patients over 75. This pattern is compatible with the clinical impression that chronic pulmonary heart disease is uncommon over the age of 75 and a real rarity over 85 years. The prevalence is in any case very patchy within the United Kingdom, because chronic obstructive airway disease is most common in large industrial cities, especially those north of a line from Bristol to the Wash.

Physiopathology

There can be few subjects on the borderline of medicine and physiology that have been investigated with the same relentless intensity given to pulmonary heart disease.

The present account will be centered around two questions: "What causes the right ventricular hypertrophy of pulmonary heart disease?" and "Is right ventricular hypertrophy the cause of edema and venous congestion, and if not, what is?"

Table 10.2 shows the abbreviations used in the text.

The immediate cause of hypertrophy of the right ventricle is an increase in its work, which is proportional to pulmonary blood flow and mean pulmonary artery pressure ($\bar{P}AP$). The $\bar{P}AP$ is linearly related to flow for increases up to 4 times the resting flow rate (Fowler 1969), each 100% increment in flow being accompanied by a rise of 25–60% in $\bar{P}AP$. Some earlier reports describe a "high" cardiac output

TABLE 10.2. Abbreviations Used in the Text

COAD	Chronic obstructive airway disease
PHD	Pulmonary heart disease
$PaCO_2$, PaO_2	Arterial blood; partial pressure[a] of carbon dioxide and oxygen
$PACO_2$, PAO_2	Alveolar partial pressure[a] of carbon dioxide and oxygen
$\bar{P}AP$	Pulmonary artery mean pressure[a]
PVR	Pulmonary vascular resistance (dyn/sec/cm^{-5})
GFR	Glomerular filtration rate (ml/min)
RPF	Renal plasma flow
FEV_1	Forced expiratory volume in one second

[a] All pressures in units of mm Hg (omitted from text).

in pulmonary heart disease, and the mistaken belief that this is common has taken firm root. Table 10.3 shows the results of three studies, each including a group of patients in heart failure, a second group recovering from it, and a third without any history of heart failure. Although the resting cardiac output of patients in pulmonary heart failure is raised, correction to a standard oxygen uptake shows

TABLE 10.3. Cardiac Output in Pulmonary Heart Disease

Research work	Number of patients	Cardiac index (liters/min/m²)		Oxygen consumption[a] (ml/min/m²)	Cardiac index corrected to oxygen consumption of 100 ml/min[b]
		Mean	Range		
Whitaker (1954)					
In heart failure	10	3.20	1.1–4.4	132 (222)	2.42
Recovering	9	3.10	2.7–3.8	145 (225)	2.14
No history of failure	13	2.60	1.7–4.8	120 (201)	2.18
Mounsey et al. (1952)					
In heart failure	13	4.20	———	182	2.30
Recovering	10	5.00	———	186	2.69
No history of failure	8	4.20	———	188	2.24
Harvey et al. (1951)					
In heart failure	4	4.65	4.04–6.06	165	2.81
Recovering	11	3.44	2.39–4.63	147	2.34
No history of failure	6	3.57	2.85–4.53	148	2.41

[a] Figures in brackets are workers' original data, uncorrected for surface area.
[b] Calculated from workers' data.

TABLE 10.4. Data on Pulmonary Circulation in COAD from Various Workers

Research work	Condition	O_2 consumption (ml/min)		$\bar{P}AP$		Cardiac index (liters/min/m²)	
		Normal	Chest disease	Normal	Chest disease	Normal	Chest disease
Burrows et al. (1972)	Rest	—	231	—	26	—	2.5
	Exercise	—	454	—	38	—	3.5
Harris et al. (1968a)	Rest	242	305	17	32	4.04	3.60
	Exercise	845	761	21	64	6.42	4.82
Cotes et al. (1963)	Rest	263	217	—	22	2.42	
	Exercise	774	899	—	44	4.18	
Hickam and Cargill[a] (1948)	Rest	157[b]	167[b]	11	18	4.26	3.88
	Exercise	315	288	13	25	6.10	4.85
Riley et al. (1948)	Rest	126[b]	146[b]	13	20	3.27	3.97
	Exercise	406	516	11	34	5.40	5.45

[a] Patient No. 24 omitted.
[b] Results are in O_2/min/m².

that the average values lie within normal limits. These high resting outputs are presumably caused by the excessive oxygen cost of quiet breathing. The term "normal output failure" is appropriate (Mounsey et al. 1952).

Patients with severe chronic obstructive airway disease not in congestive failure have a resting $\bar{P}$AP higher than normal, and also show a rise during exercise greater than can result from the normal pressure/flow relationship (Table 10.4). Since increase in flow alone cannot account for the elevated $\bar{P}$AP, other possibilities include:

1) Increase in pulmonary arteriolar tone due to hypoxia or hypercapnia, both of which undoubtedly constrict pulmonary vessels (see Bergofsky 1974). That oxygen administration has little lowering effect on $\bar{P}$AP during pulmonary heart failure (Whitaker 1954, Mounsey et al. 1952), however, argues strongly against hypoxia as the only cause of pulmonary hypertension, or even as the main cause.
2) Increased intrapulmonary pressure, which could compress pulmonary blood vessels and so increase pulmonary vascular resistance (Rodbard 1953, Harris et al. 1968b).
3) Destruction of pulmonary capillaries, which is a consistent pathological finding in chronic obstructive airway disease and can occur as a result of age alone. Emirgil et al. (1967) showed that doubling the flow through one lung caused a much larger increase in $\bar{P}$AP in normal old people than in younger men.
4) Intrinsic change in the physical properties of the pulmonary vessels.

TABLE 10.5. Renal Circulation in Pulmonary Heart Disease with and without Heart Failure[a]

Patients	Number	GFR (ml/min)	Renal plasma flow (ml/min)	Filtration fraction	Renal blood flow (ml/min)
Chronic lung disease	22	100.1 ± 19.48	400 ± 101.6	0.24	768.6 ± 180.2
Pulmonary heart failure in acute phase	26	76.7 ± 25.4	227 ± 72.54	0.31	467.3 ± 157.6
Recovery from heart failure	18	94.7 ± 18.75	381 ± 75.04	0.26	770 ± 149.8

[a] Data of Stuart-Harris et al. (1956).

TABLE 10.6. Changes in Renal Circulation with Development of Congestive Heart Failure[a]

Group	GFR (ml/min)	Renal blood flow (ml/min)	Cardiac index (liters/min/m^2)	$\bar{P}AP$	PaCO$_2$	PaO$_2$
Edematous	63	326	2.40	61.0	54.4	49.8
Nonedematous	106	650	3.06	33.0	46.9	58.9

[a] Data of Aber et al. (1963).

Factors (1), (2), and (3) all appear likely to be important in the production of pulmonary hypertension in chronic obstructive airway disease.

Edema and Salt Retention in Pulmonary Heart Disease

It was long assumed that "strain" and dilatation of the right heart must be the cause of heart failure in pulmonary heart disease, but there are other possibilities, and the renal circulation in particular has been much investigated. The same abnormal pattern of renal circulatory change occurs in both the "normal-output" failure of pulmonary heart disease and the "low-output" failure of ischemic heart disease; both the glomerular filtration rate (GFR) and renal plasma flow (RPF) are reduced (Davies and Kilpatrick 1951, Fishman et al. 1951). After effective treatment of an episode of pulmonary heart failure, the renal circulation often shows remarkable recovery (Stuart-Harris et al. 1956, Table 10.5), which does not occur after treatment of failure due to ischemic or valvular disease. Aber et al. (1963) found that RPF was correlated with PaO$_2$ and PaCO$_2$, and speculated on the possibility that the renal circulatory changes were due to the blood-gas changes (Table 10.6).

Although no clear explanation for peripheral edema in pulmonary heart failure emerges from the work reviewed, there seems to be a general inclination to believe in the importance of renal circulatory factors. In the final stages, however, right ventricular strain and dilatation must also play an important role.

Polycythemia in Pulmonary Heart Disease

The red-cell volume increases in COAD, *pari passu* with hypoxemia and to the same degree that would be expected in healthy people with hypoxemia due to living at high altitude. Arterial hypoxemia is known to stimulate the production of erythropoietin, and this mechanism probably obtains in PHD also.

Several investigators have commented, however, that the packed-cell volume in pulmonary disease with hypoxemia is not usually much raised (Shaw and Simpson 1961). Hume (1968), on the other hand, found that the logarithm of PaO_2 was reasonably well correlated with the packed-cell volume; the lowest PCV in his series was 46%, the highest 70%, and half the values were higher than 64%—levels in general much higher than those of other studies. No other similar correlation between PaO_2 and hematocrit in pulmonary heart disease has been reported.

The discrepancy between the extent of polycythemia as judged by the packed-cell volume and by the red-cell mass was attributed by Shaw and Simpson (1961) to a corresponding increase of plasma volume, but there is no consensus on this view. While changes in red-cell mass are of interest in relation to physiological adaptation to COAD, the packed-cell volume is the important factor, since it is this volume, and not the red-cell mass as such, that directly influences blood viscosity. Dintenfass and Read (1968) emphasize that acidosis increases the internal viscosity of red cells. The decreased blood pH present in most patients with hypercapnia can increase whole-blood viscosity to dangerously high levels when the hematocrit is 60% or more (see the "Treatment" section of this chapter).

Clinical Features

For many years, the diagnostic term "chronic bronchitis and emphysema" was used as if these two diseases were Siamese twins, though emphysema was usually thought of as a pathological sequel to the expiratory obstruction of chronic bronchitis. More recently, emphysema has come to be regarded as a disease in its own right—of mysterious origin, but nonetheless a separate entity. With this change, there has been a steadily growing acceptance of the idea (Fletcher et al. 1963, Burrows et al. 1966) that there are two kinds of chronic obstructive airway disease: the "emphysematous" type (also called type "A") and the "bronchial" type (type "B").

The definition of emphysema in the context of these workers' ideas is that of the WHO (1961):

> Emphysema is a condition of the lung characterized by increase beyond normal in the size of air spaces distal to the terminal bronchiole, with destruction of their walls.

The crux of this definition is the last five words, which draw the distinction between mere hyperinflation of intact alveoli, in which air distribution may be poor but there is no loss of diffusing surface, and "true" emphysema, in which coalescence of alveoli reduces the effective area for gas exchange.

This idea is of special relevance to pulmonary heart disease, since it is in type "B" that right ventricular hypertrophy and eventually heart failure are likely to develop. Evidence of a correlation between the morbid anatomical lesions and the functional disturbances in the lung and pulmonary circulation has been given by Burrows et al. (1966). The main features of the two groups are shown in Table 10.7. Type "A" corresponds, in Dornhorst's colorful phrase, to the "pink puffer"; type "B," to the "blue bloater."

While the division into two types serves a useful purpose in clarifying the natural history of the disease, it must be recognized that

TABLE 10.7. Main Distinguishing Features of the Emphysematous and Bronchial Types of COAD

Features	Type "A" (emphysematous)	Type "B" (bronchial)
Sputum	Little	Much
X-ray signs of emphysema	Yes	Little or none
Total lung capacity	Increased	Normal or slightly increased
Diffusing capacity	Reduced	Little or no reduction
$PaCO_2$	Normal at rest; may rise on exercise	Persistent hypercapnia the rule
PaO_2	Normal at rest; may fall on exercise	Persistent hypoxia the rule
Liability to heart failure	No	Yes
Physique	Asthenic	Stocky

not all patients fit neatly into one or the other category. Burrows et al. (1966) recognize an intermediate "group X," who are presumably patients with both diseases. Furthermore, patients may change, over a period of years, from one type to another. Finally, by no means all patients with significant "bronchial COAD" inevitably progress to pulmonary heart disease; many become more or less stable at a given degree of functional incapacity, and die, after a normal span, of nonrespiratory disease.

Archetypes of these two types of obstructive airway disease are easily recognized: the "emphysematous" patient hyperventilates, with such great respiratory effort and distress that in the extreme case the mere act of talking or sitting can be beyond his capacity. Respiration is gulping, erratic, and incoordinate; the shoulders are hunched; and the accessory respiratory muscles are constantly in action. The patient is usually thin, in contrast to his bulky, barrel-shaped chest. The lips are often kept pursed, and give an audible puff at the end of respiration. The whole impression is that the act of breathing is intensely laborious—which indeed it is. Central cyanosis is absent at rest (but can develop during exercise), and right ventricular hypertrophy is detectable neither clinically nor in the ECG.

The archetype of the "bronchial" variety presents a different picture. The patient is usually of heavier build, and often gives a somnolent impression. His attention and effort are much less concentrated on ventilation. Dyspnea of some degree is in fact always present (as the patient will testify), and is intensified by effort, but respiratory distress is objectively much less than one would expect from the combination of severe airway obstruction and congestive heart failure. Central cyanosis is usually detectable clinically, and is worsened by effort. If the $PaCO_2$ is much raised, there is generalized peripheral vasodilation, with abnormally warm hands in which capillary pulsation can be detected (a feature that probably contributes to the durable legend of "high-output failure" in chronic lung disease). Small-amplitude myoclonic twitching movements of the fingers and sometimes of the facial muscles are often present; when hypercapnia is severe, a coarse, flapping tremor barely distinguishable from that of liver failure is sometimes seen. In many patients, the conjunctivae are edematous and the eyes unusually bright; these conditions in combination with mild proptosis can give a superficial impression of hyperthyroidism. The patient's state is influenced by the $PaCO_2$ level. With minor degrees of hypercapnia—a $PaCO_2$ of, say, 45–60—the only change may be slight slowness of cerebration. In old people already on the verge of cerebral insufficiency, however, severe mental confusion can appear even at this level. A diurnal rhythm in which confusion, excitement, and aimless wandering develop in the evening or during the night is only too familiar in geriatric practice, and this can be the pattern in CO_2 retention. Behavior can become truculent or frankly aggressive, and such patients present a difficult nursing problem, which hampers effective therapy. In almost all patients with a $PaCO_2$ level of 60–90, some degree of drowsiness will be present; at CO_2 tensions 3 times normal, there will certainly be stupor and probably coma with depressed reflexes and small pupils. The last state is usually produced by injudicious oxygen therapy (see "Treatment").

The purely circulatory signs are rarely striking. Sinus rhythm is the rule, but auricular fibrillation occurs in a small proportion. The cardiac impulse is often impalpable, and cardiac dullness is obliterated, presumably due to lung hyperinflation. For the same reason, the left parasternal heave of right ventricular hypertrophy is often not detectable, even when there is unequivocal evidence of right ventricular enlargement in the ECG, though a powerful epigastric pulsation is usually present.

Auscultation reveals faint, occasionally inaudible heart sounds. The pulmonary second sound is often loud and can be double, but the diastolic murmur of pulmonary incompetence is very rare. A right ventricular third sound in gallop cadence and the fourth heart sound of atrial hypertension are sometimes to be heard at the lower end of the sternum and in the epigastrium.

Patients of this kind may experience many bouts of congestive heart failure. In these attacks, the general circulatory signs are the same as those seen in other kinds of heart disease: There is jugular venous congestion (often with an intrinsic, systolic venous pulsation), tender hepatic engorgement with hepatojugular reflux, and edema affecting the sacrum and dependent parts. Many patients with a protracted history of heart failure terminate with persistent edema unresponsive to diuretic therapy, permanent tricuspid incompetence, and perhaps ascites, with a "low salt syndrome" and a rising blood urea.

The ECG in Pulmonary Heart Disease

There is a bewildering mass of data available. Each successive review replaces existing sets of criteria for detecting right ventricular hypertrophy, and only general guidance can be given (see Padmavati and Raizada 1972):

1) A confident diagnosis of right ventricular hypertrophy can be made if the following two criteria are present:
   i) A dominant R wave in the right precordial leads (V_5R is the most commonly used) or in V_1. The QRS pattern can be of qR, R, or Rs conformation. An R wave of greater amplitude than 0.5 mV in V_5R or in V_1 has been widely used as a criterion.
   ii) Delayed onset of the intrinsic deflection in V_5R or V_1. If these two signs are conclusively present, it is also likely that aVR will have a qR conformation, and probable that the P-wave axis will exceed $+60°$ and have an amplitude of more than 0.2 mV.
2) If these "classic" criteria are absent, right ventricular hypertrophy will be suspected if there is electrical evidence of "clockwise rotation" in the long axis of the heart (rS pattern in V_4–V_6) and right axis deviation in the standard leads.
3) The most labile changes are seen in the T waves of V_1–V_3; these can be inverted during an attack of congestive failure and become upright during recovery.

Radiological Findings in Pulmonary Heart Disease

In many patients with the "bronchial" type of COAD, emphysema will be absent, and the lung fields can appear quite normal radiologically. The abnormalities that may be present (Simon 1970) include excessive clarity of the small blood vessels; small, ill-defined opacities presumably representing areas of bronchiolitis or zones made airless by impaction of mucus plugs; large hilar vessels without a corresponding increase in size of peripheral vessels; and relative hyperemia of the upper lung fields (a change seen in normal old people).

When the diagnosis is first made, the cardiac outline is often pear-shaped, with a narrow transverse diameter. As one attack of heart failure succeeds another, however, a progressive increase in cardiac size often occurs. Gross cardiomegaly from pulmonary heart disease alone is rare; in a substantial proportion, however, another cardiac disease will be associated by chance, and cardiac size may then be much increased.

In some patients who obstinately refuse to conform sharply to either type of COAD, emphysema will be present. To be radiologically detectable, however, it must be severe. The radiological signs are: (1) a low, flattened diaphragm; (2) a large zone of translucency in the

TABLE 10.8. Blood Gases in Pulmonary Heart Disease

Patient group	PaCO$_2$	Arterial oxygen saturation (%)	Whole blood CO$_2$ (vol %)
Normals[a]	38 ± 3	90 ± 2.9	47.5 ± 3.8
PHD not in failure[b]	54	83	59
PHD in failure[b]	64	63	66

[a] Tenney and Miller (1956): data on old people.
[b] Rounded values from Stuart-Harris et al. (1957): Table XXV, p. 167.

retrosternal region; and (3) local loss of pulmonary arterial markings—preferably identified by normal "marker" vessels in some lung regions.

Blood-Gas Abnormalities in Pulmonary Heart Disease

In advanced COAD of the "bronchial" type, many patients have a minor degree of arterial oxygen unsaturation and elevation of PaCO$_2$ at all times, but the abnormalities become much more severe when heart failure supervenes.

The rise of PaCO$_2$ causes a fall of blood pH, which eventually results in increased renal reabsorption of bicarbonate ion and a corresponding rise of plasma bicarbonate. The outcome is a partially compensated respiratory acidosis, with a fall of plasma [Cl$^-$] corresponding to the rise of [HCO$_3^-$]. Representative values would be as in Table 10.8.

Treatment

The treatment of pulmonary heart failure has two aspects: therapy that aims to minimize further progression of the underlying lung disease and so to postpone the development of heart failure, and therapy of the episodes of heart failure themselves. The main principle underlying the first aspect is reduction of respiratory work, which in COAD is chiefly expended in overcoming airflow obstruction and can be ameliorated by three measures: control of bronchial infection, relief of bronchospasm, and liquefaction of sputum.

Prolonged antibiotic therapy of *early* chronic bronchitis makes no material difference in the progress of the disease (Medical Research

Council 1966). Nor is there any substantial evidence that, in the terminal phase of COAD, antibacterial therapy will significantly delay the downward trend of ventilatory function. There is, however, a definite connection between acute exacerbations of bronchiolar infection and the development of heart failure, and treatment of lung infection is justifiable for this reason alone. Many infections are of viral origin, but the secondary bacterial invaders, almost invariably *Hemophilus influenzae* or the pneumococcus, are the immediate cause of deterioration, and they can be effectively attacked. The indication for antibacterial therapy is the appearance of pus in the sputum coupled with clinical deterioration. Treatment should not await the results of sputum culture (May 1975). Permanent eradication of infection in advanced COAD is a pipe dream, and the distinction between "cidal" and "suppressant" therapy is tenuous at this stage of the disease. A sensible approach is to give brief treatment with a bactericidal drug in sufficiently high dosage and observe whether relapse occurs at once when treatment is stopped; if it does, drug therapy will have to continue. At present, the drug of choice appears to be amoxycillin; it is absorbed better than ampicillin and is equally well concentrated in mucoid and purulent sputum. The success of therapy depends largely on the attainment of inhibitory concentrations in sputum. To achieve the necessary level of 0.2–0.6 μg/ml (May 1975) in sputum requires a dosage of ampicillin (Penbritin) of 1 g every 6 h (or 500 mg amoxycillin every 6 h).

Only slight improvement can be expected from bronchodilator drugs, but the gain can be worthwhile in terms of the relief of dyspnea. Two current widely used drugs are salbutamol (Ventolin) given by metered aerosol, and choline theophyllinate (Choledyl) or proxyphylline (Thean) by mouth. Although at least some patients have a substantial fall of $\bar{P}AP$ from long-term oxygen therapy (Abraham et al. 1968, Stark et al. 1973, Petty and Finigan 1968, Neff and Petty 1970, Anderson et al. 1973), there remains considerable doubt as to its value, especially in old people. Stark and Bishop (1973) have considered the economic factors and practical difficulties. Long-term domestic oxygen therapy presents insuperable practical problems for most old people living alone. Furthermore, the treatment causes no improvement of ventilatory function; unless the relief of hypoxia leaves a patient with reasonable functional capacity, and not simply a well-oxygenated respiratory cripple, totally dependent on others, it will be a dubious gain.

If polycythemia is sufficiently severe, it can raise the blood viscosity to a point at which right ventricular work is materially increased. There seems no reason to take any action until the packed-cell volume exceeds 60%, unless significant respiratory acidosis is also present (Dintenfass and Read 1968). Treatment by venesection of such patients carries a real risk of thrombosis, but isovolemic replacement infusion has given good results (Gregory 1971, Harrison et al. 1971). The technique is as follows:

A 10% (wt/vol) solution of "Dextran 40" in isotonic saline or glucose is infused intravenously into one arm while twice the volume of blood (up to 2 liters) is simultaneously removed from the other. Heparin, 12,500 U, is given intravenously beforehand to help maintain venesection. When venesection is completed, the other half of the dextran solution is given over 8–16 h.

Treatment During Exacerbations with Heart Failure

The aims of treatment are: (1) to relieve respiratory failure and (2) to reduce salt and water retention.

Treatment of respiratory failure has been dealt with in part above. The means of treatment are improvement of ventilatory function by vigorous treatment of infection and the use of bronchodilator drugs. Probably the best bronchodilator drug during the acute phase is aminophylline; its combined action as bronchodilator and respiratory stimulant is useful in the presence of respiratory failure.

Most patients will respond to these measures alone, but others continue to deteriorate, and the advisability of controlled oxygen therapy—the first choice—or assisted ventilation arises. Full practical details are given by Sykes et al. (1969).

That many patients with CO_2 retention will lapse into coma if given ill-controlled oxygen therapy should now be so well known as to need no emphasis, except to say that *no oxygen is better than ill-managed oxygen treatment.*

Oxygen should be given only to hypercapnic patients at controlled concentration. The possibilities are:

1) The "Ventimask," which fits over the nose and mouth and delivers a fixed O_2 concentration (28% is most commonly used), whatever the rate of flow from the cylinder (4 liters/min is recommended). The oxygen concentrations employed will cause some rise of $PaCo_2$, but not to levels that imperil consciousness.
2) The "Edinburgh mask" has the advantage of producing a variable O_2 concentration about the same as the Ventimask. The concentra-

tion of oxygen actually breathed varies inversely with minute
ventilation, and the apparatus requires more skilled nursing supervision.
3) Oxygen delivered by nasal catheter or spectacles at 2–3 liters/min is
   the simplest method. The inspired O_2 concentration can rise up to
   60%, however, and this level can cause a further elevation of $PaCO_2$
   (see results of Abraham et al. 1968, discussed above). This method
   is not suitable for patients already suffering from moderately severe
   hypercapnia, unless there is skilled nursing supervision and laboratory control of blood gases at hand.
4) Assisted ventilation requiring endotracheal intubation or tracheos-
   tomy is a last-ditch measure that is traumatic, requires special
   medical and nursing skills, and is unsuited to the treatment of
   geriatric patients, unless a special unit is available.

Respiratory Stimulants

Respiratory stimulants have their place in the emergency treatment of patients who are lapsing into hypercapnic coma as a result of
ill-controlled oxygen therapy (Bader and Bader 1965). Probably the
best is aminophylline (250–500 mg i.v. over 6–8 h). Alternatives are
amiphenazole ([Daptazole] 200–400 mg i.v. in divided doses) or the
older nikethamide (Coramine). These drugs are general analeptics and
not specific stimulants of the respiratory center; the margin between
an increased respiratory volume and excessive, general CNS stimulation is small, and the individual dosage varies considerably (Westlake
and Campbell 1959).

Diuretic Therapy

The choice of a diuretic in patients with edema and overfilling of
the vascular system will depend to some extent on the previous
history. In the initial attack of heart failure, a rapidly acting diuretic
such as frusemide (Lasix) in an oral dosage of 20–40 mg can cause a
massive diuresis. At the other end of the scale are the patients who
have suffered many previous attacks of heart failure and are already
receiving heavy dosage of potent diuretics, perhaps for the past
several months continuously; for these patients, an aldosterone antagonist is probably more appropriate therapy. Separate and adequate
replacement of iatrogenic potassium loss is essential in old people
during diuretic therapy; many exist at a level of dietary potassium
intake such that a balance of this electrolyte is only just feasible. A

supplement of 0.6 g KCl t.i.d. or q.i.d. (i.e., 24–32 mEq K$^+$ in all) is
enough.

Digitalis

The consensus is that patients with pulmonary heart disease get
little or no benefit from digitalis, and in elderly patients the risk of
provoking arrhythmias is real. In patients already receiving the drug
for coexisting ischemic heart disease with auricular fibrillation, however, it can be maintained.

Prognosis

The author has been unable to find data on the prognosis
specifically of old people once pulmonary heart disease has developed.
In a series of 110 patients (see age incidence in Table 10.1) followed for
5 years (Stuart-Harris and Hanley 1957), about one-fourth died in the
first attack of heart failure or within one year of it. By the fifth year, at
least 60% were known to have died, and many more may have done
so, as 31 patients had been lost to follow-up. Oswald et al. (1967), in a
10-year follow-up of 301 civil servants with bronchitis, found that 54%
of them had died, slightly more than half from respiratory causes.

Burrows et al. (1972), reporting on 50 patients followed for 5 years
showed successive year's survival rates of 84, 66, 56, and 44%.
Survival was fairly well negatively correlated with both the FEV$_1$ and
the pulmonary vascular resistance. All 9 patients with a PVR exceeding 600 dyn/sec/cm^{-5} died a "respiratory death," and only one survived beyond two years. During the course of Howard's (1974) 5-year
study of 178 patients with COAD, 35.5% died; of these, two-thirds
perished of pulmonary heart failure.

Clearly, patients with pulmonary heart disease of any severity
have in general no more than an even chance of surviving for 5 years,
and it is likely that the prognosis will be worse in old people, with
their added burdens of age-dependent loss of lung function and
coincidental ischemic heart disease.

Miscellaneous Causes

Diffuse Pulmonary Fibrosis

Interstitial fibrosis is a fairly common finding at autopsy in old
people, and in the largest group, no clearly identifiable cause can be

found. Many correspond to "chronic idiopathic diffuse interstitial fibrosis," or "diffuse fibrosing alveolitis," originally described in acute form by Hamman and Rich (1944).

The main findings are dyspnea, with hyperpnea, tachypnea, and finger-clubbing. Central cyanosis may be absent at rest, but is provoked by even mild exercise. Crackling "dry" rales, usually most intense at the lung bases, are characteristic, as in the absence of evidence of bronchospasm. Cardiovascular signs may never develop, as many of these patients die of severe hypoxia or intercurrent pulmonary infection, and there is surprisingly little detailed clinical information on the terminal cardiovascular state of patients with this group of diseases. The clinical signs, when present, are those of right ventricular hypertrophy and pulmonary hypertension as described for COAD.

Special Investigations. The disturbances of pulmonary function are quire different in kind from those of COAD. Obstruction to air flow plays little or no part, and the pattern of disturbance of function is "restrictive." The vital capacity is low, and lung compliance is greatly reduced, with a corresponding (2–10-fold) increase in respiratory work. There is no impairment of distribution of inspired gas, and the total lung volume is increased. The diffusing capacity of the lungs is much reduced, but whether this is due to an "alveolocapillary block" or to a diminished area of alveolar membrane, or to disturbance of the relation between ventilation and perfusion, has been a subject of warm debate (Hamer 1964, Bates et al. 1971).

Inhalation of oxygen relieves the arterial unsaturation, but barely affects the hyperpnea, which is probably due to abnormal sensory impulses from the lung, rather than to hypoxemia (Lourenco et al. 1965).

X-Ray Findings. The radiological findings are not closely correlated with either symptomatic distress or changes in pulmonary function. Positive findings on the chest film range from a normal appearance through a generalized or local "ground-glass" fine mottling, to a coarser, mottled, honeycomb pattern.

Treatment and Prognosis. The prognosis of diffuse pulmonary fibrosis is in general poor, though Scadding (1960) believed it to be better in older patients. In his group of 14 patients of average age 60, the 7 decreased had manifested symptoms from $1\frac{1}{2}$ to $7\frac{1}{2}$ years, with an average of $4\frac{1}{2}$ years.

Treatment with corticosteroids gives moderately good but clini- cally rather unpredictable results. Scadding and Hinson (1967) found that steroids suppressed the signs and symptoms in a few patients with minor alveolar wall thickening, but had no effect in the presence of gross thickening.

Obliterative Vascular Disease of the Lungs

Embolism of a pulmonary artery by a detached thrombus is a mundane event in geriatric wards and a common cause of death in the hospital. The embolus usually originates in a deep calf vein, but can come from a pelvic vein or the right auricle.

The cardiac consequences of an embolus depend largely on its size:

1) A massive embolus lodged in the main pulmonary artery or either of its large branches produces the picture of "acute cor pulmonale" with the physical signs and electrocardiographic stigmata of acute right ventricular dilatation and "strain."
2) Very small emboli, often arising in showers from the pelvic veins, can produce a progressive obstruction of the pulmonary vascular bed. The patient usually presents with dyspnea due to advancing pulmonary hypertension. This syndrome is virtually confined to pregnant women, and is of no further interest in the geriatric context.
3) A smaller but substantial embolus can lodge in a lobar or segmental branch of one pulmonary artery, usually in the lower lobes, and produce frank pulmonary infarction, though this results from only a small minority of such emboli.

The great majority of patients suffer only one pulmonary embolus; if they survive, they usually do so without any residual local impairment of lung function, though resolution takes 6–12 weeks (Duner et al. 1960). The risk of developing a persistent cardiac disability arises when there is recurrent pulmonary embolism and incomplete restoration of lung function, perhaps due to impaired fibrinolysis (Ellison and Brown 1965). Complete recovery from an embolus is much less common if there is coexisting heart or lung disease (Chait et al. 1967); in view of the ubiquity of heart disease in old people, one would expect many elderly patients to have some residual lung impairment after embolism.

The diagnosis, once in mind, depends largely on obtaining a history of repeated episodes of pain and swelling of the legs, followed by lung symptoms compatible with embolism. Since only a minority of emboli declare themselves in this way, however, one must often resort to retrospective examination of chest radiographs for evidence of past embolism. Flower (1975) gives an excellent summary of the radiographic features.

In the established case of pulmonary heart disease due to repeated thromboembolism, the major symptoms are hyperventilation at rest or on exertion, or syncopal attacks (Goodwin et al. 1963). The attacks of syncope can be due to further emboli, to a fall of blood pressure on exercise, or to brief attacks of arrhythmia. The physical signs—other than those of other intrinsic heart disease, which may well be present—are slight central cyanosis, hyperventilation, and signs of pulmonary hypertension, i.e., a parasternal heave; a loud, narrowly split pulmonary second sound; and a prominent "a-wave" in the jugular venous pulse.

The ECG. Goodwin et al. (1963) draw attention to the diagnostic value of the appearance of T-wave inversion in V_1–V_5 before the classic signs of right ventricular hypertrophy (see under COAD), and to the fact that the rS pattern with upright T waves in V_5–V_7 seen in asphyxial pulmonary heart disease does not occur in thromboembolic pulmonary heart disease.

Pulmonary Function. The abnormalities of lung function in repeated thromboembolism superficially resemble those of the "stiff lungs" of pulmonary fibrosis, in that the resting and exercising minute volume of ventilation is large, with a fast respiratory rate, but the lung volumes and vaximum breathing capacity are normal (Jones and Goodwin 1965).

Kyphoscoliosis

Although some degree of kyphoscoliosis is common in old people, severe kyphoscoliosis with "heart failure of the hunchback" is very uncommon beyond the age of 65. Pulmonary heart disease develops when the deformity has been acquired in youth, before the lungs and thoracic cage are fully grown, the essential defect being mechanical restriction of lungs already too small.

Distribution of inspired air is normal, and emphysema is not an intrinsic feature. The vital capacity is often grossly reduced and the work of breathing greatly augmented (Bergofsky et al. 1959).

Patients with severe spinal deformity often lead sheltered lives and manage well for long periods until they develop hypoxia and hypercapnia, with pulmonary hypertension, finally presenting much the same clinical and biochemical picture as asphyxial cor pulmonale (Hanley et al. 1958). They are especially sensitive to the respiratory depressant action of morphine, barbiturates, or uncontrolled oxygen therapy, and they tolerate trauma badly. The advent of a bronchial infection often precipitates the first attack of heart failure.

References

Aber, G. M., Bayley, T. J., and Bishop, J. M. (1963) *Clin. Sci.* **25**, 159.

Abraham, A. S., Cole, R. B., and Bishop, J. M. (1968) *Circ. Res.* **23**, 147.

Anderson, P. B., Cayton, R. M., Holt, P. J., and Howard, P. (1973) *Q. J. Med.*, *N.S.* **42**, 563.

Bader, M. E., and Bader, R. A. (1965) *Am. J. Med.* **38**, 165.

Bates, D. V., Macklem, P. T., and Christie, R. V. (1971) *In: Respiratory Function in Disease*, 2nd edition, W. B. Saunders and Company.

Bergofsky, E. H. (1974) *Am. J. Med.* **57**, 378.

Bergofsky, E. H., Turino, G. M., and Fishman, A. P. (1959) *Medicine*, **38**, 263.

Burrows, B., Fletcher, C. M., Heard, B. E., Jones, N. L., and Wootliff, J. S. (1966) *Lancet* **1**, 831.

Burrows, B., Kettel, L. J., Niden, A. H., Rabinowitz, M., and Diener, C. F. (1972) *N. Engl. J. Med.* **286**, 912.

Chait, A., Summers, D., Krasnow, N., and Wechsler, B. M. (1967) *Am. J. Roentgenol.* **100**, 364.

Cotes, J. E., Pisa, Z., and Thomas, A. J. (1963) *Clin. Sci.* **25**, 305.

Davies, C. E., and Kilpatrick, J. A. (1951) *Clin. Sci.* **10**, 53.

Dintenfass, L., and Read, J. (1968) *Lancet* **1**, 570.

Duner, H., Pernow, B., and Rigner, K. G. (1960) *Acta Med. Scand.* **168**, 381.

Ellison, R. C., and Brown, J. (1965) *Lancet* **1**, 786.

Emirgil, C., Sobol, B. J., Campodonico, S., Herbert, W. H., and Mechtaki, R. (1967) *J. Appl. Physiol.* **23**, 631.

Fishman, A. P., Maxwell, M. H., Crowder, C. H., and Morales, P. (1951) *Circulation* **3**, 703.

Fletcher, C. M., Hugh-Jones, P., McNicol, M. W., and Pride, N. B. (1963) *Q. J. Med.*, *N.S.* **32**, 33.

Flower, C. D. R. (1975) *Hosp. Update* **1**, 358.

Fowler, N. O. (1969) *Am. J. Med.* **47**, 1.

Goodwin, J. F., Harrison, C. V., and Wilcken, D. E. L. (1963) *Br. Med. J.* **1**, 701.

Gregory, R. J. (1971) *Lancet* **1**, 858.

Hamer, J. (1964) *Thorax* **19**, 507.

Hamman, L., and Rich, A. R. (1944) *Bull. Johns Hopkins Hosp.* **74**, 177.

Hanley, T., Platts, M. M., Clifton, M., and Morris, T. (1958) *Q. J. Med.*, *N.S.* **27**, 155.

Harris, P., Segel, N., and Bishop, J.M. (1968a) *Cardiovasc. Res.* **2**, 73.

Harris, P., Segel, N., Green, I., and Housley, E. (1968b) *Cardiovasc. Res.* **2**, 84.

Harrison, B. D. W., Gregory, R. J., Clark, T. J. H., and Scott, G. W. (1971) *Br. Med. J.* **4**, 713.

Harvey, R. M., Ferrer, M. I., Richards, D. W., Jr., and Cournand, A. (1951) *Am. J. Med.* **10**, 719.

Hickam, J. B., and Cargill, W. H. (1948) *J. Clin. Invest.* **27**, 10.

Holland, J., Milic-Emili, J., Macklem, P. T., and Bates, D. V. (1968) *J. Clin. Invest.* **47**, 81.

Howard, P. (1974) *Br. Med. J.* **1**, 89.

Hume, R. (1968) *Br. J. Haematol.* **15**, 131.

Jones, N. L., and Goodwin, J. F. (1965) *Br. Med. J.* **1**, 1089.

Kennedy, R. D., Andrews, G. R., and Caird, F. I. (1972) *In* Brocklehurst, J. C. (ed.), *Textbook of Geriatric Medicine and Gerontology,* Churchill Livingstone.

Lourenco, R. V., Turino, G. M., Davidson, L. A. G., and Fishman, A. P. (1965) *Am. J. Med.* **38**, 199.

May, J. R. (1975) *Hosp. Update* **1**, 217.

Medical Research Council Working Party (1966) *Br. Med. J.* **1**, 1317.

Mounsey, J. P. D., Ritzmann, L. W., Selverstone, N. J., Briscoe, W. A., and McLemore, G. A. (1952) *Br. Heart J.* **14**, 153.

Neff, T. A., and Petty, T. L. (1970) *Ann. Intern. Med.* **72**, 621.

Oswald, N. C., Medvei, V. C., and Waller, R. E. (1967) *Thorax* **22**, 279.

Padmavati, S., and Raizada. V. (1972) *Br. Heart J.* **34**, 658.

Petty, T. L., and Finigan, M. M. (1968) *Am. J. Med.* **45**, 242.

Riley, R. L., Himmelstein, A., Motley, H. L., Weiner, H. M., and Cournand, A. (1948) *Am. J. Physiol.* **152**, 372.

Rodbard, S. (1953) *Am. J. Med.* **15**, 356.

Scadding, J. G. (1960) *Br. Med. J.* **1**, 5171.

Scadding, J. G., and Hinson, K. F. W. (1967) *Thorax* **22**, 291.

Shaw, D. B., and Simpson, T. (1961) *Q. J. Med., N.S.* **30**, 135.

Simon, G. (1970) *In* McLaren, J. W. (ed.), *Modern Trends in Diagnostic Radiology—4,* Butterworth, London.

Stark, R. D., Finnegan, P., and Bishop, J. M. (1973) *Br. Med. J.* **3**, 467.

Stark, R. D., and Bishop, J. M. (1973) *Br. Med. J.* **2**, 105.

Stuart-Harris, C. H., and Hanley, T. (1957) *In: Chronic Bronchitis, Emphysema and Cor Pulmonale,* John Wright and Sons Ltd., Bristol.

Stuart-Harris, C. H., Mackinnon, J., Hammond, J. D. S., and Smith, W. D. (1956) *Q. J. Med., N.S.* **25**, 389.

Sykes, M. K., McNicol, M. W., and Campbell, E. J. M. (1969) *In: Respiratory Failure,* Blackwell Scientific Publications, Oxford and Edinburgh.

Tenney, S. M., and Miller, R. M. (1956) *J. Appl. Physiol.* **9**, 321.

Westlake, E. K., and Campbell, E. J. M. (1959) *Br. Med. J.* **1**, 274.

Whitaker, W. (1954) *Q. J. Med.* **23**, 57.

World Health Organization (1961) *Report of an Expert Committee, WHO Tech. Rep. Ser. No. 213,* Geneva.

11

Valvular Heart Disease

F. I. CAIRD

Introduction

The frequency and importance of valvular heart disease in old age are now well recognized. Since the problems of pathology and surgical treatment are dealt with elsewhere in this volume, this account will concentrate on clinical features, diagnosis, and natural history. It is appropriate to consider disorders of each valve separately.

Rheumatic Mitral Valve Disease

Rheumatic disease is the most common cause of mitral valve disorder in the elderly. Its frequency results from two factors: the incidence of rheumatic fever during the childhood and adolescence of the present elderly population, and the natural history of established rheumatic heart disease in middle age.

The incidence of rheumatic fever has fallen steadily during the first half of this century (Glover 1930, Cox and Schlesinger 1956, Sievers and Hall 1971), and its manifestations may also have become less severe (Cox and Schlesinger 1956). The prevalence of rheumatic heart disease in old age is thus likely to decline in future, with the death of the cohort exposed to the higher incidence of rheumatic fever in the late 19th and early 20th centuries.

About 40% of elderly patients with rheumatic mitral disease give

F. I. CAIRD · University Department of Geriatric Medicine, Southern General Hospital, Glasgow, G51 4TF, Scotland.

a history of rheumatic fever or chorea in early life (Bedford and Caird 1960). The first rheumatic manifestation occurs in over 80% under the age of 20, and in over 90% under the age of 30, an age-distribution identical to that found in large series of cases of acute rheumatic fever (e.g., Hedley 1940), but elderly patients may have suffered fewer recurrences of rheumatic activity (Hebbert and Rankin 1954). Longevity in rheumatic heart disease is thus not likely to be due to late initial rheumatic infection, though the lower frequency of recurrence may be associated with less severe valvular damage. The rate of development of rheumatic heart disease is often very slow. Clinically detectable mitral disease continues to become apparent for the first time at least up to 20 years after the initial rheumatic episode (Bland and Jones 1951), and in some cases even up to 60 years later (Currens 1967).

The natural history of mitral disease established in middle life is such that a substantial proportion of patients might be expected to survive into old age. Approximately three-quarters of middle-aged patients with asymptomatic mitral stenosis and sinus rhythm are alive 20 years later, and most have not significantly deteriorated (Wilson and Greenwood 1954, Olesen 1955). The most important single factor determining functional deterioration is undoubtedly the onset of atrial fibrillation.

Clinical Features of Rheumatic Mitral Disease in Old Age

Approximately one-third of elderly patients with rheumatic mitral disease have predominant mitral stenosis, and the remaining two-thirds predominant incompetence (Bedford and Caird 1960). About one-half also have evidence of aortic valve disease; of these, two-thirds have aortic incompetence (the common combination being mild mitral and aortic incompetence), and one-third aortic stenosis with or without incompetence. Organic tricuspid disease is distinctly rare (see below).

Of elderly patients with rheumatic mitral disease seen in the hospital, 40% have evidence of cardiac failure, and some 10% have angina, almost all of whom also have undoubted ischemic heart disease (Gardner and White 1949). Systemic embolism occurs in 6%, more commonly in those with mitral stenosis than in those with predominant incompetence (Bedford and Caird 1960). Bronchitis must be presumed, in at least some cases, to be related to mitral disease, rather than to its more common causes; it may lead to considerable diagnostic problems, since the signs of mitral disease may be obscured. Pulmonary embolism is largely a complication of cardiac failure, while subacute bacterial endocarditis occurs in the occasional case (see Chapter 12).

The physical signs are essentially the same as in the younger patients. About one-third of those seen in the hospital have atrial fibrillation, which is more common in those with mitral stenosis. A typical malar flush can sometimes be seen. Cardiac enlargement is common, and a left ventricular type of impulse is felt when mitral incompetence predominates, and occasionally a right ventricular impulse in predominant stenosis. The auscultatory signs again closely resemble those in younger patients. A loud first heart sound is common in predominant stenosis. When this sign is evident during tachycardia or cardiac failure, a very careful auscultatory search should be made at the time for other signs of mitral disease, and this search should be repeated once increase in cardiac output reveals the flow-dependent signs of mitral stenosis, such as the diastolic murmur. The opening snap has been said to be rare in the elderly (Bedford and Caird 1960), but phonocardiography clearly demonstrates its presence in many elderly patients (Caird et al. 1973). When the cardiac output is low, the opening snap may be the only sign of mitral stenosis.

The length of the apical middiastolic murmur provides some measure of the severity of stenosis. In predominant mitral incompetence, the usual pattern consists of an apical pansystolic murmur (sometimes with an apical thrill), a third heart sound, and a short middiastolic murmur. Electrocardiography is usually of little value, although in mitral stenosis, P mitrale and right ventricular hypertrophy may be found on occasions; in predominant mitral incompetence, left ventricular hypertrophy. The chest radiograph often shows left atrial enlargement, but Kerley's lines and definite evidence of pulmonary hypertension (other than increase in the upper lobe veins) are unusual. Echocardiography has been little exploited, but should prove to be valuable in the demonstration of abnormalities of mitral valve movement.

Complications of Rheumatic Mitral Disease

The most common event precipitating cardiac failure is the development of atrial fibrillation. Of elderly patients with rheumatic mitral disease and atrial fibrillation, 60% show evidence of cardiac failure, as against only a quarter of those with sinus rhythm (Bedford and Caird 1960).

Rheumatic mitral disease is not an uncommon cause of systemic embolism in the elderly, since the frequency both of atrial fibrillation and of left atrial thrombosis at autopsy increases with age (see Bedford and Caird 1960). Thrombosis, however, is a much more common cause of occlusion of systemic arteries than embolism, even in those who are potential candidates for systemic emboli.

The diagnosis of embolism thus presents considerable difficulties, since the combination of a rapid onset of symptoms of arterial occlusion, together with a manifest possible source of embolus, is not enough by itself. A firm diagnosis may be made in a patient with atrial fibrillation and mitral valve disease if more than one major vessel is occluded simultaneously or nearly so, or if the vessel occluded is a rare site for acute thrombotic occlusion and a more common one for embolism (e.g., the brachial artery or aortic bifurcation). Less reliance can be placed on features highly characteristic of embolism in younger patients, such as the abrupt onset and rapid clearing of focal cerebral disorder. Further, even if the diagnosis of embolism is established in an elderly patient with mitral disease, the source of the embolus may on occasions not be the left atrium, but mural clot overlying a cardiac infarct (especially in predominant mitral incompetence), or even the endocardial interstices of a left ventricle without evidence of infarction (Bedford and Caird 1960).

Embolism of an artery such as the brachial or femoral, or of the aortic bifurcation, is usually an indication for embolectomy regardless of the age of the patient. The operation can be carried out under local anesthesia, and the Fogarty catheter constitutes a major advance. Anticoagulant therapy should be begun and continued after embolectomy, and also in those patients in whom embolectomy is not indicated (e.g., those with cerebral emboli). Anticoagulant therapy is only likely to be of value for about 6 months (Adams et al. 1974).

Prognosis

The prognosis of rheumatic heart disease in the elderly depends on the cardiac rhythm and the presence or absence of cardiac failure. Those with sinus rhythm and no evidence of cardiac failure probably have an expectation of life little different from the elderly of the same age (Bedford and Caird 1960), but when atrial fibrillation, cardiac failure, or both, are present, survival is substantially reduced. The simultaneous presence of aortic valve disease does not seem to affect prognosis greatly.

Nonrheumatic Mitral Valve Disease

There are four varieties of nonrheumatic mitral valve disease encountered in the elderly, which must be taken into account in differential diagnosis. These are papillary muscle dysfunction, calcification of the mitral annulus, mucoid degeneration of the mitral valve, and left atrial myxoma.

Papillary Muscle Dysfunction

Rupture of a papillary muscle or of its attached chorda is a rare but spectacular complication of acute cardiac infarction, occurring some days after the infarct, and presents as dramatic clinical deterioration, accompanied by the appearance of a loud systolic murmur. It may be necessary to distinguish rupture of the papillary muscle of chorda from rupture of the ventricular septum, in which the hemodynamic consequences are often less severe, and which is certainly in some cases compatible with survival.

Dysfunction of a papillary muscle, which allows prolapse of part of the mitral valve into the left atrium during systole, and so produces mitral incompetence, is now recognized as common following acute cardiac infarction. Heikilla (1967) showed that when a pansystolic murmur is present after cardiac infarction, infarction of a papillary muscle is present in almost every case coming to autopsy. Persistent dysfunction of a papillary muscle is probably not rare (de Pasquale and Burch 1966). The diagnosis should be made from the presence of pure mitral incompetence, as evidenced by a pansystolic murmur at the apex, sometimes with a third sound, but without evidence of mitral obstruction, together with an electrocardiogram indicating past cardiac infarction. The prognosis seems to be good.

Calcification of the Mitral Annulus

This is a not infrequent pathological finding in the elderly, and is more common in women than in men (Pomerance 1967, Kirk and Russell 1969). It is usually clinically unimportant and asymptomatic, its only evidence being an obliquely-set horseshoe of calcium seen somewhat posteriorly on lateral radiographs of the chest. The calcareous shelf may prevent proper valve closure, so that incompetence, and less often stenosis, may result (Rytand and Lipsitch 1946, Simon and Liu 1954, Korn et al. 1962, Kirk and Russell 1969). The physical signs resemble those of rheumatic mitral disease, though an opening snap would not be expected. The ECG may show atrial fibrillation and atrioventricular or ventricular conduction defects.

Mucoid Degeneration of the Mitral Cusps: Mitral Valve Prolapse

This is another not infrequent autopsy finding in the elderly (Pomerance 1969). If elongation of the chordae and ballooning of part of a cusp is sufficient to allow prolapse into the left atrium during systole, mitral incompetence will result. This syndrome (the so-called "floppy valve") may occur in younger people, occasionally as a familial disorder, but is also encountered in the elderly. Some develop atrial fibrillation and cardiac failure. Ventricular ectopic beats are common, and may increase in frequency with exercise (see Winkle et al. 1975). The characteristic physical sign is a late systolic murmur, sometimes initiated by a systolic click, without evidence of mitral obstruction (Epstein and Coulshed 1973). The electrocardiogram does not show signs of cardiac infarction, as is the case with ischemic papillary muscle dysfunction, and the chest X ray does not show calcification of the mitral annulus. The echocardiogram can show the abnormal movement of the valve (Dillon et al. 1971, Popp et al. 1974).

Left Atrial Myxoma

This uncommon cardiac disorder may rarely be encountered in old age (Goodwin 1963, Harvey 1968). Its importance is greater than its frequency, because surgical treatment is urgent. The key to the diagnosis is the presence of rapidly advancing symptoms and signs of mitral obstruction, usually of 2 years' duration or less. By contrast, in elderly patients with rheumatic mitral disease, symptoms will usually have been present for a much longer period, of 10 years or more. Systemic embolic episodes are common, but syncopal episodes (due to intermittent complete obstruction of the mitral valve by the tumor) are relatively infrequent. The combination of emboli with variable mitral murmurs, a raised E.S.R., and disturbed plasma proteins may suggest bacterial endocarditis, but blood cultures are negative. Features suggesting the diagnosis should lead to detailed study by echocardiography (Nasser et al. 1972) or angiocardiography, or both, since surgical treatment must be carried out before the development of irreversible cardiac deterioration.

Aortic Valve Disease

Aortic Stenosis

This valvular lesion is common in old age. It appears to be more frequent in men under the age of 80, and in women over that age (Bedford and Caird 1960). In about 20% of clinically diagnosed cases, there is coexistent rheumatic mitral valve disease, and the aortic valve disease is presumably also rheumatic. Two more common pathological processes are calcific changes in congenitally bicuspid valves, and calcareous degeneration in tricuspid valves (Pomerance 1972). The exclusion of coexistent mitral disease is important as a surgical consideration, but in general it is neither very important nor indeed often possible to distinguish between the various varieties of aortic stenosis in old age.

Symptoms

The majority of cases of aortic stenosis in the elderly have no cardiac symptoms, but about one-third of patients seen in hospital are dyspneic, commonly because of cardiac failure. Angina pectoris is recorded in a widely varying proportion, from 10% (Bedford and Caird 1960) to 70% (Finegan et al. 1969), some of whom have coexistent ischemic heart disease. As many as 30% may have syncopal attacks (Finegan et al. 1969), usually occurring on exertion, but in patients in terminal cardiac failure, episodes of impairment of consciousness may occur at rest, accompanied by sweating, restlessness, confusion, irregular bradycardia, and hypotension (Kumpe and Bean 1948, Bedford and Caird 1960).

Physical Signs

In severe cases, most of the classic physical signs can be demonstrated: a slowly rising pulse; reduced pulse pressure; left ventricular hypertrophy with a slowly rising cardiac impulse; a long, loud, and harsh ejection murmur; and depression and reversed splitting of the second heart sound. In less severe cases, the anacrotic pulse and reduction in pulse pressure are absent (Bedford and Caird 1960). The murmur is maximum in the right second space, but is often widely audible over the precordium and at the apex. Differing pathologies in the aortic valve may produce heart patterns of murmur (Roberts et al.

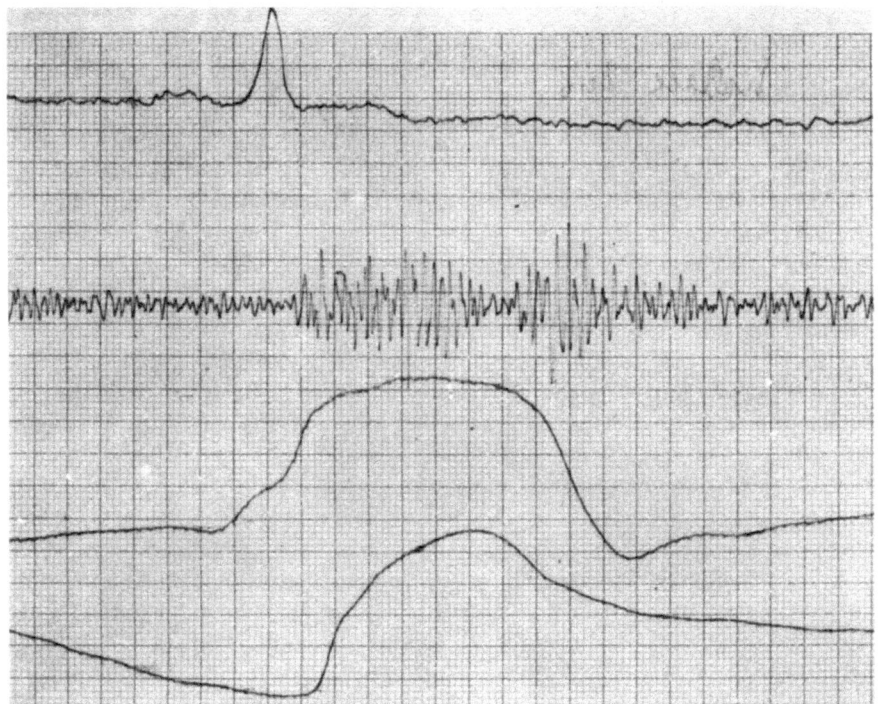

Fig. 11.1. Aortic stenosis and incompetence in a 70-year-old woman. *(Top trace)* ECG Lead II; *(2nd trace)* phonocardiogram from right second space, showing loud ejection systolic and diminuendo early diastolic murmurs; *(3rd trace)* apexcardiogram, showing square-topped shape indicating left ventricular hypertrophy; *(bottom trace)* External arterial pulse trace, showing delay in upstroke. Time: 10 and 50 msec.

1971, see Chapter 6). The murmur is sometimes accompanied by a basal thrill, commonly radiates into the neck, and on occasion shows expiratory accentuation. Approximately two-thirds have an aortic diastolic murmur (Fig. 11.1), and when incompetence is of some magnitude, the bisferiens pulse may be evident.

Investigations

The ECG usually confirms the presence of left ventricular hypertrophy, but can be normal (Bedford and Caird 1960, Forker et al. 1970). Left bundle branch block is present in 5–10% of cases, and other conduction defects are also occasionally encountered. Unless mitral disease coexists, sinus rhythm is usually preserved, even with the development of congestive failure.

The chest X ray shows left ventricular enlargement, particularly if there is aortic incompetence or cardiac failure. Calcification of the aortic valve may be demonstrable on lateral radiographs, on screening, or on tomography; when present, it is well correlated with the presence of severe stenosis (Glancy et al. 1969). Other investigations have relatively little to contribute, since the echocardiographic demonstration of aortic valve movement is difficult (Gramiak and Shah 1970, Gibson 1973, Popp and Harrison 1974). If cardiac surgery is contemplated, left heart catheterization may be necessary to confirm the presence of a major systolic gradient. The magnitude of such gradients, and the peak left ventricular systolic pressures generated, are as high in the elderly as in younger patients (Table 11.1)—a striking tribute to the powers of compensation of the elderly heart (Finegan et al. 1969, Roberts et al. 1971).

Diagnosis

The principal diagnostic problems are those of distinguishing between aortic stenosis and aortic valvular sclerosis without obstruction, between aortic stenosis and incompetence and other causes of aortic incompetence, and between aortic stenosis and the relatively rare case of hypertrophic obstructive cardiomyopathy in old age (see p. 245).

The distinction from aortic valvular sclerosis is essentially based on the loudness and length of the systolic murmur, the presence of changes in the second heart sound, and evidence of left ventricular hypertrophy. In aortic stenosis, the systolic murmur is for practical purposes invariably louder than grade 2/4, and is longer than that of aortic valvular sclerosis (Aravanis and Luisada 1957). A longer murmur, with a peak reached later in systole, implies obstruction to ejection. The phonocardiogram may be of value in this connection, but the reduction in duration and the earlier peak of the murmur when cardiac failure develops must be remembered. Reduction in intensity and reversal in splitting of the second heart sound (Gray 1956) can usually be demonstrated in aortic stenosis at least phonocardiographically, and provide an important distinguishing feature. Left ventricular hypertrophy must be present for aortic stenosis to be confidently diagnosed, but may be absent (Forker et al. 1970); also, of course, it may have other causes in the elderly, coexisting with aortic valvular sclerosis.

TABLE 11.1. Clinical, Hemodynamic, and Pathological Findings in 5 Elderly Women with Aortic Stenosis[a]

	Clinical						Hemodynamics						Pathology		
							Pressures		Gradient			Aortic			Coro-
	Chronic							BA (mm			CO	valve	Heart	Commis-	nary
	cardiac	Angina									(liters/	area	weight	sural	calcifi-
Age	failure	pectoris	Syncope	AF	DM	LVH	LV	Hg)	Peak	Mean	min)	(cm²)	(g)	fusion	cation
76	0	+	+	0	+	+	256/12	126/55	130	102	2.0	0.2	480	0	+
75	0	+	+	0	+	+	280/8	120/50	160	—	2.2	0.2	390	+	+
83	0	0	+	+	0	+	180/4	115/40	65	55	3.6	0.5	380	0	+
81	0	+	0	0	0	+	265/25	172/78	93	59			400	0	+
74	+	0	0	0	+	0	205/20	135/44	70	55	1.8	0.3	530	0	0

[a] Roberts et al. (1971). All had systolic murmurs, calcification of the mitral annulus, and left ventricular hypertrophy at autopsy. Abbreviations: AF, atrial fibrillation; DM, diastolic murmur; LVH, left ventricular hypertrophy; LV, left ventricle; BA, brachial artery; CO, cardiac output.

Most errors of diagnosis are still those of omission (Anderson et al. 1975), but certain diagnosis may at times be impossible (Rodstein and Zeman 1967).

Aortic Incompetence

Aortic incompetence is probably the most common valvular lesion encountered in old age. It has many causes, most of them rare, and only four are common. The rare causes, which personal experience shows do in fact occasionally occur in old age, include rupture of an aortic cusp (Carroll 1951), bacterial endocarditis, dissecting aneurysm of the aorta (Levine et al. 1951), incomplete aortic rupture [in which a tear in the aortic intima just above the aortic valve, similar to that in dissecting aneurysm, allows the adjacent aortic cusp to prolapse into the left ventricle in diastole (Peery 1942)], and aortitis in ankylosing spondylitis (Clark et al. 1957). The four common causes are rheumatic heart disease, calcareous disease of the aortic valve, syphilitic heart disease, and what has been termed "isolated nonsyphilitic aortic incompetence" (Bedford and Caird 1960).

Approximately 40% of cases of rheumatic heart disease in old age show aortic incompetence in addition to signs of mitral disease. As in younger patients, the combination is somewhat more common in men than in women (Bedford and Caird 1960). The early diastolic murmur is heard in the usual site, at the base of the heart, down the left sternal edge, and at the apex. It is almost always soft and short. Evidence of hemodynamically severe aortic incompetence, such as a collapsing pulse and capillary pulsation, is unusual, but left ventricular hypertrophy may be present.

Aortic incompetence occurring in calcareous aortic valve disease is usually also slight, and the features of aortic stenosis described above will be present. Particular importance should be attached to depression of the aortic component of the second heart sound.

Syphilitic heart disease is now a relative rarity at any age, but in recent years, a substantial proportion of cases have occurred in the elderly (Heggtveit 1964, Prewitt 1970). A past history of syphilis or of antisyphilitic treatment is rarely obtainable, but there is often clinical evidence of neurosyphilis, especially tabes dorsalis or taboparesis (Bedford and Caird 1960). Cardiac symptoms are frequent, and the aortic incompetence is usually clinically severe, with a collapsing pulse, high pulse pressure, and left ventricular hypertrophy and dilatation. There is usually an aortic ejection murmur, the aortic

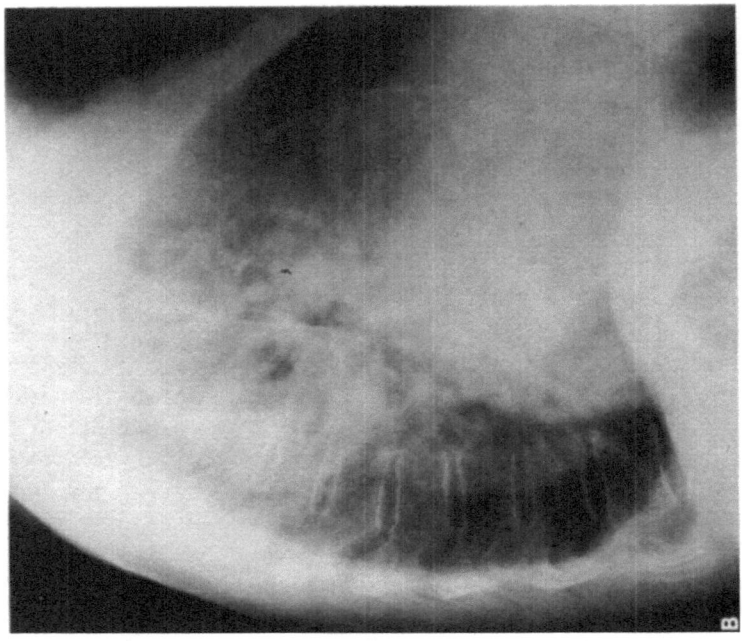

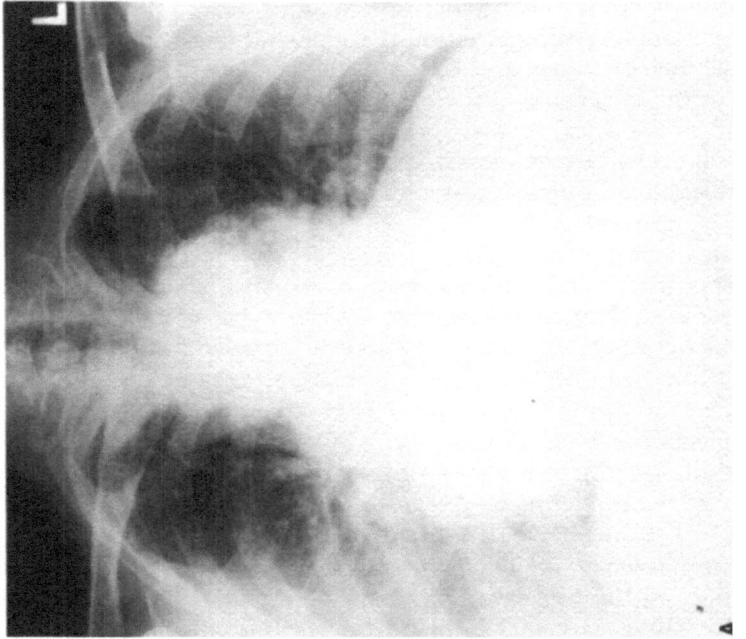

Fig. 11.2. Syphilitic aortitis with incompetence in a 65-year-old woman (Bedford and Caird 1960). Posteroanterior and lateral chest radiographs showing calcification in the ascending aorta.

component of the second sound is loud and ringing (Potain's *bruit de tabourka*), and there is a long aortic diastolic murmur widely heard over the precordium. The electrocardiogram is not of great value, though it is usually abnormal (Storey 1958), but the chest X-ray is of great diagnostic significance, since irregular dilatation of the aorta, occasionally with frank aneurysm formation, and calcification of the ascending aorta are frequent (Fig. 11.2). The serological tests for syphilis are usually positive, or are known to have been so in the recent past, either in the blood or in the cerebrospinal fluid.

The diagnosis of syphilitic aortic incompetence is thus not usually difficult in the elderly. Its prognosis is in general poor (Bedford and Caird 1960).

Isolated Aortic Incompetence

Aortic incompetence in old age may not be due to any of the more common causes mentioned, and may indeed lack a clearly defined pathological basis. Thus, Ruffin et al. (1941), Gouley and Sickel (1943), Fenichel (1950), and Bedford and Caird (1960) described cases of aortic incompetence in old age that they regarded as due to dilatation of the aorta in which there was no evidence of syphilis, and the aortic valves were normal. The nomenclature is confused, but the term "functional aortic incompetence" would seem inappropriate for a condition that is permanent once it develops, while "arteriosclerotic" carries connotations that are certainly imprecise and probably incorrect. The term "isolated aortic incompetence" may be used to refer to cases of pure aortic incompetence, without aortic stenosis or disease of other valves, occurring in elderly patients in whom there is no evidence of syphilis (Bedford and Caird 1960).

The prevalence of this condition is not certainly known, since the figure of 4% of hospital admissions (Bedford and Caird 1960) is almost certainly too high. Only one case was encountered in 500 randomly selected old people (Kennedy, Andrews, and Caird, unpublished). Isolated aortic incompetence is almost always asymptomatic, and indeed the frequency of cardiac failure is no greater than in elderly hospital patients without aortic valve disease (Bedford and Caird 1960). Signs of hemodynamically severe aortic incompetence are rare, and the pulse and pulse pressure are commonly normal. Only rarely is there clinical evidence of left ventricular hypertrophy. An aortic ejection murmur is common, but in contrast with aortic stenosis is usually soft, and the aortic component of the second sound is normal or loud. The early diastolic murmur is usually short.

The electrocardiogram on occasion shows left ventricular hypertrophy, but the chest X ray is unhelpful, because aortic dilatation is rarely gross enough to be clearly recognizable radiologically.

The prognosis is excellent, and indeed the condition is more important as a problem in differential diagnosis, which may give rise to considerable difficulty. In general, however, rheumatic aortic incompetence is distinguished by the presence of signs of mitral valve disease, calcareous aortic valve disease by the evidence of aortic obstruction, and syphilitic aortic incompetence by signs of neurosyphilis and the characteristic radiological and serological changes. The rare causes mentioned may give rise to difficulty, and there will inevitably be errors. Attention to the points mentioned, however, will allow correct diagnosis in the great majority of cases.

Tricuspid Valve Disease

Tricuspid stenosis is almost always part of severe multivalvular rheumatic heart disease, and is thus not common in old age. The occasional case will be manifest by gross elevation of the venous pressure, with hepatomegaly but without frank cardiac failure, and often without severe dyspnea or orthopnea. Superior mediastinal obstruction is excluded by the absence of evidence of a collateral circulation. The electrocardiogram is usually unhelpful, unless sinus rhythm is still present, when the tall pointed P wave of right atrial hypertrophy may be combined with first degree heart block (Goodwin et al. 1957, Kitchin and Turner 1964, El-Sherif 1971). The chest X ray shows evidence of gross enlargement of the right atrium.

By comparison, tricuspid incompetence is common in old age. Functional incompetence may complicate right heart failure of any etiology, as it is almost always present when the right ventricular diastolic pressures, and thus the right atrial pressures, are grossly elevated (Korner and Shillingford 1957). The diagnosis is made from the presence in the venous pulse of a large positive systolic wave, together with a pansystolic murmur maximal at the left lower sternal border, and usually showing clear accentuation on inspiration. Attention to these details will distinguish the murmur from that of mitral incompetence.

Organic tricuspid incompetence due to destructive changes in the valve is usually associated with tricuspid stenosis, and thus is decidedly rare in old people.

Pulmonary Valve Disease

Pulmonary valve disease is most uncommon in old people. Virtually the only cause of undoubted right-sided ejection murmurs is atrial septal defect, carcinoid heart disease being extremely rare in the elderly (Roberts and Sjoerdsma 1964).

Pulmonary incompetence is confined to very rare cases of severe chronic pulmonary hypertension, whether due to mitral valve disease, chronic lung disease, or thromboembolism. Personal experience is only of a single case, secondary to chronic diffuse interstitial fibrosis of the lungs. The diagnosis is possible only when there is evidence of severe pulmonary hypertension, with clinical, electrocardiographic, and radiological signs of gross right ventricular hypertrophy, and dilatation of the main pulmonary arteries.

Multivalvular Disease

Multivalvular heart disease is not rare in the elderly, common combinations being mitral and aortic valve disease, in particular combined mitral and aortic incompetence. In one series of 130 cases of rheumatic heart disease in old age, there were 38 cases of mitral disease and aortic incompetence, and 18 of mitral disease and aortic stenosis (Bedford and Caird 1960).

The principal problems presented are those of diagnosis of mitral disease, since the signs of aortic valve disease, whether obstructive or regurgitant, may mask the characteristic signs of mitral disorder. From the prognostic point of view, there appears to be relatively little difference between these forms of multivalvular heart disease and pure mitral disease; as Mitchell et al. (1954) comment, however, mitral disease complicated by aortic stenosis behaves more like isolated aortic stenosis than isolated mitral disease.

One rare but potentially important differential diagnosis of multivalvular heart disease is hypertrophic obstructive cardiomyopathy, which is occasionally encountered in the elderly. Obstruction to ejection gives rise to a loud ejection murmur, but characteristically the pulse is rapidly rising, and the aortic component of the second heart sound is normal. There is usually mitral regurgitation, associated with papillary muscle dysfunction, and the clinical picture is thus very like that of rheumatic heart disease. Radiological examination, however, will fail to detect calcification of the aortic valve. The potential importance of this diagnosis lies in the fact that β-adrenergic blockade may help less severe cases and surgical treatment more severe cases of obstructive cardiomyopathy (Goodwin 1970, Swan et al. 1971).

References

Adams, G. F., Merrett, J. D., Hutchinson, W. M., and Pollock, A. M. (1974) *J. Neurol. Neurosurg. Psychiatry* **37**, 378.

Andersen, J. A., Hansen, B. F., and Lyngborg, K. (1975) *Acta Med. Scand.* **197**, 61.

Aravanis, C., and Luisada, A. A. (1957) *Am. Heart J.* **54**, 32.

Bedford, P. D., and Caird, F. I. (1960) *Valvular Disease of the Heart in Old Age*, J.&A. Churchill, London.

Bland, E. F., and Jones, T. D. (1951) *Circulation* **4**, 836.

Caird, F. I., Kennedy, R. D., and Kelly, J. C. C. (1973) *Gerontol. Clin.* **15**, 366.

Carroll, D. (1951) *Bull. Johns Hopkins Hosp.* **89**, 309.

Clark, W. S., Kulka, J. P., and Bauer, W. (1957) *Am. J. Med.* **22**, 580.

Cox, T. J. N., and Schlesinger, B. R. (1956) *Great Ormond St. J.* **11**, 38.

Currens, J. H. (1967) *J. Am. Med. Assoc.* **199**, 849.

Dillon, J. C., Haine, C. L., Chang, S., and Feigenbaum, H. (1971) *Circulation* **43**, 503.

El-Sherif, N. (1971) *Br.Heart J.* **33**, 16.

Epstein, E. J., and Coulshed, N. (1964) *Br. Heart J.* **26**, 84.

Epstein, E. J., and Coulshed, N. (1973) *Br. Heart J.* **35**, 260.

Fenichel, N. M. (1950) *Am. Heart J.* **40**, 117.

Finegan, R. E., Gianelly, R. E., and Harrison, D. C. (1969) *N. Engl. J. Med.* **281**, 1261.

Forker, A. D., McCallister, B. D., Giuliani, E. R., and Osmundson, P. J. (1970) *J. Am. Med. Assoc.* **212**, 774.

Garner, F. E., and White, P. D. (1949) *Ann. Intern. Med.* **31**, 1,003.

Gibson, D. (1973) *In* Hamer, J. (ed.), *Recent Advances in Cardiology*, 6th edition, Churchill Livingston, London and Edinburgh, p. 266.

Glancy, D. L., Freed, T. A., O'Brien, K. P., and Epstein, S. E. (1969) *Ann. Intern. Med.* **71**, 245.

Glover, J. A. (1930) *Lancet* **1**, 499.

Goodwin, J. F. (1963) *Lancet* **1**, 464.

Goodwin, J. F. (1970) *Lancet* **1**, 731.

Goodwin, J. F., Rab, S. M., Sinha, A. K., and Zoob, M. (1957) *Br. Med. J.* **2**, 1383.

Gouley, B. A., and Sickel, E. M. (1943) *Am. Heart J.* **26**, 24.

Gramiak, R., and Shah, P. M. (1970) *Radiology* **96**, 1.

Gray, I. R. (1956) *Br. Heart J.* **18**, 21.

Harvey, W. P. (1968) *Am. J. Cardiol.* **21**, 328.

Hebbert, F. J., and Rankin, J. (1954) *Acta Med. Scand.* **150**, 101.

Hedley, C. F. (1940) *U.S. Publ. Health Rep.* **55**, 1657.

Heggtveit, H. A. (1964) *Circulation* **29**, 346.

Heikilla, J. (1967) *Br. Heart J.* **29**, 162.

Kirk, R. S., and Russell, J. G. B. (1969) *Br. Heart J.* **31**, 684.

Kitchin, A., and Turner, R. (1964) *Br. Heart J.* **26**, 354.

Korn, D., de Sanctis, R. W., and Sell, S. (1962) *N. Engl. J. Med.* **267**, 900.

Korner, P., and Shillingford, J. P. (1957) *Br. Heart J.* **19,** 1.

Kumpe, C. W., and Bean, W. B. (1948) *Medicine (Baltimore)* **27,** 139.

Levine, E., Stein, M., Gordon, G., and Mitchell, N. (1951) *N. Engl. J. Med.* **224,** 902.

Mitchell, A. M., Sackett, C. H., Hunzicker, W. F., and Levine, S. A. (1954) *Am. Heart J.* **48,** 684.

Nasser, W. K., Davis, R. H., Dillon, J. C., Tavel, M. E., Helmen, C. H., Feigenbaum, H., and Fisch, C. (1972) *Am. Heart J.* **83,** 810.

Olesen, K. H. (1955) *Mitral Stenosis: A Follow-up of 351 Patients,* Munksgaard, Copenhagen.

de Pasquale, N. P., and Burch, G. E. (1966) *Am. J. Cardiol.* **17,** 169.

Peery, T. M. (1942) *Arch. Intern. Med.* **70,** 689.

Pomerance, A. (1967) *Br. Heart J.* **29,** 222.

Pomerance, A. (1969) *Br. Heart J.* **31,** 343.

Pomerance, A. (1972) *Gerontol. Clin.* **14,** 1.

Popp, R. L., and Harrison, D. C. (1974) *In* Weissler, A. M. (ed.), *Non-Invasive Cardiology,* Grune and Stratton, New York and London, p. 149.

Popp, R. L., Brown, O. W., Silverman, J. F., and Harrison, D. C. (1974) *Circulation* **49,** 428.

Prewitt, T. A. (1970) *J. Am. Med. Assoc.* **211,** 637.

Roberts, W. C., and Sjoerdsma, A. (1964) *Am. J. Med.* **36,** 5.

Roberts, W. C., Perloff, J. K., and Constantino, T. (1971) *Am. J. Cardiol.* **27,** 497.

Rodstein, M., and Zeman, F. D. (1967) *Am. J. Med. Sci.* **254,** 577.

Ruffin, N. de G., Castleman, B., and White, P. D. (1941) *Am. Heart J.* **22,** 458.

Rytand, D. A., and Lipsitch, L. S. (1946) *Arch. Intern. Med.* **78,** 544.

Sievers, J., and Hall, P. (1971) *Br. Heart J.* **33,** 833.

Simon, M. A., and Liu, S. F. (1954) *Am. Heart J.* **48,** 497.

Storey, G. (1958) *Br. Heart J.* **20,** 483.

Swan, D. A., Bell, B., Oakley, C. M., and Goodwin, J. F. (1971) *Br. Heart J.* **33,** 671.

Wilson, J. K., and Greenwood, W. F. (1954) *Can. Med. Assoc. J.* **71,** 723.

Winkle, R. A., Lopes, M. G., Fitzgerald, J. W., Goodman, D. J., Schroeder, J. S., and Harrison, D. C. (1975) *Circulation* **52,** 73.

12

Remediable Heart Disease
BACTERIAL ENDOCARDITIS, HEART DISEASE AND THE
THYROID, HEART DISEASE AND ANEMIA, PERICARDIAL
DISEASE

JOHN WEDGWOOD

Bacterial Endocarditis

Bacterial endocarditis in both its acute and subacute forms is increasingly common in the elderly. It is usually possible to distinguish the two forms of the disease on clinical grounds. The distinction is valuable and will be used in this chapter, although its limitations are recognized.

For convenience, the abbreviations *SBE*, *ABE,* and *BE* will be used for subacute, acute, and bacterial endocarditis, respectively, and *NBTE* for nonbacterial thrombotic endocarditis.

Subacute Bacterial Endocarditis

This disease was first described in the elderly by Gibson (1896). Although the total annual number of cases has apparently changed very little since 1939 (Hayward 1973), the incidence of SBE in the old has increased dramatically in the last 30 years. In a large series of cases from different authors reported in 1936 (Perry 1936), only 6% were over 60, and the peak incidence was in the third decade. Ten years postwar, the peak incidence was in the fourth decade, and 17–18% were over 60 (Anderson and Staffurth 1955, Wedgwood 1955). At

JOHN WEDGWOOD   ·   The Middlesex Hospital, London, W.1., England.

present, the peak incidence appears to be in the sixth and seventh decades (Shinebourne et al. 1969), and 28% are over 60 (Staffurth 1969). Lerner and Weinstein (1966) reported 30% over the age of 60 and a similar general trend. In England and Wales, there were 259 recorded deaths from BE in 1973. Of these, 157, or 60.6%, were over 60 years of age; of these, in turn, 70, or 44.6%, were over 75 years old (Registrar General 1975).

Sex Incidence. In general, there is a preponderance of male over female cases, particularly in old age, where ratios of 3:1 or 5:1 have been reported (Kerr 1964), and even 8:1 in the age group 51–70 years (Lerner and Weinstein 1966). Staffurth (1969) found about equal numbers of male and female cases, but this finding must be taken in the context of the marked preponderance of females in the elderly population of the United Kingdom, where, by the age of 85, the ratio of women to men is itself almost 3:1 (Wedderburn 1973).

Underlying Heart Disease. It is generally accepted that SBE develops in patients with underlying valvular or congenital heart disease, but there has always been a number of cases in which the evidence, particularly in the old, has been uncertain. Staffurth (1969) found that between 31 and 59 years of age, 79% of cases had known previous heart disease; over 60 years, however, the proportion was only 31–42%. Over the 20-year period 1945–1964, *pari passu* with the increasing age incidence of SBE and the decrease in rheumatic fever, the number of cases of SBE giving a history of "miscellaneous" heart disease (as opposed to rheumatic, congenital, or syphilitic) increased from 7.7% to 53.6%. The mean age of the cases giving a past history of rheumatic heart disease was 40.0 years; of "miscellaneous" heart disease, 66.2 years (Hughes and Gauld 1966).

In elderly cases of SBE, the various forms of degenerative and arteriosclerotic heart disease (Chapter 2) are likely to be found underlying the infection. Nodular arteriosclerotic changes on the valves, insufficiency of the posterior mitral valve cusp, calcific aortic sclerosis or stenosis, and calcification of the mitral valve ring (Burnside and Desanctis 1972) are all predisposing lesions. A minimal valve deficiency causing a jet effect is likely to predispose to the disease (Rodbard 1963).

Ejection systolic murmurs are frequently found in elderly patients. Late systolic murmurs from posterior mitral valve cusp defects, particularly vulnerable to SBE (Hayward 1973), mitral pansystolic murmurs, and early diastolic murmurs due to aortic valve ectasia (Bedford and Caird 1960) form a galaxy of murmurs often heard. They are frequently difficult to hear or hemodynamically insignificant, and hence are ignored. It is probable that in many elderly patients with SBE, the evidence of previous heart disease will not have been recorded. Setting aside speculation, the main significance of these lesions is in the prophylaxis and early diagnosis of subacute bacterial endocarditis.

Source of Infection and Bacteriology. An obvious source of infection is relatively uncommon in elderly cases of SBE, and is becoming less common at all ages. In particular, dental sepsis and extraction is a less common cause. Shinebourne et al. (1969) found dental sepsis as a factor in 34% of cases of all ages, but in another 35%, no cause could be found. In the elderly, Wedgwood (1961) found a source of infection in 6 of 13 cases, including 4 with dental sepsis and 2 with recent dental extraction. Staffurth (1969) found a source of infection in only 8 of 47 cases, 1 with dental sepsis. Gastrointestinal and genitourinary sources of infection are more common in the old, particularly in enterococcal infections (Koenig and Kaye 1961). A history of symptoms of respiratory infection is common, but these symptoms may indicate a focus of infection or be symptoms of SBE itself. In general, elderly patients with SBE have a high incidence of carcinoma, surgical or manipulative procedures, and genitourinary infections (Guze and Pearce 1963).

The incidence of *Streptococcus viridans* infection is diminishing, and has fallen from 95% in the pre-penicillin era to 56% (Hayward 1973). The number of cases due to nonhemolytic or microaerophilic streptococci and enterococci is increasing. In the elderly, 42% of cases of SBE were due to *Str. viridans*, 17% to nonhemolytic streptococci, 6% (2 cases) to enterococci, and 10% (3 cases) to *Staphylococcus albus* (Staffurth 1969). The wide spectrum of bacterial and mycotic infections that may cause SBE does not appear to be exclusive to any age group, except for the cases that follow cardiotomy or "mainline" drug addiction. In a series of 400 cases of BE at the Boston City Hospital between 1933 and 1965, Finland and Barnes (1969) found fewer cases over the age of 60 due to hemolytic streptococcus, *Str. viridans, Staph. albus,* and miscellaneous organisms, and more cases due to *Staph. aureus, Str. faecalis,* and gram-negative bacilli.

Persistent Negative Cultures. Cases of SBE with persistently negative blood cultures have been reported in 7–28% of cases in many series since 1951 (Lerner and Weinstein 1966). Shinebourne et al. (1969) reported an incidence of 26% in BE. Their series included a group of 13 cases of SBE with sterile blood cultures and is of particular significance. Cases with negative cultures (or unavailable evidence) were more common over the age of 60 (Finland and Barnes 1969).

Information about SBE with negative cultures is difficult to obtain, because it is influenced by the criteria of selection and diagnosis. Negative cultures may be due to failure to provide specialized growth requirements, to the prior use of antibiotics, or to the presence of infection for prolonged periods when organisms may no longer be released into the bloodstream (Shinebourne et al. 1969), to unusual organisms or fungi, or to the presence of "L forms" of bacteria (Hamburger 1968). The remainder may be cases of nonbacterial thrombotic endocarditis (Barry and Scarpelli 1962, Angrist et al. 1967), a condition that is most common in the aged or in those with terminal disease.

Cases with persistent negative cultures from whatever cause produce major problems of diagnosis and treatment.

Symptoms. The length of history before diagnosis in SBE in the elderly appears to be diminishing. In 13 cases, it varied between 2 and 23 weeks, the mean being 9.3 weeks (Wedgwood 1961). Anderson and Staffurth (1955) found an average of 5.6 months in the seventh decade. Recently, however, it was less than 1 month in 55% of elderly cases (Staffurth 1969). This decrease may be due to increased recognition of the disease in old age, but there is a considerable variation of host response (Hayward 1973). *Streptococcus viridans* can cause a very acute illness in the elderly (Staffurth 1969), and a *Staph. aureus* infection may follow a subacute course. Shinebourne et al. (1969) were unable to show any correlation between length of history before treatment and prognosis. The insidious onset and misleading symptomatology of SBE are well known (Wedgwood 1955). The problem of diagnosis is considerable in the elderly, in whom nonspecific illness is common.

The constitutional symptoms of SBE can be classified as toxemic and febrile (Cates and Christie 1951). Febrile symptoms are not usually

TABLE 12.1. Incidence of Symptoms of SBE in 13 Cases 60–81 Years Old[a]

Toxemic	12	Febrile	7
Loss of weight	11	Fever	4
Anorexia	10	Sweats	4
Weakness	9	Chills	2
Malaise	3	Dyspnea	4
Psychiatric disturbance	6	Cough	4
Pain	6	Hemorrhage (G.U. tract)	1

[a] Wedgwood (1961).

Case Report of SBE

An 80-year-old widow who had had a laparotomy for division of adhesions for small-bowel obstruction on 12/24/73, and who also had a hiatus hernia and iron deficieny anemia, remained in ill health throughout the following nine months with no specific symptoms. She had no appetite and lost weight. She was admitted to the hospital on 9/30/74, at which time she weighed 46.4 kg.

On examination, she appeared tired and ill; she had early finger-clubbing, a petechial hemorrhage in the left lower conjunctiva (see Fig. 12.3) and on the hard palate. There was a soft pansystolic murmur audible at the mitral area and left sternal edge (Figure 12.2).

Her investigations showed: Hb 7.8 g%, WBC 4,800 mm³, and ESR (Westergren) 130 mm/h. Blood cultures on 10/1/74 and 10/2/74 gave a heavy growth of a penicillin-sensitive *Str. viridans* in one of two bottles.

Subsequent laboratory studies indicated a requirement for crystalline penicillin, 12 MU daily, which was given by continuous i.v. drip, and streptomycin, 0.75 g daily. Therapy was continued for 6 weeks.

It was about a year before she returned to her normal health and her sedimentation rate to a normal level.

Fig. 12.1. Case history of SBE.

obvious, although a surprising degree of fever may in fact be present, and toxemic symptoms, usually of weakness, "failure to cope," and weight loss, predominate. Loss of appetite is usually present and may be marked.

Psychiatric symptoms of depression, toxiconfusional states, or paranoid states are common, and may dominate the clinical picture. Persistent pain, often in the back, rather than frank embolism, is another relatively common symptom.

The incidence of the more common symptoms in SBE over the age of 60 is shown in Table 12.1 (Wedgwood 1961). Three common patterns emerge: (1) a combination of weakness, loss of appetite, and loss of weight, likely to be attributed to "carcinoma" (case history: Fig. 12.1); (2) confusional or depressive states, likely to be mistaken for manifestations of cerebral arteriosclerosis; (3) pain in the back or trunk, likely to be confused with symptoms of osteoporosis, spondylitis, or spinal metastases.

Physical Signs. Fever and a heart murmur are the cardinal physical signs, but may be absent on presentation or difficult to elicit. Fortunately, it is rare for both to be absent at the same time.

Fever may be slight or intermittent, unless diligently sought with 4-hourly temperature charts (Fig. 12.2). Even a slight degree of fever is

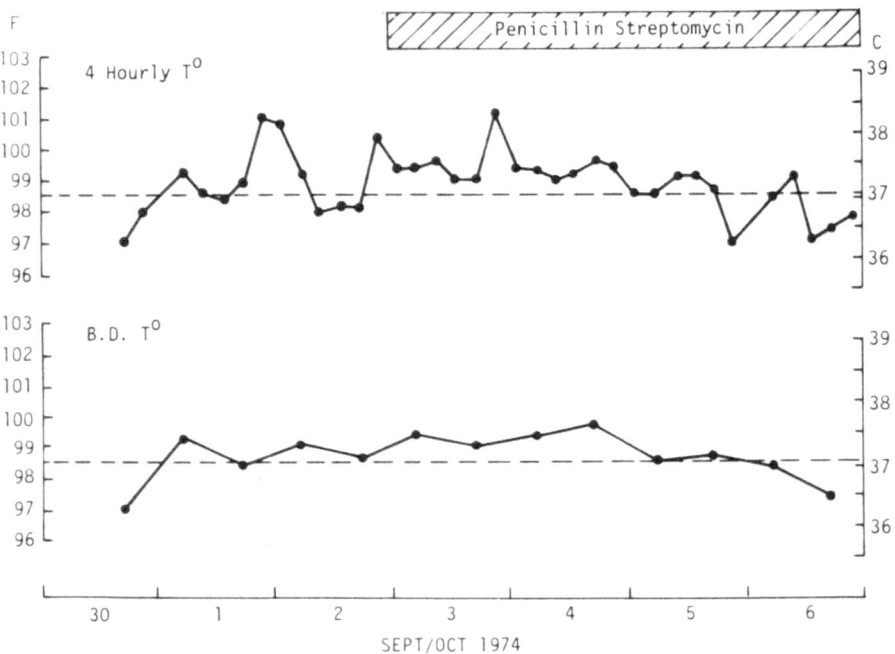

Fig. 12.2. Temperature chart in SBE.

significant in an elderly patient. Conversely, the degree of fever may be surprisingly high and unexpected.

Heart murmurs are usually present, but may be absent when the patient is first seen. No murmur was heard at presentation in 7 of 31 cases (Staffurth 1969). The murmur may also be soft or, because it is of the ejection systolic type, regarded as of no significance. Early diastolic murmurs of aortic incompetence may be absent or easily missed. The most common murmur is a mitral pansystolic or late systolic due to mitral incompetence. An aortic ejection systolic or early diastolic murmur is common, but less frequent.

Further examination of the cardiovascular system may show congestive heart failure, sometimes a presenting symptom, and atrial fibrillation is not rare. The cardiovascular signs in two series of cases are shown in Table 12.2 (Staffurth 1969, Wedgwood 1961).

The classic signs of SBE—café au lait pallor, clubbing, petechiae, Osler's nodes, and embolism—are found singly or in varying combination in about 60% of cases (Staffurth 1969, Wedgwood 1961, (Table 12.3), but cannot be relied on if the diagnosis is to be made early.

TABLE 12.2. Cardiovascular Signs in SBE in the
Elderly on Presentation

Signs	Wedgwood (1961)	Staffurth (1969)
No murmur	0	7 (23%)
Mitral incompetence	11 (85%)	16 (52%)
Aortic incompetence	4 (31%)	8 (26%)
Mitral stenosis	1 (8%)	2 (6%)
Aortic ejection systolic	0	3 (10%)
Atrial fibrillation	2 (16%)	5 (16%)
TOTAL CASES:	11	31

Clubbing is helpful and can appear quickly (Hayward 1973). Petechial hemorrhages are more helpful, particularly in the conjunctivae or oral mucosa (Fig. 12.3), when they are easily found and appear quite early in the disease. Splinter hemorrhages in the nails, unless they are obviously recent and unrelated to trauma, are misleading.

Investigations. Blood cultures are of paramount importance both in diagnosis and in the initiation and control of therapy. Bacteremia, if present, is usually persistent and unrelated to fever (Ridley 1969). There is no advantage in delaying cultures for fever, spacing them

TABLE 12.3. Signs of SBE on Presentation[a]

Signs	Wedgwood (1961) (13 cases over 60)	Staffurth (1969) (31 cases over 60)
Heart murmur	13 (100)	24 (77.4)
Fever	11 (85)	31 (100)
Pallor	8 (62)	—
Clubbing	5 (38)	6 (20)
Splenomegaly	4 (31)	3 (10)
Petechiae	4 (31)	8 (26)
Embolism	2 (15.5)	5 (16)
Osler's nodes	—	2 (6)
Meningitis	—	2 (6)

[a] With acknowledgment to Dr. J. S. Staffurth, Beecham Research, and *Gerontologia Clinica.* Percentages are given in parentheses.

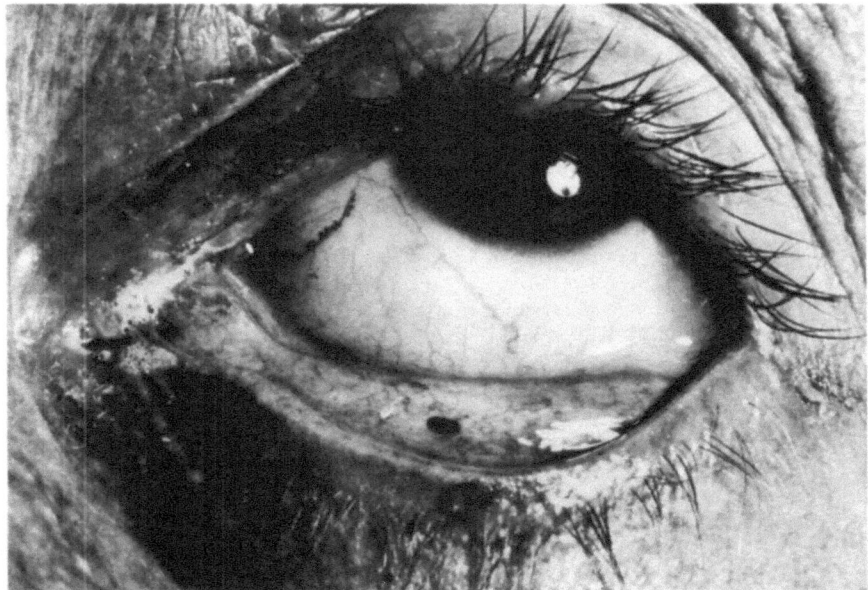

Fig. 12.3. Petechial hemorrhage in conjunctiva in SBE (Wedgwood 1955).

apart by several days, or taking them in excessive numbers. Four to six cultures should be taken within the first two or three days of suspicion of the disease. In most cases, if a positive result is going to be obtained, some growth will be evident within a few days, and treatment can be started pending the final result. The technique of culture, the determination of antibiotic sensitivity, and the control of treatment are highly specialized and require close collaboration between the clinician and the bacteriologist. A helpful discussion is given by Ridley (1969). A brief account of the organisms encountered in the elderly and the problem of persistently negative cultures has been given. Staffurth (1969) emphasizes the importance of treating so-called "contaminants" with suspicion. In difficult cases, estimation of the antibody response to the suspected organism may be helpful.

Other investigations are chiefly of importance in excluding diseases with similar symptoms. A full blood count and sedimentation rate may also be of some use as a screening test, since a normal hemoglobin and a low sedimentation rate are rare. Staffurth (1969) found only 1 case out of 35 with an ESR below 10 mm/h. The ESR may also be unusually high in association with immune complex disease (Hayward 1973).

Examination of the urinary spun deposit for microscopic hematuria was positive in practically all cases of SBE (Shinebourne et al. 1969). It is important to use fresh specimens of urine, which is not always easy in confused, incontinent elderly patients.

Diagnosis. The main difficulty in diagnosis is due to failure to suspect the presence of the disease. The importance of a high "index of suspicion" for this treatable disease cannot be overemphasized for elderly patients with nonspecific symptoms, fever, and a heart murmur, even if the latter is "insignificant."

The small proportion of cases with persistent negative cultures, however, may present a formidable problem. In these cases, diagnosis must rely on clinical criteria, exclusion of other diseases, and well-balanced judgment.

Treatment. It is not within the scope of this chapter to discuss the details of antibiotic therapy. Reference has already been made to the need for close collaboration with the bacteriologist in this area. Similar principles apply to the treatment of SBE at all ages, but there are certain points of particular importance in the older patient. The temptation to depart from recognized therapeutic regimes on the grounds of age should be resisted. Parenteral therapy is necessary in nearly all cases. Crystalline penicillin is still the first choice, but should usually be combined with a second antibiotic.

Continuous intravenous infusion is well tolerated, with proper precautions. It is often preferable to repeated intramuscular injections because of the diminished buttock muscle in elderly, often emaciated patients, and the problem of pressure areas. The duration of treatment should not be curtailed below the usually accepted figure of 4 weeks (Hayward 1973).

The choice of antibacterial agent depends on the organism and its sensitivity. Because of the high incidence of resistant organisms and the occurrence of cases with persistent negative cultures, penicillin and streptomycin are still the most commonly used combination of drugs. The old, with their small body mass and impaired renal function, are particularly at risk. Penicillin in large doses may cause toxic effects, particularly convulsions (Hayward 1973); streptomycin causes ototoxicity in doses as small as 0.25 g. Careful monitoring of blood levels is essential, as is regular observation of auditory function.

Once a therapeutic program is decided on, with proper bacteriological control and satisfactory blood levels of antibiotic, it should be continued. The temperature may persist for one or two weeks with satisfactory treatment, and a low-grade fever may persist throughout the course of treatment if intramuscular injection is used (Hayward 1973). Frequent changes, without proper control, are one of the more common causes of failure in antibacterial treatment. The patient's appetite, weight, mental state, and general well-being are usually a satisfactory guide to success. The ESR, in particular, may not fall until treatment is concluded. Occasional petechiae and minor emboli may also occur in the early stages of a satisfactory regime.

Bacteriologically negative cases present a considerable therapeutic problem. Treatment should be given as for a penicillin-resistant organism, and it is necessary for the clinician to maintain a firm conviction that his diagnosis is correct.

In young patients, particularly those with congenital heart disease, cardiac surgery has greatly improved the outlook in cases with resistant organisms or severe valvular damage and heart failure (Mills et al. 1974). Its possible use in elderly cases, with obvious reservations, should not be entirely ignored.

The therapeutic regime outlined here is prolonged and arduous. Very careful attention must be paid to the patient's mobilization and nutrition, and to the prevention of pressure sores. Proper treatment of associated heart failure and anemia, and attention to electrolyte balance, are also essential to a satisfactory outcome.

Prophylaxis. There is surprisingly little evidence that prophylactic antibiotic cover for dental procedures or minor surgery is effective (Hayward 1973), but it ought nevertheless to be practiced. Elderly patients at risk should be covered for dental extraction or minor surgery by penicillin 600,000 U i.m., 2 h before operation, or ampicillin if an enterococcal infection is likely. Prophylactic treatment for longer periods is contraindicated, because it may produce penicillin-resistant organisms.

The antibiotic treatment of an acute infection in a patient with a heart murmur should not be delayed because of the possibility of SBE. Staffurth (1973) found no evidence that such treatment caused delays in diagnosis.

Prognosis. The mortality of SBE has declined steadily since the advent of the antibiotic era. The overall mortality in bacteriologically positive cases between 1966 and 1972 was 14% (Hayward 1973). The mortality in the elderly is higher. Staffurth (1973) found a mortality of 30% in 31 cases diagnosed during life. Mortality figures are difficult to evaluate in the elderly, particularly in advanced old age, when the actuarial expectation of life is short and the occurrence of associated terminal disease common. Attention should be given to the survivors of an otherwise fatal disease with prolonged preterminal invalidism. A 70% survival rate in this age group is not unsatisfactory.

Acute Bacterial Endocarditis

In the elderly, acute and subacute bacterial endocarditis merge. An acute course, or cases in which the duration of symptoms is short, is being more often recognized. A clinically acute illness can be caused by *Str. viridans* (Staffurth 1973); most commonly, though, ABE is a relatively rare disease caused by a virulent organism, particularly *Staph. aureus*. The history is short. Severe toxemic and febrile symptoms predominate, and pyemic abscesses may occur. Intracutaneous hemorrhages or Janeway lesions (Janeway 1899) are characteristic. In other cases, the evidence of endocarditis in life is equivocal, and the picture is of acute septicemia, often due to a gram-negative organism. Diagnosis and treatment are a matter of great urgency.

Nonbacterial Thrombotic Endocarditis

Traditionally, NBTE occurs as an associated finding at autopsy in patients dying of carcinomatosis or other terminal illness—so-called "marantic" endocarditis. It may also occur in elderly patients, in whom it resembles the "endocarditis lenta" described in young adults exposed to prolonged deprivation and stress, particularly after World War I (Starling 1923, Coombs 1923). The disease has a prolonged course, sometimes several years, with fever and embolization. The aortic valve is usually affected. Some cases with persistently negative cultures may belong in this group (Hayward 1973), but confirmation can be made only by finding bacteria-free vegetations at autopsy.

The possibility that NBTE is a stage in the development of SBE has been suggested and the subject reviewed by Angrist et al. (1967).

Heart Disease and the Thyroid

Heart disease can result from both hyperthyroidism and hypothyroidism. Both conditions present diagnostic problems in the elderly, because the systemic manifestations of the endocrine disease may be masked or absent and the cardiac effects may therefore dominate the clinical picture.

Thyroid disease is not uncommon in geriatric hospitals. Lloyd and Goldberg (1961) reported an incidence of 1.7% of new admissions with hypothyroidism and 0.5% with hyperthyroidism.

Thyrotoxic Heart Disease

Thyrotoxicosis can be associated with atrial fibrillation, cardiac enlargement, and cardiac failure in all age groups. Cardiac involvement increases with age: The concept of the young woman with typical Graves disease and the middle-aged one with an established thyroid nodule and atrial fibrillation is familiar. Thyrotoxicosis becomes less common over the age of 70, but is nevertheless an important disease because the general symptomatology is so variable and "masked" thyrotoxicosis or "apathetic hyperthyroidism" (Lahey 1931) becomes more common. Cardiovascular involvement is more frequent in this age group, and may dominate the clinical picture, with or without coexistent coronary heart disease.

Bartels (1965) stressed the variability of the symptoms of thyrotoxicosis in the elderly and the occurrence of "masked" forms. Atrial fibrillation was present in 32% of their cases, congestive failure in 15%. "Apathetic" thyrotoxicosis is described by Thomas et al. (1970). Weight loss was an important age-related symptom. Myxedema was the diagnosis on admission in 3 of 9 cases. The majority of their cases were elderly; all had congestive failure and cardiac enlargement. Atrial fibrillation was present in 7 of 9 cases.

Atrial fibrillation is a common finding in elderly patients without thyrotoxicosis, occurring in as many as 15% of elderly patients in the hospital (Bedford and Caird 1960). In thyrotoxicosis, atrial fibrillation may be paroxysmal rather than established, but its chief characteristic is the failure of the ventricular rate to respond to digitalis. Evidence of a hyperkinetic circulatory state is not usually impressive (Symons et al. 1971).

A palpable enlarged thyroid gland or nodule was found in 97% of cases of thyrotoxicosis over 60 (Bartels 1965), but in the elderly, particularly with "masked" or "apathetic" thyrotoxicosis, it is much less common.

If the disease is suspected, confirmation can be obtained in most cases by the serum T_4, the T_4 index, and if necessary the serum T_3 values. Slight elevations of the serum T_4 may be equivocal, because they may be found in euthyroid elderly patients (Britton et al. 1975); in doubtful cases, more sophisticated investigations such as the T.R.H. test (Hall et al. 1975) may be required. The difficulties of interpreting thyroid function tests, and the inaccessability or delay involved in the more sophisticated procedures, may indicate the need for a therapeutic trial of antithyroid drugs if the clinical evidence is strong. A carefully supervised trial of carbimazole (Neomercazole) is often of considerable help in diagnosis.

The choice of treatment, among antithyroid drugs, radioiodine and surgery, depends on a careful assessment. Antithyroid drugs, sometimes with propanalol (Inderal) in the first instance, have much to recommend them, unless there is a clear-cut reason for the alternative. Diuretics, sometimes with digitalis, will be required routinely. Care must be taken not to be misled by the failure of the ventricular rate to respond to digitalis, lest overdosage of digitalis result. Atrial fibrillation due to thyrotoxicosis by itself may revert to sinus rhythm after antithyroid treatment, but this reversion does not always occur in the elderly because of the presence of coincident coronary heart disease.

Hypothyroidism

The diagnosis of hypothyroidism is difficult and often unsuspected without laboratory investigation. The disease may present with any of its characteristic symptoms: mental confusion, apathy, myxedema coma or hypothermia, or unexplained ascites or pleural effusions. Congestive heart failure and pericardial effusion are the cardiac manifestations, and are common and important in the old.

The cardiac signs are sinus bradycardia, cardiomegaly, and low-output failure, usually associated with pericardial effusion inferred from the large size of the cardiac silhouette on chest X ray. The classic signs of pericardial effusion are usually equivocal, and the relative contribution of failure and effusion debatable. There is occasionally a pericardial rub. The heart sounds are quiet. Pleural effusion is often present.

The ECG is characteristic, showing generalized low-voltage complexes and flat or inverted T waves. The presence of sinus bradycardia helps to distinguish the electrocardiographic findings from those due to other forms of pericardial disease (Fig. 12.4). The typical findings may occur when there is little clinical evidence of cardiac involvement.

The pathological changes in the heart are variable and not always specific. Coexistent coronary heart disease often complicates the picture, as may the presence of pericardial effusion. The problem is discussed by McKeown (1965). The complexity of the association with coronary artery disease is increased by the occurrence of secondary hyperlipidemia in hypothyroidism.

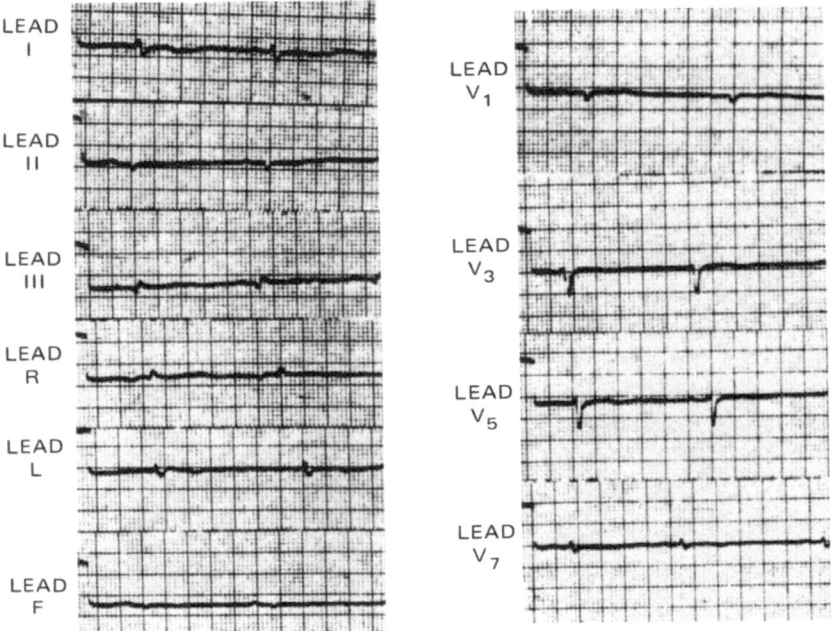

Fig. 12.4. ECG in hypothyroidism. (By courtesy of Dr. G. W. Hayward.)

The presence of delayed relaxation of the deep reflexes is an important aid to clinical diagnosis, and the electrocardiographic findings are often most helpful. Confirmation of the diagnosis can usually be obtained from thyroid function tests, but in equivocal cases, measurement of the serum T.S.H. may be necessary (Hall et al. 1971).

When clinical evidence is suggestive, but laboratory evidence is equivocal, a cautious therapeutic trial of L-thyroxine (Eltroxin) may be indicated. Treatment is often difficult because of the danger of precipitating cardiac failure or cardiac arrhythmias. In the presence of coronary artery disease, cardiac infarction may occur or angina be aggravated. Treatment with L-thyroxin must therefore be very cautious. An initial dose of 0.05 mg, or at most 0.1 mg, increased by similar amounts at weekly intervals, is usually as much as the patient can tolerate, and will have to be reduced with any unfavorable reaction. The patient must be under careful observation until there is obvious clinical improvement, particularly in the ECG changes. Sometimes the patient cannot tolerate the full replacement dose, particularly if symptoms of angina are present, and a compromise must be reached.

Heart Disease and Anemia

Congestive heart failure due to anemia is more common in the old because of coexistent coronary heart disease. It appears to be related to the degree and duration of anemia, and is therefore a more common problem in pernicious anemia. Anemia may also aggravate the symptoms of angina of effort in patients with coronary artery disease. The presence of anemia in patients with signs of valvular heart disease should raise the suspicion of SBE. Typical high-output failure with a hyperkinetic circulation may occur, but congestive failure is often nonspecific due to a mixed pathology.

It is urgent that in the presence of heart failure anemia be diagnosed and treated. The cause of the anemia should be corrected and appropriate hematinics given as soon as possible. If the anemia cannot easily be corrected with reasonable speed, or the symptoms are severe, blood transfusion using packed cells from 1 liter of blood given over 6–8 h at 2- to 3-day intervals, combined with a diuretic such as frusemide (Lasix), and under careful supervision, is well tolerated and should not be witheld (Bedford and Caird 1960).

In severe megaloblastic anemia, particularly in B_{12} deficiency but also in folic acid deficiency, sudden death of cardiac origin may occur in the early stages of specific therapy. Cases particularly at risk are those with a packed-cell volume below 25% and an initial platelet count below 90,000/μl; these findings are thought to be related to a depletion of whole-body potassium. Following specific therapy, usually at the onset of the reticulocyte response, there is a fall in serum potassium that may further embarrass myocardial function. The start of hematinic therapy in severe megaloblastic anemia, particularly if failure is present, should therefore be under close supervision, with a careful watch on the serum potassium and the administration of potassium supplements (Lawson et al. 1972, Leading article 1972).

Pericardial Disease

The Registrar General's returns for 1973 (Registrar General 1975), subject to the reservations of death certification, show a surprisingly high incidence of pericardial disease in the older age groups. Taking acute and chronic nonrheumatic pericardial disease together, there were 152 deaths, of which 81 (53%) were over 70 years of age and 18 (15%) over 85 years.

Clinically, pericarditis is uncommon in the old, except in association with terminal illness, particularly carcinomatosis. It may also occur in uremia. In severe hypothyroidism, a pericardial effusion is common and may be the presenting symptom. Rarely, a purulent pericarditis occurs in association with lobar pneumonia. A pericardial friction rub may be heard after cardiac infarction or later as a result of the postcardiac injury syndrome; it may also be a useful sign of unsuspected rupture of the esophagus. Pericarditis occasionally occurs in elderly patients with severe rheumatoid arthritis. Benign viral pericarditis is rare but not unknown in the old, and confirmed cases of pericarditis due to Coxsackie-group viruses have been recognized in the seventh decade.

Pericardial effusion is more than usually difficult to diagnose in the old. Distortion of the rib cage and senile kyphosis make the physical signs difficult to interpret. It should be suspected, however, if the characteristic venous pulse is observed, an obvious pulsus paradoxus is present, or the cardiac outline is unusually large and the ECG shows the characteristic pattern of low-voltage and flat or inverted T waves. Echocardiography is a valid and noninvasive confirmatory investigation. Aspiration of the pericardium is unlikely to be necessary unless tamponade is present or pyogenic pericarditis suspected.

Constrictive pericarditis is uncommon, but occurs in old age. Two cases over 60 were reported in a successful surgical series (Portal et al. 1966). The condition should be suspected when signs similar to those in pericardial effusion are found with a relatively small heart, particularly if the liver is unusually enlarged and ascites is present. The raised jugular venous pressure is often missed in these cases, who are at first thought to be suffering from liver disease and ascites. The ECG changes are similar to those in pericardial effusion, but atrial fibrillation is common or the P waves in sinus rhythm are conspicuous or bifid. The ECG may be normal (Wood 1962). Calcification may be seen in the pericardium on chest X ray. Age alone should not be a contraindication to surgery. More common in the old is the X-ray finding of patches of calcification in the pericardium, without evidence of constriction, and apparently of no significance.

References

Anderson, H. J., and Staffurth, J. S. (1955) *Lancet* **2**, 1055.
Angrist, A. A., Oka, M., and Na Kao, K. (1967) *In* Sommers, S. C. (ed.), *Pathology Annual*, Butterworth, London.
Barry W. E., and Scarpelli, D. (1962) *Arch. Intern. Med.* **109**, 151.

Bartels, E. C. (1965) *Geriatrics* **20,** 459.

Bedford, P. D., and Caird, F. I. (1960) *In: Valvular Disease of the Heart in Old Age,* Churchill, London.

Britton, K. E., Quinn, V., Ellis, S., Cayley, A. C. D., Miralles, J. M., Brown, B. C., and Ekins, R. P. (1975) *Lancet* **2,** 141.

Burnside, J. W., and Desanctis, R. W. (1972) *Ann. Intern. Med.* **76,** 615.

Cates, J. E., and Christie, R. V. (1951) *Q. J. Med. N.S.* **20,** 93.

Coombs, C. F. (1923) *Q. J. Med., N.S.* **16,** 309.

Finland, M., and Barnes, M. W. (1969) *Bacterial Endocarditis, Proceedings of a National Symposium,* Beecham Research Laboratory, p. 66.

Gibson, W. M. (1896) *Trans. Am. Clin. Climatol. Assoc.* **12,** 174.

Guze, L. B., and Pearce, M. L. (1963) *Arch. Intern. Med.* **112,** 56.

Hall, R., Amos, J., and Ormston, B. J. (1971) *Br. Med. J.* **1,** 582.

Hall, R., Sachdev, Y., and Evered, D. C. (1975) *J. Clin. Pathol.* **28,** 248.

Hamburger, M. (1968) *Arch. Intern. Med.* **122,** 175.

Hayward, G. W. (1973) *Br. Med. J.* **2,** 706, 764.

Hughes, P., and Gauld, W. R. (1966) *Q. J. Med. N.S.* **35,** 511.

Janeway, E. (1899) *Med. News* **75,** 257.

Kerr, A., Jr. (1964) *Mod. Concepts Cardiovasc. Dis.* **33,** 831.

Koenig, M. G., and Kaye, D. (1961) *N. Engl. J. Med.* **264,** 257.

Lahey, F. H. (1931) *Ann. Surg.* **93,** 1026.

Lawson, D. H., Murray, R. M., and Parker, J. L. W. (1972) *Q. J. Med. N.S.* **41,** 1.

Leading Article (1972) *Lancet* **1,** 415.

Lerner, P. I., and Weinstein, L. (1966) *N. Engl. J. Med.* **274,** 199, 259, 323, 338.

Lloyd, W. H., and Goldberg, I. J. L. (1961) *Br. Med. J.* **2,** 1256.

McKeown, F. (1965) *Pathology of the Aged,* Butterworth, London.

Mills, J., Utley, J., and Abbott, J. (1974) *Chest* **66,** 151.

Perry, C. B. (1936) *Bacterial Endocarditis,* John Wright, Bristol.

Portal, R. W., Besterman, E. M. M., Chambers, R. J., Sellors, T. H., and Somerville, W. (1966) *Br. Med. J.* **1,** 563.

Registrar General's Statistical Review of England and Wales for the Year 1973, Part 1(A) (1975) H.M.S.O., pp. 88, 89.

Ridley, M. (1969) *Bacterial Endocarditis, Proceedings of a National Symposium,* Beecham Research Laboratory, p. 49.

Rodbard, S. (1963) *Circulation* **27,** 18.

Shinebourne, E. A., Cripps, C. M., Hayward, G. W., and Shooter, R. A. (1969) *Br. Heart J.* **31,** 536.

Staffurth, J. S. (1969) *Bacterial Endocarditis, Proceedings of a National Symposium,* Beecham Research Laboratory, p. 30.

Starling, H. J. (1923) *Q. J. Med., N.S.* **16,** 263.

Symons, C., Richardson, P. J., and Wood, J. B. (1971) *Lancet* **2,** 7735.

Thomas, F. B., Mazzaferri, E. L., and Skillman, T. G. (1970) *Ann. Intern. Med.* **72,** 679.

Wedderburn, D. (1973) *In* Brocklehurst, J. C. (ed.), *Textbook of Geriatric Medicine and Gerontology,* Churchill Livingstone, Edinburgh and London, p. 692.

Wedgwood, J. (1955) *Lancet* **2,** 1058.

Wedgwood, J. (1961) *Gerontol. Clin. Suppl.* **3,** 11.

Wood, P. (1962) *Disease of the Heart and Circulation,* 2nd edition, Eyre and Spottiswoode, London.

13

Cardiac Glycosides

J. L. C. DALL

Introduction

The cardiac glycosides are the active principles of the plants *Digitalis purpurea,* from which we obtain digitoxin, gitoxin, and gitalin, and *Digitalis lanata,* which yields digoxin. Digoxin is a degradation product of acetyl-digoxin (Lanatoside C). All the glycosides break down to form combinations of sugars with genins (sterol derivates), or aglycones. Glycosides from *Strophanthus* (acetylstrophanthidin, ouabain) are poorly absorbed from the gastrointestinal tract, but may be prepared as pure crystalline substances and given by injection.

The desire to improve prescribing by the use of pure substances led to the change to glycosides in place of digitalis-leaf preparations, which were of variable potency and oftenly poorly absorbed. Recent work on the bioavailability of drugs has shown that chemical purity alone is of relatively little importance (Shaw 1973), and that particle size and formulation determine the rate of dissolution and absorption. Wide variations in commercial preparations have been demonstrated, so that one digoxin preparation may yield serum levels 7 times greater than another. Recent legislation now ensures more standardized bioavailability in digoxin tablets; one of the variables in the problem of maintenance therapy is resolved.

Digoxin is preferred to the other glycosides because it is excreted by the kidney, absorbed well, and acts rapidly. Digitoxin is also well absorbed, but has a long half-life and relatively slow excretion,

J. L. C. DALL · Victoria Infirmary, Glasgow, G42 9TY, Scotland.

because its enterohepatic phase and metabolic degradation are slower than direct renal excretion.

Another important consideration is the level of protein binding. Digitoxin is 98% bound to serum albumin (Schick and Sheurer 1974), so that its therapeutic effect is achieved by the 2% of free drug. Many other drugs in common clinical use—e.g., phenylbutazone (Butazolidin), fenamates, sulfonamides, warfarin, and clofibrate (Atromid-S)— will compete more avidly for the protein-binding sites. A 10% reduction in the protein-binding capacity, which can readily occur, will increase the amount of free digitoxin 5-fold. In these circumstances, maintenance treatment would be difficult, and frequent changes of dose required. Digoxin, on the other hand, is only 25% protein bound, and the therapeutic effect is that of 75% of free drug. An equivalent 10% reduction in protein-binding will increase the free digoxin by only 2.5%. The effect in clinical terms will be negligible, and the need for frequent changes of dosage for this reason should thus not arise.

Much of the information now available has resulted from the development of techniques for measuring the serum level of digoxin. Methods evolved include isotope dilution (Lukas and Peterson 1966), gas chromatography (Watson and Kalman 1971), inhibition of red-cell rubidium uptake (Grahame-Smith and Everest 1969), and radioimmunoassay (Evered et al. 1970). These techniques can be varied to measure glycosides other than digoxin. Radioimmunoassay seems most likely to be adopted by clinical laboratories as the method of choice. Inaccurate results may arise because of preexisting radioactivity in the serum sample, or because of therapy with steroids or steroid antagonists (e.g., spironolactone) at the time of sampling.

Many authors have contributed to the wealth of papers that have helped to establish a "normal" therapeutic range of serum levels, as

TABLE 13.1. Serum Digoxin Levels Related to Toxic Effects

Authors	(Year)	Toxic (mean, ng/ml)	Nontoxic (mean, ng/ml)
Chamberlain et al.	(1970)	3.1	1.4
Smith and Haber	(1970)	3.7	1.4
Evered and Chapman	(1971)	3.36	1.38
Oliver et al.	(1971)	3.0	1.6

opposed to levels associated with toxic effects (see Table 13.1). Many factors are involved in digitalis toxicity, however, of which the serum level of the drug is only one. Simple measurement of the serum level in isolation is thus of little value unless the other factors are known.

Action of Cardiac Glycosides

It is now established that glycosides increase the force and velocity of contraction of cardiac muscle. This positive inotropic effect does not occur in skeletal muscle, and the precise mechanism of action at the subcellular level is still not clear. Nevertheless, there appears to be an optimum value of positive inotropy, which is dependent on the cellular content of sodium, potassium, magnesium, and calcium (Farah 1969).

For some years, it has been appreciated that the cardioactive glycosides could influence the cation content of myocardial cells, and it has been suggested that sodium–potassium adenosine triphosphatase ($Na^+ + K^+$ ATPase) might be a receptor (Glynn 1969, Langer 1971, Schwartz et al. 1969). There is evidence that the positive inotropic responses induced by glycosides are accompanied by a net cellular loss of potassium and a gain of sodium and calcium (Langer and Serena 1970). High extracellular concentrations of potassium and low concentrations of sodium have an inhibitory effect on glycoside activity (Caprio and Farah 1967). Clinical experience suggests that the converse may also be true, since many of the reported toxic effects of glycosides are associated with hypokalemia. The importance of calcium in myocardial cellular activity was appreciated by Ringer (1883), but its exact role is not yet defined. Its importance in cardiac excitation–contraction coupling and the contractility of heart muscle is accepted, and it has been shown that a small labile pool of calcium is closely linked with the contractile activity of the cell (Langer and Serena 1970). The overall ionic change associated with contraction appears to be influx of sodium and calcium, and a loss of potassium and probably magnesium from the cell. Digoxin may act in part by facilitating this transfer. Since the gradients of extra- to intracellular levels of these cations will influence the rate of movement across the cell membrane, the importance of alterations in extracellular electrolyte concentrations by diuretics can be appreciated.

The effect of the glycosides on cardiac muscle is not uniform, but varies with the site studied. It is influenced not only by electrolyte activity, but also by hypoxia and pH. Atrial and ventricular myocardial cells show an increase in force and velocity of contraction, coupled with a shortened refractory period, which is reflected in the shortening of the Q–T interval on the ECG. In the specialized conducting tissues, on the other hand, the refractory period is increased, and conduction velocity decreased, so that in sinus rhythm the P–R interval is prolonged, and in atrial fibrillation the ventricular response rate is reduced.

The hemodynamic effects of these biophysical actions have been observed in the normal and failing heart. The effects on the nonfailing heart have been difficult to interpret, but most authors now agree that the administration of glycosides to normal subjects has an effect on the myocardium. The cardiac output is unchanged because of compensating effects on peripheral arterial resistance, carotid baroreceptors, and ventricular filling pressures (Rodman et al. 1961). In the failing heart, the same effects on the myocardial cells result in shortening of fiber length, increased cardiac output, fall in ventricular end-diastolic pressure, improved cardiac filling, and a fall in the central venous pressure. This sequence of events has made the cardioactive glycosides the cornerstone of treatment of heart failure.

Where cardiac failure is complicated by atrial fibrillation, the selective action on conducting tissue reduces the ventricular rate, improves coronary flow and myocardial oxygenation, and improves ventricular filling, as well as increasing the force and velocity of contraction, and so improving the cardiac output. It is in this situation that the action of glycosides is seen to best advantage.

Although digitalis is a powerful vagal stimulant, the bradycardia it induces is not vagus-dependent and can be induced in the fully atropinized subject.

Use of Glycosides

Heart Failure

The cardiac glycosides are the drugs of choice where there is evidence of heart failure. Where failure has resulted from primary cardiac disease (see Chapter 6), maintenance therapy is likely to be required after compensation has been achieved, but the situation should be reviewed, since digitalis is a toxic drug with serious side effects, and can be withdrawn completely in many elderly patients (Dall 1970). When atrial fibrillation is present, the ventricular rate is a good guide to the adequacy of digitalization, and may be used to control maintenance therapy. Excessive slowing of the ventricular rate below 60 beats/minute is an indication for reducing dosage. An increase in ventricular rate usually requires an increased dose of glycoside. It is at this point that many other factors—including electrolyte balance, pH, thyroid activity, hypoxia, and renal function—come into play, and the safety margin between therapeutic and toxic effects is blurred. When the heart is in sinus rhythm, the clinician gets little guidance from the rate alone, and must use the level of central venous pressure as his best guide to whether compensation has been achieved or not. Tachycardia and edema per se are poor indicators, since each has many other causes in the elderly that are unrelated to heart disease.

Arrhythmias

It is important to note that digitalis poisoning can induce all abnormal rhythms. It must always be established that no glycoside has been given before treatment is started.

Atrial Fibrillation. Atrial fibrillation is the most common abnormal rhythm and the one in which the glycosides are most easily seen to be effective. When rapid atrial fibrillation fails to respond readily to digitalization, thyrotoxicosis should be suspected.

Atrial Flutter. Digitalization slows the heart rate and may cause the rhythm to change to atrial fibrillation. Once the heart is adequately digitalized, if the patient is not in cardiac failure, treatment should be stopped to see whether sinus rhythm will return. Failing this, cardioversion is justified if the flutter is of recent onset, before maintenance digoxin is decided on.

Paroxysmal Atrial Tachycardia. Paroxysmal atrial tachycardia with a rapid ventricular rate is an indication for rapid digitalization; recurring attacks may be suppressed by maintenance digoxin therapy. It should be noted that atrial tachycardia with A-V block and slow ventricular rate is a sign of digitalis toxicity detectable only by ECG appearances.

Supraventricular Tachycardia. In supraventricular tachycardia, as in the other tachyarrhythmias, the blocking action on the A-V conducting tissue protects the ventricle and slows the ventricular response. This blocking will allow improved coronary filling and reduce myocardial hypoxia, which may be a factor in the production or maintenance of the abnormal rhythm.

Bradyarrhythmias. Progressive increase in digitalization will lengthen the P–R interval of the normal heart, but not usually to more than 0.25 s. Where there is already some degree of conduction defect, such as first or second degree heart block, digitalization may accentuate the delay and cause atrioventricular dissociation. It is probably best to avoid the use of the glycosides in this situation. Where complete heart block and cardiac failure coexist, digitalization will improve cardiac output without affecting the conduction defect, and is not contraindicated.

Choice of Preparation

Digoxin is the glycoside in most common use, and is one of the four most frequently prescribed drugs. It is well absorbed from the gastrointestinal tract (75%), and effective within 1 to 3 h. It has a half-life of 36 h when renal function is normal (Smith and Haber 1973). The absorption of digoxin is enhanced by drugs that reduce gastric motility, such as anticholinergic drugs, but the efficiency of absorption is reduced by diarrhea, intestinal hurry, or the malabsorption syndrome, or when the drug is taken with food. Nonabsorbed substances like antacids, kaolin, neomycin, and cholestyramine interfere with digoxin absorption (Manninen et al. 1973; White et al. 1971). These should therefore be given some time after digoxin.

Acetyl strophanthidin and ouabain may be given intravenously and are rapidly effective, but there is seldom justification for using them in the elderly. The prolonged half-life of digitoxin increases the risk of toxic effects during maintenance therapy if excretion is impaired.

Influence of Cations

The introduction of the thiazide group of diuretics into common clinical use in 1959 was marked by an abrupt increase in the number of communications in the medical press relating to digoxin or digitalis glycoside poisoning. The clinical importance of potassium in this situation was quickly appreciated, and the association of toxic arrhythmias in those who became hypokalemic and the value of potassium administration to correct these arrhythmias was established (von Capeller et al. 1959, Soffer 1961, Caird 1963).

Further experimental work has shown that serum magnesium levels are closely related to potassium levels, and that magnesium is also lost during thiazide diuresis. Animal experiments show that pretreatment with magnesium increases the tolerance of digoxin by the myocardium, and when abnormal rhythms have been induced by digoxin in magnesium-depleted animals, these rhythms can be corrected by the administration of magnesium (Neff et al. 1972).

While the effects of potassium loss and magnesium depletion are parallel, and it seems likely that potassium is the more important of the two, the possibility of magnesium depletion must not be overlooked in the difficult clinical situation where extreme sensitivity to digitalis glycosides hinders maintenance therapy.

Whereas a reduction in potassium levels increases the sensitivity to digoxin, an increase to hyperkalemic levels interferes with the utilization of digoxin by the myocardial cell, and in consequence digoxin is less effective. A similar situation arises in hyponatremia, and in these circumstances, the heart is apparently unresponsive to normal dosage levels of glycosides.

The relationship between calcium ions and the myocardial cell is still to be clarified, but it is reasonable to assume that in hypokalemia, the relative excess of calcium ions within the cell may result in increased irritability, and so induce the toxic arrhythmias of clinical experience. Administration of potassium ions is known to correct the situation, but it has also been shown that reduction in extracellular calcium levels by administration of disodium EDTA is equally effective (Szekely and Wynne 1963). In both therapeutic endeavors, the balance between potassium and calcium is being restored and myocardial irritability is reduced.

Arrhythmias apparently due to digitalis toxicity can occur when the serum level of digoxin is in the therapeutic range, and the cause of the arrhythmias is a matter for debate (Fogelman et al. 1971). Animal experiments have shown that the maintenance of normal cation balance increases tolerance to digitalis glycosides. If cardiotoxicity is linked to disturbed calcium and potassium balance, this linking would explain why the toxic arrhythmias, which were relatively uncommon before the introduction of thiazide diuretics, are now accepted as the most common single "toxic" effect of digitalis, and the one most likely to occur first as the toxic state develops (Dall 1970).

Since digitalis toxicity is the result of the interaction of many factors, the serum levels of the glycoside must be interpreted as part of the whole clinical picture. Nevertheless, many investigations have shown that although there is an overlap between "nontoxic" and "toxic" values of serum digoxin levels, levels of less than 2 ng/ml are not usually associated with toxic signs, and point to one of the previously mentioned factors that increase sensitivity to digoxin—

e.g., hypokalemia, hypomagnesemia, hypothyroidism, or hypoxia—as a contributory factor, whereas levels greater than 2 ng/ml suggest that excessive dosage or impaired renal excretion is responsible.

The toxic effects of digoxin may be divided into cardiac and noncardiac. All forms of abnormal rhythm may occur, from occasional to frequent ectopic beats, coupled rhythms, supraventricular tachycardia with or without atrioventricular block, ventricular tachycardia, and ventricular fibrillation. The last is thought to be responsible for death associated with tachyarrhythmia. At the other end of the spectrum, bradycardia, prolonged P–R interval, with latent or second or third degree heart block, may occur. Chung (1971) has provided a very detailed account of the cardiac dysrhythmias associated with digitalis toxicity. It is important to remember that no single feature identifies these abnormal rhythms as induced by digitalis; all can occur in patients who have established cardiac damage and are not taking digitalis. The availability of a rapid estimation of serum digoxin levels may be most helpful in establishing whether digoxin is the cause.

The noncardiac features of glycoside toxicity include anorexia and nausea, which appear to be due to a central action on the medulla and are dose-related. Gastric irritation is less frequent with the purified glycosides, but intestinal necrosis with diarrhea may occur. In the elderly, confusion, delirium, and psychotic disturbances occur as frequently as gastrointestinal symptoms (Dall 1970), and may be the presenting feature. Yellow vision and gynecomastia are recorded, but are rare (Le Winn 1953, Dall 1965).

Treatment of Digitalis Toxicity

The noncardiac features appear to be dose-related (Beller et al. 1971); when they are present, therapy should be interrupted until serum levels have been measured. When symptoms are minimal, it can be difficult to differentiate the nausea of hepatic congestion in congestive cardiac failure from that due to digoxin, and other features such as the heart rate and the ECG can be used as a guide. A rapid arrhythmia constitutes an urgent situation. Potassium or magnesium deficiency must be assumed, even if the serum levels of these electrolytes are normal. Oral potassium therapy is safe, and potassium chloride and magnesium sulphate should be given. Life-threatening ectopic rhythms require urgent treatment with phenytoin sodium, lignocaine, or propanolol, all of which may be slowly given intravenously, under the control of continuous ECG monitoring. If there is no response, DC countershock may be tried. Since the arrhythmia is due to digitalis toxicity, however, reversal with countershock is likely to be temporary until the basic cause is corrected. In the face of a massive overdosage, cholestyramine, given orally, will inhibit absorption of digoxin and the other glycosides from the gut; phenytoin sodium will enhance liver enzyme handling, especially where digitoxin or digitalis leaf has been taken. These measures should be used as adjuavants to the measures already described.

Recently, glycoside-specific antibodies produced in sensitized animals have been shown to be useful in protection from large doses of glycosides, and may prove to have a place in the management of the toxic arrhythmias (Smith and Haber 1973).

When digoxin causes severe depression of A–V conduction with bradycardia, atropine is usually effective, but occasionally electrical pacing may be required temporarily for extreme bradycardia (Biggar and Strauss 1972).

In the elderly, these toxic disturbances of rhythm are of serious consequence, and a fatal outcome is not infrequent (Dreifus et al. 1963). Age is often cited as a factor in digitalis toxicity, but it is probably relevant only in that elderly patients have poorer hearts, take a diet that is low in potassium (Judge et al. 1974, Dall and Gardiner 1971), and have impaired renal function. Nevertheless, if age serves to remind clinicians to consider these factors, it is worth preserving the status quo.

Digitalization Program

It is well established that digitalis glycosides should be used with caution in the elderly patient. There must be an absolute indication for starting treatment. Cardiac failure and rapid atrial fibrillation are the only good reasons, and there should be at least one trial period without therapy before the need for a maintenance regime is accepted as proved. Without proceeding to computer assistance (Peck et al. 1973), it is prudent to review renal function and electrolyte status regularly, as well as the serum digoxin level when this can readily be done.

Since the glomerular filtration rate can be expected to be less than normal in most elderly subjects, even when the serum urea concentration is normal, the half-life of digoxin is likely to be prolonged. Digitalization can usually be effected by 0.25 mg digoxin daily over a period of 3 to 4 days (Taylor et al. 1974). A more rapid effect can be achieved by a parenteral loading dose of 0.25 mg initially, but intravenous therapy is seldom justified in heart failure. In all cases, it is important to establish whether digoxin has already been given within the preceding 5 days, and whether the patient has been receiving thiazide diuretics, which may have already caused a degree of potassium deficiency. In either of these circumstances, 0.25 mg digoxin should be given as a single dose in the first 24 h until the effect on the ECG can be observed, and there is an opportunity to evaluate the electrolyte status.

Maintenance dosage should seldom exceed 0.25 mg digoxin daily 7 days each week. Signs of intolerance to this regime suggest potassium or magnesium deficiency, or both, or severe renal failure. Under these circumstances, the maintenance dose should be 0.125 mg or 0.0625 mg digoxin daily. Conversely, failure to achieve a therapeutic effect on a dosage of 0.25 mg daily may indicate hyponatremia, hyperkalemia, or thyrotoxicosis.

Conclusion

Digoxin is a potent and effective drug, and toxic effects reflect on the prescribing physician, rather than on the glycoside.

References

Beller, G. A., Smith, T. W., Abelman, W. H. (1971) *N. Engl. J. Med.* **284**, 989.

Bigger, J. R., Jr., Strauss, H. C. (1972) *Semin. Drug Treat.* **2**, 147.

Caird, F. I. (1963) *Postgrad. Med. J.* **39**, 408.

Caprio, A., and Farah, A. (1967) *J. Pharmacol. Exp. Ther.* **155**, 403.

Chamberlain, D. A., White, R. J., Howard, M. R. (1970) *Br. Med. J.* **3**, 429.

Chung, E. K. (1971) *Principles of Cardiac Arrhythmias*, Williams and Wilkins, Baltimore.

von Capeller, D., Copeland, G. D., and Stern, T. N. (1959) *Ann. Intern. Med.* **50**, 869.

Dall, J. L. C. (1965) *Lancet* **1**, 194.

Dall, J. L. C. (1970) *Br. Med. J.* **2**, 705.

Dall, J. L. C., and Gardiner, M. (1971) *Gerontol. Clin.* **13**, 119.

Dreifus, L. S., McNight, E. H., Katz, N., and Likoff, W. (1963) *Geriatrics* **18**, 494.

Evered, D. C., and Chapman, C. (1971) *Br. Heart J.* **33**, 540.

Evered, D. C., Chapman, C., Hayter, C. J. (1970) *Br. Med. J.* **3**, 427.

Farah, A. (1969), *In* Fisch, C., and Surawicz, B. (eds.), *Digitalis*, Grune and Stratton, New York, p. 55.

Fogelman, A. M., La Mont, J. T., and Finkelstein, S. (1971) *Lancet* **2**, 727.

Glynn, M. (1969) *In* Fisch, C., and Surawicz, B. (eds.), *Digitalis*, Grune and Stratton, New York, p. 30.

Grahame-Smith, D. G., and Everest, M. S. (1969) *Br. Med. J.* **1**, 286.

Judge, T. G., Caird, F. I., Leask, R. G. S., and Macleod, C. (1974) *Age and Ageing* **3**, 158.

Langer, G. H. (1971) *N. Engl. J. Med.* **285**, 1065.

Langer, G. H., and Serena, S. D. (1970) *J. Mol. Cell. Cardiol.* **1**, 65.

Le Winn, E. B. (1953) *N. Engl. J. Med.* **248**, 316.

Lukas, D. J., and Peterson, R. E. (1966) *J. Clin. Invest.* **45**, 782.

Manninen, V., Apajalahti, A., and Melin, J. (1973) *Lancet* **1**, 398.

Neff, M. S., Mendelssohn, S. Kim, K. E., Banach, A., Swatz, C., and Seller, R. E. (1972) *Am. J. Cardiol.* **29**, 377.

Oliver, G. C., Parker, B. M., and Parker, C. W. (1971) *Am. J. Med.* **51**, 186.

Peck, C. C., Sheiner, L. B., Martin, C. M., Darrel, T., Coomb, M. D., and Melmon, K. L. (1973) *N. Engl. J. Med.* **289**, 441.

Ringer, S. (1883) *J. Physiol. (London)* **4**, 222.

Rodman, T., Gorczyca, C. A., and Pastor, B. H. (1961) *Ann. Intern. Med.* **55**, 620.

Schwartz, A., Allen, J. C., Harigaya, S. (1969) *J. Pharmacol. Exp. Ther.* **168**, 31.

Shaw, T. R. D. (1973) *Lancet* **2**, 209.

Shick, D., and Sheuer, J. (1974) *Am. Heart J.* **87**, 253.

Smith, T. W., and Haber, E. (1970) *J. Clin. Invest.* **49**, 2377.

Smith, T. W., and Haber, E. (1973) *N. Engl. J. Med.* **289**, 1063, 1125.

Soffer, A. (1961) *Arch. Intern. Med.* **107**, 681.

Szekeley, P., and Wynne, N. A. (1963) *Br. Heart J.* **25**, 589.

Taylor, B. B., Kennedy, R. D., and Caird, F. I. (1974) *Age and Ageing* **3**, 79.

Watson, E., and Kalman, S. M. (1971) *J. Chromatograph.* **56**, 209.

White, R. J., Chamberlain, D. H., and Howard, M. (1971) *Br. Med. J.* **1**, 380.

14

Diuretics

J. L. C. DALL

Introduction

Urine formation starts with ultrafiltration at the glomerulus. The ultrafiltrate is then subjected to osmotic effects and the influence of electropotential gradients as it passes through to the collecting ducts. Sodium is reabsorbed from at least three sites, the proximal convoluted tubule, the ascending limb of the loop of Henle, and the distal convoluted tubule. The purpose of diuretic therapy is to obtain sodium and water loss, and the various drugs in clinical use interfere with sodium reabsorption and conservation at one or more of these sites in the nephron.

Sites of Action

Digoxin exerts its diuretic effect primarily by improvement in *glomerular filtration*, although it is also thought to have a weak inhibitory effect on distal tubular sodium reabsorption (Strickler and Kessler 1961). The xanthine derivatives such as aminophylline act in a similar manner.

In the proximal convoluted tubule, sodium reabsorption is active; the consequent secondary reabsorption of chloride and water keeps the filtrate isosmotic. The mercurial diuretics and the thiazides act at this point (Beyer and Baer 1962), but their main site of action is more

J. L. C. DALL · Victoria Infirmary, Glasgow, G42 9TY, Scotland.

likely to be in the distal tubule (Levitt and Goldstein 1962), or at several points.

Ethacrynic acid (Edecrin) appears to act on the *loop of Henle,* and possibly on the proximal tubule (Cannon et al. 1963, Goldberg et al. 1964). Frusemide (Lasix) also appears to act primarily on the loop of Henle, although actions on the proximal tubule have been postulated (Seldin et al. 1966).

Most diuretics can be shown to act on the *distal convoluted tubule,* where effects on ion exchange result in potassium loss. The aldosterone antagonist spironolactone (Aldactone), and also triamterene (Dytac) and amiloride (Midamor), have a weak action on the distal tubule, and achieve sodium loss by inhibiting cation exchange, with consequent potassium conservation. Their principal place is in combination with thiazides.

Groups of Diuretic Drugs

Mercurial diuretics have been superseded by oral drugs, which are more potent and need not be given by injection. The mercurial diuretics were nephrotoxic, the injections were painful, and skin rashes not uncommon.

Benzothiadiazines (thiazides) are available in many preparations (Table 14.1), which have little to differentiate them from the original chlorothiazide (Saluric), except for more efficient absorption and therefore smaller relative dose. They are effective in all but resistant edema resulting from renal failure or severe electrolyte disorder. In the normal subject, their duration of action is about 8–12 h. Potassium loss occurs because of distal tubular inhibition and stimulation of aldosterone secretion (Laragh 1962), and a potassium supplement or combination with a potassium-sparing agent is therefore required. They are to be regarded as moderately potent diuretics, useful for maintenance therapy in cardiac failure and in the treatment of hypertension.

Chlorthalidone (Hygroton), a nonthiazide, has a prolonged action (18–24 h), which limits its usefulness, as its diuretic effect is not greater than that of the thiazides.

Frusemide is an analogue of the thiazides. It is a more potent and rapidly acting diuretic. Although over 24 h it causes no greater loss of sodium and water than the thiazides (Forrester and Shiriffs 1965), its prompt action within minutes when given intravenously has estab-

TABLE 14.1. Diuretics in Common Use

Action	Diuretic	Usual dose (mg/day)
Powerful	frusemide (furosemide)[a]	40–80
	bumetanide[a]	0.5–1
	ethacrynic acid	50–100
Moderate	Thiazides	500–1000
	chlorothiazide	50–100
	hydrochlorothiazide[a]	5–10
	bendrofluazide (bendroflumethiazide)[a]	50–100
	hydroflumethiazide	
	Analogues	50–100
	chlorthalidone[a]	0.25–1
	cyclopenthiazide[a]	20–60
	clopamide[a]	25–50
	mefruside	
Weak	spironolactone[b]	100[c]
	triamterene[b]	100–200
Potassium-sparing	amiloride[b]	5–10

[a] Also available with added potassium.
[b] Also available with added thiazide.
[c] As Aldactone-A.

lished it as the drug of choice in acute left ventricular failure. When renal function is normal, its duration of action when given by mouth is estimated as 4–8 h. Its powerful action results in greatly increased urinary frequency, which may make it unacceptable as maintenance therapy in many patients. In established severe cardiac failure, it is superior to the thiazides, and if incremental doses up to 500 mg/day are used, resistant edema is seldom encountered, even in the presence of renal failure. Potassium loss is significant, and should always be replaced.

Ethacrynic acid is unrelated to the thiazides. Like frusemide, it is most effective when rapid diuresis is required in an emergency (Ledingham 1964), or when edema has become refractory to thiazides. It can then be used alone, or in conjunction with thiazides to add the "loop" effect and augment the distal tubular effect of the thiazides. Massive diuresis may be dangerous (Daley and Evans 1963), and potassium loss is severe.

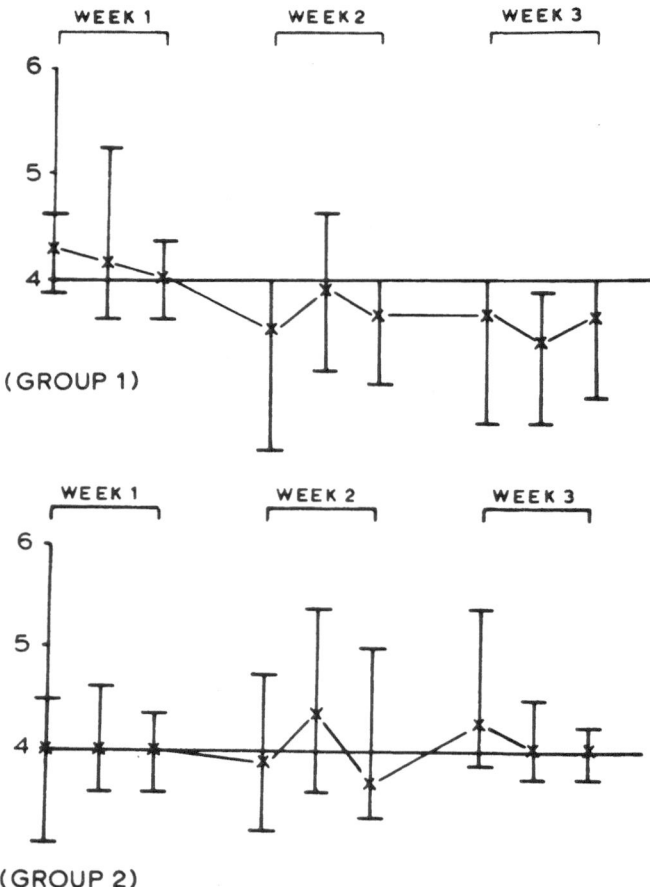

Fig. 14.1. Mean serum potassium levels (mmol/liter) in 12 elderly patients on frusemide, 40 mg daily, alone (*Group 1*), and frusemide, 40 mg, plus amiloride, 5 mg (*Group 2*). Dall, MacFarlane, and Kennedy (1971).

Spironolactone is structurally similar to aldosterone, and blocks its action on the distal tubule. It has a short duration of action and a cumulative effect, so that it must be given every 6 h over a period of days to achieve its effect. It is seldom of value on its own, but may be used with a thiazide or frusemide in resistant cardiac edema, in a dose of 250 mg every 6 h (Aldactone) or 25 mg every 6 h (Aldactone A).

Triamterene has a weak natriuretic effect, and may be used in combination with thiazides to minimize potassium loss in maintenance therapy (Wilson 1963).

Amiloride has a similar action to triamterene on the distal tubule, blocking the exchange of potassium for sodium. It is thus a weak natriuretic, and its potassium-sparing effect appears to be more potent than that of its predecessors (Lant et al. 1969). It has been shown to be of value in the elderly (MacFarlane and Kennedy 1972). A daily dose of 5 mg protects against potassium depletion resulting from thiazides or frusemide (Dall et al. 1971a; Fig. 14.1).

Side Effects

Skin rashes were frequent with mercurial diuretics, and all the more modern oral diuretics have the same potential, but sufficient preparations are now available to allow a change of regime without interruption of treatment.

Potassium depletion is not so much a side-effect as an inevitable consequence of diuretic therapy, even when there is no abrupt diuresis, as during hypotensive therapy. It is particularly a consequence of treatment with diuretics acting on the loop of Henle and of the thiazides. Potassium loss is greatest in patients with cirrhosis and the nephrotic syndrome, in whom aldosterone secretion contributes to overall potassium loss (Laragh 1962); in young patients eating a good diet containing perhaps 100 mEq potassium/day, depletion may occur only after prolonged therapy. Even normal elderly patients, however, may have a low dietary potassium intake of 50 mEq/day or less (Judge and Macleod 1968, Dall and Gardiner 1971, Judge et al. 1974), and in them potassium depletion is readily produced. The clinical picture is one of muscular weakness, constipation, depression, and increased sensitivity to digitalis. This picture may occur early in diuretic therapy, and the state of deficiency may be concealed by a normal serum potassium level. Values of less than 4 mmol K should be taken as evidence of potassium depletion. Either a potassium-sparing regime or adequate supplements must be given from the outset, and continued until the diuretic is stopped.

Since there is evidence that potassium depletion is accompanied by intracellular alkalosis (Aber et al. 1962), replacement therapy should include chloride ion. Unfortunately, an acceptable formulation of potassium chloride is still awaited, and default on potassium supple-

mentation is frequent. The average requirement of potassium supplement for elderly patients on maintenance diuretic regimes has been
estimated as 24 mEq K^+ per day (Dall *et al.* 1971*b*), or more if the
patient is ill or subjected to intense diuresis. "Slow-K" (600 mg KCl =
8.5 mEq K^+) is relatively well tolerated, and should be given 3 times a
day. Ulceration of the small bowel attributed to potassium chloride
has been described in debilitated patients with poor diet. In these
circumstances, potassium supplementation should be achieved with
effervescent preparations (e.g., Kloref − 500 mg KCl = 6.7 mEq K^+) or
with tomato or fruit juice concentrates.

Hyperuricemia is common to all diuretic regimes, but precipitation
of acute gout is rare (Leading article 1975), and the serum uric acid
falls when treatment is withdrawn.

Hyperglycemia is of greater concern. All the potent thiazide
diuretics can uncover latent diabetes, can aggravate preexisting mild
diabetes, and can even induce diabetic ketosis or nonketotic coma
(Toivonen and Mustala 1966, Hicks 1973, Lavender and McGill 1974).
The effect may or may not be reversible by discontinuance of the
diuretic.

Choice of Diuretic

In *emergencies* or in severe cardiac failure, the potent "loop"
diuretics such as frusemide or ethacrynic acid should be used unless
contraindicated by known previous sensitivity. The response to oral
therapy is prompt, and intravenous therapy with frusemide, 20 mg, or
ethacrynic acid, 25 mg, is needed only in urgent clinical situations.
Oral frusemide (40–80 mg daily) or ethacrynic acid (50–100 mg daily)
should be adequate, but if renal failure is severe or edema refractory,
doses of 500 mg frusemide or 250–500 mg ethacrynic acid may be
needed. Close supervision of the blood pressure and serum urea and
electrolyte concentrations is necessary, as a fall in systolic blood
pressure and an abrupt rise in serum urea may indicate a significant
fall in glomerular filtration rate, and so necessitate at least temporary
interruption of therapy.

For *maintenance* regimes, the thiazides are to be preferred, since
their more gentle if more prolonged action need not be socially
upsetting, except when a degree of renal failure prolongs their effect
from 8–12 to 24 h, and diuresis continues at night and interferes with

sleep. It is a good rule that no elderly patient should be labeled as persistently incontinent while on a diuretic. Nocturia is an indication for the use of a shorter-acting diuretic, even in a maintenance regime. A special case can also be made for a shorter-acting drug given in the evening to prevent nocturnal dyspnea.

In *hypertension*, no study of the very potent diuretics has shown any clear superiority to the thiazides; in fact, the latter are to be preferred, since they allow a single daily dose (Anderson 1971).

In established *renal failure*, the thiazides are less effective, and only the very potent "loop" diuretics are of value. Large doses may be needed when renal function is less than 20% of normal (Berliner 1966).

Combination Therapy

There are 40 diuretic preparations available at present, half of which are combinations of diuretics and potassium. None, however, contains sufficient potassium to allow its safe use in the elderly without additional supplements.

In refractory edema, after correction of obvious electrolyte imbalance, the addition of ethacrynic acid or spironolactone to a thiazide or frusemide will result in further response. Parenteral aminophylline will potentiate diuretic action by increasing the glomerular filtration rate (Domenet et al. 1961).

Moduretic offers a combination of hydrochlorothiazide, 50 mg, and amiloride, 5 mg, to prevent hypokalemia. In elderly patients with impaired renal function, experience suggests that 5 mg amiloride given in a separate tablet is preferable, and may be combined with more potent diuretics.

References

Aber, G. M., Sampson, P. A., Whitehead, T. B., and Brooke, B. N. (1962) *Lancet* **2**, 1028.

Anderson, J. (1971) *Q. J. Med. N.S.* **40**, 541.

Berliner, R. W. (1966) *Circulation* **33**, 802.

Beyer, K. H., and Baer, J. E. (1962) *Enzymes and Drug Action,* Churchill, London.

Cannon, P. J., Ames, R. P., and Laragh, J. H. (1963) *J. Am. Med. Assoc.* **185**, 854.

Daley, D., and, Evans, B. (1963) *Br. Med. J.* **2**, 1169.

Dall, J. L. C., and Gardiner, H. S. (1971) *Gerontol. Clin.* **113**, 119.

Dall, J. L. C., MacFarlane, J. P. R., and Kennedy, R. D. (1971a) *Proceedings of the Sixth European Congress of Gerontology,* Huber, Berne.

Dall, J. L. C., Paulose, S., and Ferguson, J. A. (1971*b*) *Gerontol. Clin.* **13,** 114.

Domenet, J. G., Evans, D. W., and Brenner, O. (1961) *Br. Med. J.* **1,** 1130.

Forrester, T. M., and Shirriffs, G. G. (1965) *Lancet* **1,** 409.

Goldberg, M., McCurdy, D. K., Foltz, E. L., and Bluemle, L. W. (1964) *J. Clin. Invest.* **43,** 201.

Hicks, B. H. (1973) *Metabolism* **22,** 101.

Judge, T. G., and Macleod, C. C. (1968) *Proceedings of the Fifth European Congress of Gerontology,* Brussels.

Judge, T. G., MacLeod, C. C., Leask,

Lant, K. F., Smith, A. J., and Wilson, G. M. (1969) *Clin. Pharmacol. Ther.* **10,** 50.

Laragh, J. H. (1962) *Circulation* **25,** 1015.

Lavender, S., and McGill, R. J. (1974) *Diabetes* **23,** 247.

Leading Article (1975) *Br. Med. J.* **2,** 521.

Ledingham, J. G. G. (1964) *Lancet* **1,** 952.

Levitt, M. F., and Goldstein, M. H. (1962) *Bull. N.Y. Acad. Med.* **38,** 249.

MacFarlane, J. P. R., and Kennedy, R. D. (1972) *Age and Ageing* **1,** 103.

Seldin, D. W., Eknoyan, G., Suki, W. N., and Rectir, F. C. (1966) *Ann. N.Y. Acad. Sci.* **139,** 328.

Strickler, J. C., and Kessler, R. H. (1961) *J. Clin. Invest.* **40,** 311.

Toivonen, S., and Mustala, O. (1966) *Br. Med. J.* **1,** 920.

Wilson, G. M. (1963) *Br. Med. J.* **1,** 285.

15

Management of Cardiac Failure

J. L. C. DALL and F. I. CAIRD

Introduction

Cardiac failure is a common problem in clinical geriatrics. Moreover, its importance is much increased because proper treatment can probably benefit the patient more than treatment for any other condition of equal severity in old age, while improper treatment can lead to disaster.

Diagnosis

Proper management begins with diagnosis, which depends essentially on demonstration of the appropriate physical signs (Bedford and Caird 1960).

Left heart failure is signaled by dyspnea on effort, paroxysmal nocturnal dyspnea, or orthopnea; bilateral pulmonary signs (usually basal rales, but occasionally patchy bronchial breathing); and gallop rhythm. Signs of the causal disease of the left heart may be present. The diagnosis of left heart failure in the elderly may be difficult when there is coexistent airway obstruction resulting from chronic bronchi-

J. L. C. DALL · Victoria Infirmary, Glasgow, G42 9TY, Scotland. F. I. CAIRD · University Department of Geriatric Medicine, Southern General Hospital, Glasgow, G51 4TF, Scotland.

tis. Orthopnea, left-sided gallop rhythm, and in particular nonpurulence of the sputum, will establish the presence of cardiac dyspnea. The degree of airway obstruction will be inadequate to account for the severity of dyspnea, as, for instance, when the peak expiratory flow rate is more than 250 liters/min. The chest radiograph will show cardiomegaly, pulmonary congestion, and on occasion Kerley's lines; the ECG will show signs of left heart disease. Other investigations are in general unhelpful in establishing the diagnosis of left heart failure, but may be of importance in establishing its cause.

Congestive cardiac failure is signaled by dyspnea, which is often less urgent than in left heart failure, and may be replaced as a leading symptom by fatigue. The first symptom is often edema of the legs, but hepatic congestion may lead to abdominal pain, congestion of the gut to nausea and vomiting, and hypoxemia and reduction in cerebral blood flow to confusion. The cardinal signs are the presence of objectively demonstrable dyspnea, symmetrical elevation of the venous pressure in all phases of respiration, positive hepatojugular reflux, bilateral pulmonary signs, smooth hepatomegaly, and edema of both legs or sacrum. If edema is asymmetrical, it cannot be due solely to cardiac failure, and venous disease in the legs is by far the most likely cause. The bilateral pulmonary signs are usually basal rales, but sometimes are those of effusion. If all these signs are present, the diagnosis of congestive heart failure is correct. If any one is absent, it is most unlikely.

In addition to the correct diagnosis of the presence of cardiac failure, two further points must be established: the *type of heart disease* responsible, and the reason the patient is in cardiac failure at the time in question (i.e., *the precipitating cause* of failure).

The reason for the importance of establishing the nature of the underlying heart disease is that in old age, cardiac failure may develop either because there is primary disease of the heart, or because the heart cannot achieve the output demanded of it by extracardiac circumstances. In the first instance ("primary cardiac failure"), treatment may need to be continued for life; in the second ("secondary cardiac failure"), treatment of the extracardiac disease, especially severe anemia or thyrotoxicosis, often results in the return of normal cardiac function, and removes the need for potentially hazardous continuing maintenance therapy (Dall 1970).

The reason for the importance of establishing the precipitating cause of the episode of cardiac failure is that many such causes are treatable (e.g., respiratory infections; Flint 1954), or may tend to natural improvement (e.g., myocardial infarction or pulmonary embolism), or may be guarded against (e.g., physical overexertion or discontinuance of necessary therapy). Cardiac failure precipitated by a definite diagnosable event carries a better prognosis, if the event is not likely to recur, than failure occurring without such a precipitating cause in the course of relentlessly progressive heart disease. The implication is that the heart disease is more serious in the second situation than in the first. These long-established principles apply as much to heart failure in the elderly as to failure in the middle-aged.

Principles of Management

The basic principles of management of cardiac failure are essentially the same at all ages, but special allowance must be made for particular circumstances in old age. The management of an acute episode of cardiac failure depends on rest, digitalis, and diuretic therapy.

Although the emphasis on the dangers of bed rest in the elderly has been entirely correct and necessary, it has nevertheless led to neglect of its crucial importance in certain circumstances, one of which is cardiac failure. Adequate rest must be ensured in the initial stages. This requirement may not necessarily mean rest in bed, since orthopnea often makes rest in a chair more comfortable. Walking must be prohibited, if only because of the clearly demonstrated deleterious effect of even minor effort on the renal circulation and sodium excretion in cardiac patients (Sinclair-Smith et al. 1949). The common cause of unnecessary exercise is getting out of bed and walking to the toilet. At home, a commode by the bedside may be all that is necessary, and in the hospital, clear instructions to the nursing staff. Sedation may be necessary to produce adequate rest; diazepam (Valium), 5 mg, or thioridazine (Melleril), 25–50 mg, 1 to 3 times daily is usually adequate. Small doses of morphine (e.g., 10 mg) may be used for the first few nights. The best sedative for the elderly patient with cardiac failure, however, is control of the failure. Severe and uncontrollable restlessness carries a very poor prognosis, and whatever is done, the patient usually dies within a few days.

Fluid restriction by itself is unnecessary, and with modern diuretic therapy, salt restriction need not be severe; it is sufficient not to add salt to food.

Digitalis and diuretic therapy, and the particular problems of management of pulmonary heart failure, are discussed in Chapters 13, 14, and 10, respectively.

Assessment of Progress

The observations required for the control of treatment of cardiac failure in its early stages are simple and few. Clinical improvement constitutes the most important criterion of successful treatment of congestive failure. There is reduction of breathlessness and diminution of edema, a fall in venous pressure, and often improvement in mental state. Much assistance may be gained from a regularly kept weight chart (Fig. 15.1). Unless virtually moribund, no elderly patient is too ill to weigh, and the information obtained is much more valuable than that provided by records of the fluid input and output of an incontinent patient. Diuresis and loss of edema result in a fall in weight—often of 10 kg or more, over a period of a week or so—until a steady weight without edema is attained and maintained. In left ventricular failure, weight loss will be less, and the best guide is disappearance of nocturnal breathlessness and of basal rales.

It is useful to measure blood urea and electrolyte concentrations weekly; more frequent observations are not necessary, unless there is evidence of severe electrolyte disorder. The serum urea concentration is often raised in cardiac failure, and a further rise may occur during the first few days of treatment. This rise need not indicate a deterioration of renal function; urea production is often increased, particularly in pulmonary heart failure, and also when the cardiac output is very low, and the peripheral circulation much reduced (Domenet and Evans 1969).

A minor fall in serum sodium concentration, to 132–135 mmol/liter, and in chloride to 90–95 mmol/liter, should not be regarded as important, but a fall in serum potassium level below 3.5 mmol/liter should be taken as an indication for increasing potassium supplements.

Once the patient is free of formal signs of cardiac failure, and weight loss has ceased, gradual mobilization should begin (see Fig. 15.1). The patient should initially walk only to the toilet and back, and later, further about the ward or the house. Finally, climbing stairs should be allowed. Changes in the amount of exercise allowed should not in general be made oftener than weekly, and drug therapy (with the important exception of digitalis if there is evidence of toxicity) should not usually be altered during this phase, so that the effects of only one change in treatment at a time can be observed. Watch should be kept for weight gain, or the recurrence of edema, nocturnal breathlessness, or fatigue.

When a moderate degree of physical activity has been achieved,

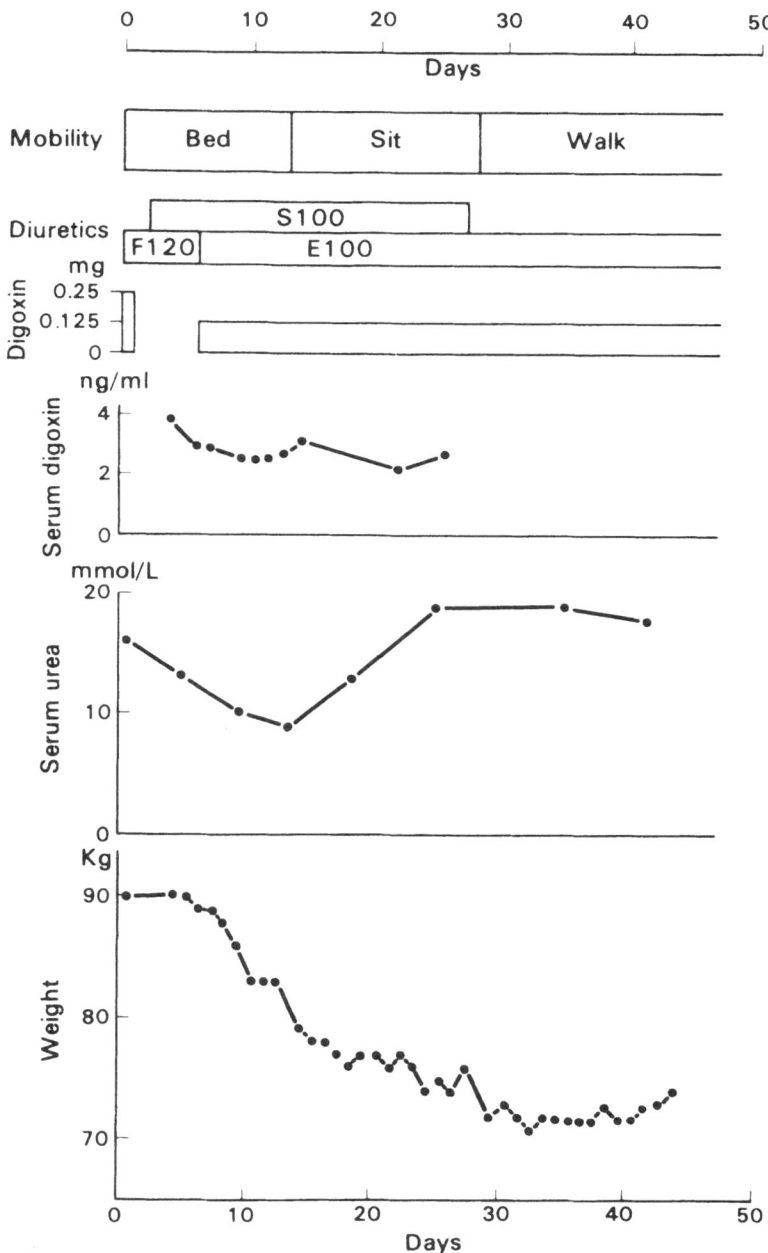

Fig. 15.1. Course of an episode of cardiac failure in a 77-year-old man. S Spironolactone, F frusemide, E ethacrynic acid; figures are mg/day.

and the patient is walking about the ward or the house, the next phase of alteration of treatment may begin. This phase consists in an attempt to reduce the drug regime to the simplest compatible with adequate control of the cardiac failure. In particular, the diuretic regime should be reviewed, and if at all possible, multiple diuretics reduced to a single one. The minimum therapy usually consists of a single daily dose of digoxin, a single dose of a diuretic, and potassium supplements.

The final phase of rehabilitation may now begin, with the patient gradually increasing his exercise until he is out of the house and going for short walks. After about 3 months, therapy should be reviewed again, and its complexity again reduced. It is probably best to discontinue diuretics before digitalis, and it is usually possible to stop all cardiac therapy in patients with "secondary cardiac failure" as defined above. Apart from those patients whose failure was the result of a proven recent myocardial infarct, however, most elderly patients who have been in "primary" congestive heart failure require continuation of digitalis and diuretics indefinitely (Dall 1970).

Psychological rehabilitation is as important as physical, if only because cardiac neurosis can be as crippling to an old person as cardiac failure. An optimistic outlook is essential, with encouragement that prolonged invalidism is not in question—but bear in mind that the need to restrict physical effort and the danger of overexertion as a precipitating factor in relapse necessitates moderation in advising increase in activities. Regular review is of much supportive value, and should always include clinical examination and consideration of current drug therapy.

Resistant Cardiac Failure

A small proportion of elderly patients with congestive failure do not respond rapidly to conventional therapy as outlined above. Hope should not be abandoned, but a detailed review made of a number of key problems, including: (1) the correctness and completeness of the diagnosis of cardiac failure, (2) the presence or absence of complications, and (3) the correctness of therapy.

The correctness of the diagnosis of congestive failure should be checked against the criteria set out above. The completeness of the diagnosis must be assessed in the light of possible additional diagnoses that might contribute to cardiac failure. These include anemia, hyperthyroidism, and bacterial endocarditis.

A search should be made for possible complications of cardiac failure or additional complicating factors, including pulmonary embolism, respiratory infection, chronic venous disease, hypoproteinemia, and electrolyte disorder. Pulmonary embolism is likely to be signaled by episodic fever and tachypnea, hemoptysis (often persistent or recurrent), pleurisy, unexplained tachycardia resistant to digitalis, digitalis toxicity (Tench 1955), and changing pulmonary signs, including the development of a pleural effusion, or the enlargement of one of two preexisting effusions. The ESR may be raised, and signs of recent venous thrombosis in the legs should be looked for. Fever, leucocytosis, and purulent sputum will be evidence of respiratory infection. Chronic venous disease in the legs is usually clinically obvious, and hypoproteinemia (a further cause of persistent edema unlikely to respond easily to diuretics) will be evident on biochemical investigation.

Common electrolyte abnormalities include potassium depletion, hyponatremia, and hypochloremic alkalosis. Potassium depletion is usually present in elderly patients with cardiac failure even before therapy (Cox et al. 1971), and is increased by almost all diuretic regimes, including so-called potassium-sparing diuretics (Cox and Porthouse 1974). Potassium supplements should therefore be given to all elderly patients with cardiac failure.

Hyponatremia has a variety of causal mechanisms (Edelman 1956, Fuisz 1963). Its least usual cause is true sodium depletion, consequent on excessive diuresis; this depletion is manifested by weakness, lethargy, anorexia, hypotension, and oliguria. The serum urea concentration is high, there is no edema, and weight loss has been persistent and severe. It responds rapidly and dramatically to sodium repletion (Schroeder 1949, Black and Litchfield 1951). Hyponatremia may result from inadequate water excretion (Hanenson et al. 1956), when as a rule it is associated with severe congestive failure. There is increasing edema and weight gain, but the blood pressure is normal, and the serum urea is normal or only slightly raised. The hyponatremia responds to selective water restriction combined with improvement in myocardial function. Hyponatremia is probably most commonly due to potassium depletion, since this depletion results in reduction in cellular osmolarity, and the extracellular sodium concentration falls to maintain osmotic equilibrium (Edelman et al. 1958).

These conditions require recognition and proper treatment before cardiac failure will respond. Pulmonary embolism should be treated with anticoagulants, bearing in mind the sensitivity to anticoagulants of elderly patients, particularly those with cardiac failure (Stats and

Davison 1949, Harvey and Finch 1950). Therapy should never be begun without an initial estimation of the prothrombin time, and loading doses should always be small (see Bedford and Caird 1960). Respiratory infection should be treated with the appropriate antibiotic. Chronic venous disease and hypoproteinemia should be recognized, and some edema seen to be an essential part of the patient's condition, rather than evidence of persistent cardiac failure; elastic stockings are better therapy than more powerful diuretics.

Treatment should be reviewed, with particular reference to the choice of diuretic and the evidence of adequacy or excess of digitalis therapy. Measurement of the serum digoxin level can be very helpful in this context.

If none of these factors is present, or all have been remedied as far as possible, and the patient remains in cardiac failure, then the prognosis is bad. The most satisfactory method of management is to insist on a prolonged period of absolute bed rest, with prophylactic anticoagulant therapy at least in some cases. Bed rest may be needed for a period of 4 weeks, during which time the patient's weight will slowly fall and signs of cardiac failure disappear. Mobilization should then begin, but very slowly and cautiously. Consideration should be given to the use of therapeutic hypothyroidism, which is best begun with an antithyroid drug, and completed with radioiodine therapy (Blumgart and Freedberg 1952). This form of treatment is probably underused, but seems of greatest value in patients with severe pulmonary heart failure, who may benefit most from reduction in oxygen requirements.

Prognosis

There has been relatively little study of the prognosis of cardiac failure in the elderly. Twenty years ago, 28% of elderly patients admitted to a geriatric unit with congestive heart failure survived for 2 years, and 16% for 4 years (Bedford and Caird 1956). Prognosis was worst in patients with pulmonary heart disease, virtually all of whom were dead within 2 years; in syphilitic aortic incompetence; and, somewhat surprisingly, in hypertensive heart disease with atrial fibrillation. It was relatively better in patients with coronary artery disease and other forms of valvular disease.

The principal cause of death was respiratory infection, but as many as 1 death in 7 was due to pulmonary embolism.

Prognosis may have improved in recent years, because of earlier therapy with oral diuretics, while earlier mobilization may perhaps have reduced the frequency of venous thrombosis and pulmonary embolism, and so reduced the early mortality. It may be that what has improved is not survival, but quality of life. Clearly, congestive heart failure is not a terminal event in many old people (Leading article 1956). It should always be correctly diagnosed and actively treated.

References

Bedford, P. D., and Caird, F. I. (1956) *Q. J. Med., N.S.* **25**, 406.

Bedford, P. D., and Caird, F. I. (1960) *Vascular Disease of the Heart in Old Age*, J&A Churchill, London.

Black, A. B., and Litchfield, J. A. (1951) *Q. J. Med., N.S.* **20**, 149.

Blumgart, H. L., and Freedberg, A. S. (1952) *Circulation* **6**, 222.

Cox, J. R., Horrocks, P., Speight, C. J., Pearson, R. E., and Hobson, N. (1971) *Clin. Sci.* **41**, 55.

Cox, J. R., and Porthouse, A. (1974) *Gerontol. Clin.* **16**, 157.

Dall, J. L. C. (1970) *Br. Med. J.* **1**, 705.

Domenet, J. G., and Evans, D. W. (1969) *Q. J. Med., N.S.* **38**, 117.

Edelman, I. S. (1956) *Metabolism* **5**, 500.

Edelman, I. S., Leibman, J. O'Meara, M. P., and Birkenfeld, L. W. (1958) *J. Clin. Invest.* **37**, 1236.

Flint, F. J. (1954) *Br. Med. J.* **2**, 1018.

Fuisz, R. E. (1963) *Medicine (Baltimore)* **42**, 149.

Hanenson, I. O., Goluboff, B., Grossman, J., Weston, R. E., and Leiter, L. (1956) *Circulation* **13**, 242.

Harvey, W. P., and Finch, C. A. (1950) *N. Engl. J. Med.* **242**, 208.

Leading Article (1956) *Lancet* **1**, 255.

Schroeder, H. A. (1949) *J. Am. Med. Assoc.* **141**, 117.

Sinclair-Smith, B., Kattus, A. A., Genest, J., and Newman, E. V. (1949) *Bull. Johns Hopkins Hosp.* **84**, 369.

Stats, D., and Davison, S. (1949) *Am. J. Med. Sci.* **218**, 318.

Tench, W. R. (1955) *Am. J. Med.* **19**, 869.

16

Coronary Care for the Elderly

T. SEMPLE and B. O. WILLIAMS

Introduction

Although many facts about coronary heart disease (CHD) and about acute myocardial infarction have emerged from intensive observations made in modern coronary care units (CCU), many sophisticated units capable of undertaking clinical research have operated with an age barrier for admission, usually 70 years (Lawrie et al. 1967). Thus, our knowledge of the natural history of the disease, and of its presentations and progress after this age, is less firmly established than for younger patients. Teaching has tended to be based on clinical and anecdotal impressions—for instance, that heart attacks in elderly females are uncommon, but severe and fatal. In contrast to "myocarditis" and to cardiac failure, acute myocardial infarct as a diagnosis has been less frequent in the aged. Cardiac failure and sudden death tend to be accepted with some equanimity in this group of patients as not unexpected terminal events, and thus precision of cardiac diagnosis sometimes seems less important. Fewer hospital autopsies may be requested; when they are performed, the frequency, distribution, and significance of atheromatous occlusion affecting the coronary arteries and of old and fresh muscle infarction may receive superficial attention.

   The object of this chapter is to review present-day knowledge of

T. SEMPLE and B. O. WILLIAMS · Victoria Infirmary, Glasgow, G42 9TY, Scotland.

TABLE 16.1. Previous History

History	Age: Group: No.:	<60 Y 210	60–69 O 189	70+ E 104	χ^2 Analysis
Angina		46.7%	50.3%	52.9%	N.S.
Definite myocardial infarct		23.8%	24.3%	21.2%	N.S.
Systemic hypertension		15.7%	25.9%	25%	Y vs. O, $P < 0.05$; Y vs. E, $P < 0.05$
Diabetes mellitus		3.8%	4.2%	2.9%	N.S.

how myocardial infarction affects the elderly, as compared with younger people, and how these patients should be cared for and rehabilitated.

The Aged in Coronary Care Units

Chaturvedi et al. (1972) have reported on a series of elderly patients admitted to a CCU, and have indicated that age should not debar a patient from the benefits of hospital coronary care. The present authors, as part of a study of 918 patients admitted to a teaching hospital CCU, have made a similar analysis (Williams et al. 1976). Altogether, there were 503 patients with proven infarcts. For comparison, these 503 were divided into 210 younger patients (Y

TABLE 16.2. Circumstances of Onset of Main Attack

Circumstances	Y (210)	O (189)	E (104)
At rest	55.8%	55%	52.9%
Sleeping	18.6%	20.6%	29.8%
Exertion	22.9%	18.5%	11.5%
Other	2.7%	5.9%	5.8%

χ^2 Analysis: Y vs. O and O vs. E, no significant difference;
Y vs. E, $P < 0.01$.

Group), under 60 years of age; 189 older, 60–69 years (O Group); and the 104 elderly patients 70 years of age and over (E Group).

Findings on Admission

The previous medical history of the three groups was similar (Table 16.1). Almost exactly half had suffered angina, quite apart from preceding "buildup" and "crescendo" angina, and more of the older people for longer than 5 years. Rather surprisingly, there was no significant difference in the proportions having had previous infarction and previous ischemic attacks. Known hypertension was found to be more prevalent in the E Group only in comparison with the Y Group, which was still not true of angina, nor did the elderly have a higher incidence of diabetes.

Of the E Group, 83% had experienced their presenting symptoms at rest; rather more were asleep and fewer were active at the time than in the younger groups (Table 16.2), but this could be a reflection of life patterns.

Previous studies (Rodstein 1956, Pathy 1967, Ristic et al. 1971) had reported a high incidence of painless infarction in the elderly. Excluding confused patients, Pathy found that about 60% had had no pain. As can be seen in Table 16.3, however, elderly patients selected for admission to a CCU, often by the family doctor, usually do present with chest pain or discomfort, although as often as not it is accompanied by breathlessness. Only 11.5% had an atypical presentation, without chest pain or discomfort. These apparently conflicting findings are probably explained by (a) the greater tendency of patients thus selected for CCU admission to have more classic presentations, (b) the better opportunities available for eliciting an accurate history, and (c) the labeling of tightness and chest discomfort without tachypnea as pain rather than dyspnea.

TABLE 16.3. Main Symptoms

Symptoms	Y (210)	O (189)	E (104)	χ^2 Analysis
Chest pain and breathlessness	37.2%	42.6%	45.2%	No significant differences
Chest pain	57.5%	52.5%	43.3%	
Breathlessness	3.8%	4.3%	7.7%	
Neither	1.4%	0.6%	3.8%	

TABLE 16.4. Source of Admission

Source	Y (210)	O (189)	E (104)
Family doctor or deputy	64.8%	70.9%	80.8%
Via Casualty Department	23.8%	16.4%	11.5%
From Outpatient Clinic of other ward	11.4%	12.7%	7.7%

χ^2 Analysis: Y vs. O and O vs. E, not significant; Y vs. E, $P < 0.05$.

A high proportion of the elderly group was admitted from home, with fewer self-referrals (Table 16.4). Admission to the unit was not associated with an undue proportion of "false alarms"; the diagnosis of infarct made before admission, usually by the family doctor, was confirmed in a similar proportion (58.5%) to the younger groups (Table 16.5).

Infarct Complications

Conduction defects related to infarction are more common in older patients (Table 16.6). Mortality associated with complete heart block is unrelated to age in this series. Atrial fibrillation and atrial flutter are the only arrhythmias to show increased incidence with age. Systolic pressure on admission, which has been shown to be an important prognostic factor (Norris et al. 1969), was below 100 mm Hg in 17.3% of Group E, 9% of Group O, and 10% of Group Y (the only significant difference being between Groups E and Y, where $P < .05$).

TABLE 16.5. Main Diagnosis—All Admissions

Main diagnosis	Y (423)	O (317)	E (178)
Proven myocardial infarct	49.4%	59.5%	58.5%
Ischemic incident	24.5%	18.4%	19.1%
Dysrhythmia	5.4%	9.8%	10.1%
Other	20.7%	12.3%	12.3%

χ^2 Analysis: Y vs. O, $P < 0.001$; O vs. E, P not significant; Y vs. E, $P < 0.01$.

TABLE 16.6. Dysrhythmias and Conduction Defects

ECG findings	Y (210)	O (189)	E (104)	χ^2 Analysis
Atrial flutter or atrial fibrillation	5.25%	11.6%	14.4%	Y vs. O, $P < 0.05$; Y vs. E, $P < 0.01$
Ventricular fibrillation	5.25%	5.8%	3.8%	
Heart block and conduction defects	20%	22.2%	34.6%	O vs. E, $P < 0.05$; Y vs. E, $P < 0.01$

Pulmonary edema, the "shock picture," and congestive failure, all recognized as strong determinants of severity and mortality, were more common in Group E (Table 16.7); pericarditis, which does not have such a grave reputation (Thadani et al. 1971), showed no such predominance.

Infarct Severity

Assessment of the severity of infarction and of consequent myocardial dysfunction is as important in the elderly as it is in younger patients. It can be done using either a prognostic index (Peel et al. 1962, Norris et al. 1969) or a simple system, e.g.: Grade 1—mild and uncomplicated; Grade 2—moderate, slightly, or temporarily complicated; Grade 3—severe, with complications and evidence of myocardial damage. Suggestions for defining the grades are appended in Table 16.8; reference to the significance and value of the gradings is

TABLE 16.7. Other Complications

Complications	Y (210)	O (189)	E (104)	χ^2 Analysis
"Shock" picture	13.8%	15.3%	25%	O vs. E, $P < 0.05$; Y vs. E, $P < 0.05$
Pericarditis	10.5%	10.6%	8.7%	
Pulmonary edema	47.1%	59.2%	74%	Y vs. O, $P < 0.05$; O vs. E, $P < 0.01$; Y vs. E, $P < 0.001$
Right heart failure	6.2%	11.1%	22.1%	O vs. E, $P < 0.05$; Y vs. E, $P < 0.001$

TABLE 16.8. Assessment of Infarct Severity—Suggested Grading Procedure, Perhaps at 48 Hours and 14 Days Postinfarct

Grade 1: Mild, uncomplicated myocardial infarction; absence throughout of any of the features mentioned under Grades 2 and 3.

Grade 2: Absence of the features mentioned in Grade 3, but any of the following features occurring only temporarily or responding to treatment:
a) Sinus tachycardia (over 100 beats/min) at rest, persisting longer than 1 h but less than 48 h.
b) Temporary arrhythmia, e.g., significant ectopics, supraventricular tachycardia, atrial fibrillation, atrial flutter, or ventricular arrhythmia.
c) Dyspnea during ordinary activities.
d) Temporary abnormal cardiac impulse (dyskinesia).
e) Moist sounds persisting after coughing, or pulmonary venous engorgement on X ray, calling for oral diuretic therapy.

Grade 3: Occurrence of one of the following features:
  a) Sinus tachycardia at rest, persisting longer than 48 h.
  b) Arrhythmia still present at time of grading.
  c) Dyspnea at rest.
  d) Alveolar or interstitial pulmonary edema on X ray.
  e) Third heart sound.
  f) Continuing palpable dyskinesia or ventricular aneurysm.
  g) Definite cardiac enlargement.
  h) Persisting heart block, left bundle branch block, or bifascicular block.

made in later paragraphs. Briefly, it is important to remember that early and late patient management will differ from group to group, and that a substantial proportion of elderly survivors remain in Grade 1. Such patients have an excellent prognosis, late complications are rare, and rapid mobilization and return to an active way of life are indicated (Working Party 1975).

The prognostic index and the simple grading procedure each reflect a considerably increased severity of infarction with aging, and Table 16.9 shows that, despite a considerable initial loss by deaths in the CCU, severe Grade 3 infarcts remain prevalent among the E Group CCU survivors. It has been shown (Nagle and Williams 1974, Norris et al. 1970) that while survival at 3 years is usual (about 80%) in mild cases, it is much less common (around 25%) in the severe group. A recent report from Gothenburg (Wihelmsen et al. 1975) confirms that late mortality is 3 times higher with repeat infarcts. The degree of myocardial damage and of disability, as well as the prognosis, will

TABLE 16.9. Severity of Infarction in CCU Survivors

Severity	Y (186[a])	O (160)	E (75[a])	χ^2 Analysis
Grade 1	43.6%	39.4%	30%	No
Grade 2	40.9%	51.2%	48%	significant
Grade 3	15.5%	9.4%	22%	differences

[a] Of the 190 CCU survivors in the Y Group and the 77 in the E Group, 4 and 2, respectively, had no severity grading.

depend on the severity of each of these infarcts, especially that of the most recent one.

Mortality

The contrast in severity with aging is reflected in a considerable difference in hospital mortality, which was 21.3% for the whole series of 503 infarct patients, 15.2% for Group Y, 19% for Group O, and 37.5% for Group E (Table 16.10). Coronary care units have reduced mortality in patients with acute myocardial infarction, and the elderly are no exception. A total of 2,074 patients with acute myocardial infarction admitted directly to general medical wards of the same hospital, in the 5 years preceding the opening of the CCU, are perhaps not wholly comparable, but hospital mortality then was 28% for the whole series, 17% for the group equivalent to Group Y, 30% for the group equivalent to Group O, and 43% for the elderly.

TABLE 16.10. Mortality

	Y (210)	O (189)	E (104)	χ^2 Analysis
CCU mortality	9.5%	15.3%	26%	O vs. E, $P < 0.05$; Y vs. E, $P < 0.001$
Late hospital mortality	5.7%	3.7%	11 .5%	O vs. E, $P < 0.01$; Y vs. E, $P < 0.05$
TOTAL hospital mortality	15.2%	19%	37.5%	O vs. E, $P < 0.001$; Y vs. E, $P < 0.001$

It is found that death in the CCU and later in the ward is rare even in elderly patients when they have been graded mild and uncomplicated. The incidence of reversible primary ventricular fibrillation is about the same (4–6%), and immediate defibrillation is as successful in the aged as in the younger groups.

Influence of Sex

There is a mean male:female ratio of 2:1 for all myocardial infarct patients in the hospital. This ratio drops from about 6:1 below the age of 50 to 3.5:1 in the sixth decade, 2.0:1 in the seventh decade, and to less than 1:1 in the elderly (Peel and Semple 1972). Chaturvedi et al. (1972) had 52 males and 53 females in their elderly series; our Group E consisted of 50 males and 54 females.

This later age incidence of myocardial infarction in women produces an apparent anomaly in studies of infarct mortality in relation to sex. The percentage mortality in comparable age groups is the same for both sexes, but as mortality increases with age, it is higher among women as a whole (Norris et al. 1969, Peel and Semple 1972).

Management in the Coronary Care Unit

Most deaths in acute myocardial infarction occur before the patient can be admitted to the hospital, but intensive coronary care facilities offer benefits to the patient who has survived thus far, with some reduction in mortality due to control of arrhythmias, especially ventricular fibrillation, and of temporary complete heart block.

In the CCU, patients are usually nursed in single rooms with bed rest maintained throughout, although they are permitted to use the commode under nursing supervision. The unit is staffed by physicians and nurses who have special skills in recognizing ECG abnormalities and in using antiarrhythmic measures. Continuous ECG tracings are displayed at a control monitor, where there is an auditory tachycardia/bradycardia alarm device; at the bedside, there is an ECG monitor with defibrillator immediately available. A reassuring, optimistic atmosphere of calm, disciplined care prevails in the unit. Psychological rehabilitation commences at the time of admission, simple explanatory discussion helping to dissolve fears of the strange environment, of sudden death, and of permanent invalidism.

Elderly patients are more vulnerable to cerebral dysfunction and confusion as a result of hypotension, cardiac arrhythmia, or the injudicious use of narcotic analgesics. The staff can help orient these patients by explaining and by encouraging access to a clock and calendar. Occasionally, confusion may be the only clinical indication of acute myocardial infarction, but these patients, in the absence of more classic features, are rarely admitted to such a unit.

Patients usually remain in the CCU for a minimum period of 72 h; Semple et al. (1972) have shown they can by this time be transferred if necessary, even to another nearby hospital, without added risk. However, transfer to a general medical ward may be delayed when complications merit further special management.

Each patient has an intravenous infusion line, and in the absence of contraindications, anticoagulant therapy is administered, commencing with intravenous heparin in a dose of 20,000 U in 12-h bottles for 36 h and continuing with oral once-daily warfarin at least until the stage of mobilization is reached. Although anticoagulants are of limited value in reducing mortality, they reduce the incidence of thromboembolism, particularly venous thromboembolism, to which the elderly are especially prone. Ill effects of anticoagulant therapy are uncommon in hospital patients without such contraindications as active ulceration of the gastrointestinal tract, severe renal or hepatic insufficiency, anemia, pericarditis, or significant systemic hypertension.

Where chest pain is a commanding feature, analgesia should be rapid in action. As yet, there is no firm evidence that there is a better alternative to morphine (Kerr and Donald 1974), although a proportion of individuals will have an emetic or a vagal response, and some may require atropine. Diamorphine (heroin) is marginally more satisfactory in these respects, and in such a special unit, the dangers of keeping this extremely addictive drug at hand may be acceptable. Pentazocine (Fortral) is not a satisfactory alternative for this purpose, because it tends to have an adverse effect on cardiac function, as manifested by an increase in left ventricular end-diastolic pressure and in pulmonary artery pressure. General sedation is achieved by the use of chlordiazepoxide (Librium), which has a satisfactory anxiolytic action without an excessive hypnotic side effect.

Concentrated oxygen therapy is indicated on admission. An increase in arterial PO_2, which affords special benefit in pulmonary edema, may increase the oxygen supply to the ischemic zone bordering the infarct and reduce the extension of the developing infarct zone. The elderly, however, may not tolerate the tight-fitting oxygen mask necessary for administering 100% oxygen.

The elderly are particularly afraid of illness and of death, and admission to the hospital, and in particular to special units, may produce unusual stresses, when they fail to understand the concept of monitoring devices and the need for the numerous uniformed personnel required in modern coronary care. Bladder care is a special problem, particularly in the male. The use of potent diuretics, perhaps atropine, and enforced bed rest may lead to retention, necessitating early temporary urethral catheterization with full aseptic technique. The daily use of an oral aperient, of the stool-softening and lubricant form, will avoid fecal impaction and resultant isometric straining, which produces excessive cardiovascular stress. Use of the commode is standard practice in such units, but bowel movement need not be actively encouraged during the first 48 h.

Diet should be in a soft, digestible form. Assistance in feeding may sometimes be indicated, but is not routine practice.

Management of Complications

The special aims of the CCU are to reduce mortality by the rapid treatment of complications and to minimize resultant cardiovascular disability in the survivors. The staff are skilled in recognizing the presence and significance of rhythm and conduction disturbances. Almost all patients have a temporary disturbance of rhythm after acute myocardial infarction. The tendency to myocardial irritability and vulnerability to life-threatening ventricular arrhythmias falls steadily to near zero within 72 h.

Most supraventricular arrhythmias are not life-threatening, and immediate management depends on the patient's ability to maintain cardiac output. In uncontrolled atrial fibrillation, atrial flutter, or supraventricular tachycardia, oral digitalization is the treatment of choice; if, however, the general hemodynamic status is compromised, with resultant hypotension, cardiac pain, or cardiac failure, synchronized electric shock (cardioversion), commencing with a small shock of 25 W·sec, is indicated to regain sinus rhythm. Some centers administer intravenous beta-blocking agents such as practolol (Eraldin, up to 20 mg) in supraventricular arrhythmias, using digitalization or synchronized shock only for refractory cases. Cardiac glycosides must be administered with care in the elderly, who are most sensitive to their toxic effects, especially when myocardial irritability is already present following the infarction. The likelihood of digitalis poisoning is reduced by careful attention to renal function and to serum potassium levels, which may affect initial dosage and maintenance therapy.

Sinus bradycardia may result from increased vagal tone, sometimes related to cardiac pain or to morphia administration. When untreated, bradycardia may further aggravate existing hypotension and lead to life-threatening ventricular arrhythmia or even asystole. Adequate analgesia may be helpful in reducing vagal tone, and intravenous bolus injections of atropine (0.65 mg) are usually successful in abolishing sinus bradycardia. Care must be taken, however, that injudicious or repeated inappropriate doses of this drug do not precipitate acute glaucoma or aggravate existing urinary retention or confusion. In resistant bradycardia, intravenous isoprenaline (Isuprel) titration may be helpful in maintaining sinus rate, but tachycardia, with resultant increased myocardial oxygen demands, must be avoided. The ventricular bradycardia of complete heart block may also respond to atropine or isoprenaline. Here again the main dangers are ventricular arrhythmias and ventricular standstill. The latter can always be reversed, at least temporarily, by precordial thump as an emergency measure prior to transvenous pacing, which, as in younger patients, is most effective in controlling ventricular rate.

The main indication for acute pacing is ventricular bradycardia that does not respond to medication. With inferior infarction, where complete heart block is neither a permanent nor necessarily a very serious complication when well managed, such temporary transvenous pacing can be a life-saving measure, by maintaining a satisfactory ventricular rate and cardiac output until normal conduction ensues spontaneously within hours or days. With anterior infarction, however, major conduction defects usually signify multiple bundle branch involvement from extensive infarction. The prognosis is necessarily poor, and pacing rarely confers permanent benefit.

Early management of significant ventricular ectopic activity reduces the risk of ventricular arrhythmias and cardiac arrest. Immediate treatment with intravenous lignocaine (Xylocaine) is often effective and largely free from side effects, although excessive doses may produce confusion and aggravate hypotension. Ventricular tachycardia (VT), when it is producing disturbance of consciousness or cardiac failure, should be treated by synchronized shock. When VT is recurrent, a number of therapeutic agents, usually lignocaine or procainamide (Pronestyl), are employed.

Unexpected cardiac arrest in ventricular fibrillation (primary VF) in the mild, as yet uncomplicated, infarct patient responds to immediate unsynchronized shock in full dose (400 W·sec) administered within 40 sec. In such circumstances within a CCU, the elderly respond as well as do younger patients (Linn and Yurt 1976). In the present series of 104 patients, there were 4 examples of primary VF, and 3 left the CCU. In the 399 patients under the age of 70, there were 22 examples

(5.5%), and 12 survived. Even more so than in younger patients, however, when cardiac arrest occurs in those already having complications, a resuscitation attempt is rarely a worthwhile exercise.

Acute pulmonary edema and congestive cardiac failure are controlled with potent "loop" diuretics like frusemide (Lasix) or ethacrynic acid (Edecrin), and by a cardiac glycoside, usually digoxin, particularly if there is concurrent atrial fibrillation. Oral digitalization is generally satisfactory and should be titrated and carefully supervised, and adequate blood potassium levels ensured.

Cardiogenic shock due to the loss of live myocardial tissue and resulting "pump failure" is the major cause of death in the CCU. A successful method of managing this complication remains elusive, and superfluous attempts in the elderly to reverse it should be discouraged.

Economics of the Elderly in the Coronary Care Unit

When there is no age barrier to CCU admission, it is found that one-fifth of all admissions are 70 years of age and over. Although there is the same dramatic saving of life by primary defibrillation, mortality is substantially higher, and indeed hospital mortality is double that of all those under 70. The average infarct severity of aged survivors is greater, and there is a rather longer average stay in the special unit and later in the wards. There is more residual cardiac invalidism, and there are more late deaths. On the other hand, the proportion of Grade 1 mild, uncomplicated infarcts among survivors is substantial, although it is less than in younger patients (see Table 16.9).

Thus, any rule for excluding the elderly from the CCU militates against the occasional individual with a first infarct of moderate severity who is unfortunate enough to have a primary reversible ventricular fibrillation. Apart from this occasional exception, however, there seems little medical advantage in the CCU for the aged infarct patient. On economic grounds, intensive coronary care beds may be best reserved for those of working age, but ethically a barrier age limit is not easy to decide. Numerous hospitals with a cutoff age of 70 may be justified in their decision, even if erring slightly on the elderly side from the economic standpoint. For the mild to moderate elderly infarct patient who has been admitted to a hospital general medical ward, it remains good practice to monitor the ECG and to be prepared to treat primary ventricular fibrillation.

Research

There is merit in having one or more sophisticated intensive coronary units continuing to accept older infarct patients, so that the cost and benefit of new techniques can be assessed at all ages and coronary heart disease can be studied in depth—clinically, hemodynamically, and at autopsy—in well-documented, aged patients.

Coronary arteriography in the working population has contributed much to our knowledge of the natural history of coronary heart disease, but is seldom undertaken in the aged. Fortunately, a similar technique, using X-ray image-intensification, can provide equally satisfactory selective coronary arteriograms, using the isolated autopsy heart (Semple 1973). Additional information not available at coronary angiography in life is obtained by palpation of the main coronary arteries and branches in their length for atheroma and by careful radiological inspection of the coronary orifices, as well as the valves and uninjected arteries, for calcium. This type of examination can usefully be included as an essential part of cardiac autopsy of those who die in such a unit. Correlation of the angiograms with the clinical, hemodynamic, and radiological events in life adds much to our understanding of the condition and of nature's compensatory efforts to bypass obstructive disease, be they successful or unsuccessful.

Management of Acute Myocardial Infarction in the Home

Most elderly survivors of myocardial infarction will be managed at home eventually, and many will be treated there from the start as elective policy. The role of the family doctor is crucial in early management, aftercare, and rehabilitation. A hospital discharge letter should be more than a terse statement of diagnosis, drug treatment, and date of discharge. Ideally, it should refer to psychological and social circumstances, and to the severity of the infarct, complications, and expected degree of disability, so that physical rehabilitative measures of suitable gradation and vigor can be prescribed.

In the home, diagnosis and assessment are based on the assumption that anterior chest pain or tightness usually means myocardial ischemia of coronary origin. If the symptoms are severe and prolonged, and if the patient is clearly ill, the diagnosis of acute infarction is usually self-evident, even without confirmatory ECG and enzyme rise. Occasionally, acute infarction may be heralded by acute left ventricular failure, without appreciable chest pain. If pain or discomfort is of short duration or repetitive, and there is no constitutional upset, the diagnosis often lies between mild infarct and an ischemic episode. As in the middle-aged patient, such an episode will usually be uncomplicated and the risk of early ventricular fibrillation slight. An initial ECG may be unhelpful (McGuinness et al. 1976). Serial blood specimens for enzyme estimation are valuable, but daily ECG tracings are usually not practical in the home situation. A tracing taken at the third day is likely to be most helpful.

As in the CCU, assessment of severity is as important in early and late management as is diagnosis. In each situation, the simple grading system can be used (see Table 16.8). All degrees of infarct severity are seen, but, for convenience, reference will be made below to the home management of the Grade 1 mild, uncomplicated infarct patient, and to the Grade 3 severe, complicated, and invalided patient.

The Mild Case

In the absence of failure, cardiac enlargement, and rate and rhythm disturbance, the most important aim of management is to prevent unnecessary invalidism and to have the patient back to a normal way of life within a week or two (Myocardial Infarction—How to Prevent—How to Rehabilitate 1973). The rate of mobilization, although perhaps not its vigor, should be almost the same as for mild infarction in younger patients. The elderly patient should be out of bed in a week, and getting around in the house on the flat within two weeks.

Coronary risk factors have less relevance at this age. It is still worthwhile to stop smoking cigarettes, now that we have the evidence from Dublin and Gothenburg (Mulcahy et al. 1975, Wilhelmsson et al. 1975) that smoking has an effect on postinfarct mortality; it is even more important to stop smoking if bronchitis is already present. Graded walking exercise will help to extend the patient's physical horizon and, it is to be hoped, retard his physical aging process. As in younger coronary subjects, a degree of physical fitness will counteract angina and depression (Working Party 1975). Less than severe hypertension should be managed conservatively. There does appear to be some danger in reducing pressure to low normal levels, because myocardial viability may depend on the adequacy of collateral vessel perfusion pressures. Rarely will the hyperlipidemias be sought at this

age; control of substantial obesity and of diabetes mellitus are probably the only reasons for special dietetic advice.

As always, the doctor's psychological approach to the patient and
to the family is vital. Hospital admission by itself may have encouraged them to take an overpessimistic view of the heart attack, with
resulting homecoming depression on the patient's part and overpro-
tection by the family. Advice in such circumstances should be optimistic and not too guarded, and guidance about physical activity will
help to promote a healthier psychological climate.

The aging coronary myocardium, although it will benefit from
regular, graded, slightly vigorous exercise, requires intervening rest
periods. At no time thereafter should the patient undertake even
slightly strenuous, prolonged sports and recreation on successive
days. Although cardiac rehabilitation in general cannot be expected to
contribute much to prevention of coronary mortality and further
infarction, it can counteract many other important and common
sequelae of infarct, such as cardiac neurosis and iatrogenic invalidism
and inertia, anxiety and depression, cessation of social and recrea-
tional activities, giving up a beneficial and interesting light job, and
false beliefs about sexual abstinence and types of food and alcoholic
beverages.

Clearly, the family doctor, once he is confident about the assessment of severity, must take the opportunity and time to advise on
such matters, which may not be self-evident or volunteered as
problems by the patient. The patient's well-being, and his future
happiness and usefulness, may all depend on receiving this proper
advice and having it reinforced at intervals. An advisory booklet, the
contents of which are familiar to the practitioner, can be of great help
to some. Fortunately, people in this age group take rather more kindly
than do younger individuals to being told they have had a mild heart
attack, which may interrupt their way of life for only a few weeks—
little more, indeed, than an attack of flu. They should be warned not
to pay too much attention to the experiences and well-meaning advice
of ex-patient friends.

The More Disabled Elderly Cardiac Patient

A Grade 3 infarct patient will have a large heart and barely
controlled cardiac failure. He will be having to take tablets—diuretic,
potassium, and possibly digoxin, perhaps even warfarin—and sleeping tablets in addition. Modern diuretics have done much to prolong

the comfort and life of such patients, and repetitive, distressing nocturnal cardiac asthma is now rare. The taking of a multiplicity of tablets, however, raises new problems for the elderly cardiac invalid. Balance is so delicate and vital that many instances of relapse are caused by failure to take the correct daily medication.

In the home situation, thiazides are preferable to frusemide; digoxin is probably best reserved in elderly cardiac invalids for those requiring it to control atrial fibrillation, because adjustment of dose with sinus rhythm is fraught with difficulty, even with dependable administration. Tactful daily supervision of medication by a friend or community nurse is sometimes essential.

Immobilization and lack of encouragement in themselves create rehabilitation problems, so that patients quickly become excessively dependent. Elderly patients and their relatives are often unduly pessimistic after a heart attack, and it is well to assure them that permanent severe invalidism is now an uncommon sequela. Chair nursing for part of the day should be instituted early, perhaps within a matter of days of the infarction, and limb movements encouraged at least daily.

The elderly tend to suffer from multiple, often degenerative, pathology, especially of the special senses and of the autonomic and muscle joint systems, and from a combination of medical, psychological, and social problems (Brocklehurst 1975). Anxiety and depression are common. Confusion and lack of insight are barriers to recovery, while clarity of intellect and motivation greatly facilitate all aspects of rehabilitation. Adverse social circumstances in the home may make demands on the doctor, the relatives, and the community services. In some instances, day hospital reeducation facilities may be indicated to retrieve confidence and to help the cardiac patient adapt to living alone again and to regaining a measure of independence in the community.

References

Brocklehurst, J. C. (1975) *Hosp. Update* **1**, 435.

Chaturvedi, N. C., Shivalingappa, G., Shanks, P., McKay, A., Cumming, K., Walsh, M. J., Scaria, K., Lynas, P., Courtney, D., Barber, J. M., and Boyle, D. M. (1972) *Lancet* **1**, 280.

Kerr, F., and Donald, K. W. (1974) *Br. Heart J.* **36**, 117.

Lawrie, D. M., Greenwood, T. W., Goddard, M., Harvey, A. C., Donald, K. W., Julian, D. G., and Oliver, M. F. (1967) *Lancet* **2**, 109.

Linn, B. S., and Yurt, R. W. (1970) *Br. Med. J.* **2**, 25.

Mulcahy, R., Hickey, H., McKenzie, G., and Graham, I. (1975) *Br. Heart J.* **37**, 158.

Myocardial Infarction—How to Prevent—How to Rehabilitate (1973) *In* Semple, B. et al. (eds.), *ISC Handbook 1973*, Boehringer, Mannheim, p. 000.

McGuinness, J. B., Begg, T. B., and Semple, T. (1976) *Br. Med. J.* (in press).

Nagle, R. E., and Williams, D. O. (1974) *Br. Heart J.* **36**, 1037 (abstract).

Norris, R. M., Brandt, P. W. T., Caughey, D. E., Lee, A. J., and Scott, P. J. (1969) *Lancet* **1**, 274.

Norris, R. M., Caughey, D. E., Deeming, L. W., Mercer, C. J., and Scott, P. J. (1970) *Lancet* **2**, 485.

Pathy, M. S. (1967) *Br. Heart J.* **29**, 190.

Peel, A. A. F., and Semple, T. (1972) *In* Meltzer, L. E., and Dunning, A. J. (eds.), *Textbook of Coronary Care*, Excerpta Medica, Amsterdam.

Peel, A. A. F., Semple, T., Wang, I., Lancaster, W. M., and Dall, J. L. C. (1962) *Br. Heart J.* **24**, 745.

Ristic, V., Najdanovic, B., Ivankovik, D., Korolja, P., and Gavrilovic, D. (1971) *Proceedings of the Sixth European Congress of Clinical Gerontology*, Huber, Berne.

Rodstein, M. (1956) *Arch. Intern. Med.* **98**, 84.

Semple, T. (1973) *In: Das chronisch kranke Herz*, Proc. Symp. Bad Krozingen 1972, F. K. Schattauer Verlag, Stuttgart and New York, p. 39.

Semple, T., Williams, B. O., Begg, T. B., and McGuinness, J. B. (1974) *Br. Heart J.* **36**, 536.

Thadani, U., Chopin, M. P., Aber, C. P., and Portal, R. W. (1971) *Br. Med. J.* **2**, 135.

Wilhelmsen, L., Sanne, H., Elmfeldt, D., Grimby, G., and Tibblin, G., and Wedel, H. J. (1975) *Preventive Medicine* **4**, 491.

Wilhelmsson, G., Vedin, J. A., Elmfeldt, E., Tibblin, G., and Wilhelmsen, L. (1975) *Lancet* **1**, 415.

Williams, B. O., Begg, T. B., Semple, T., and McGuinness, J. B. (1976) *Br. Med. J.* (in press).

Working Party (1975) *J. R. Coll. Physicians London* **9**, 281.

17

Cardiac Arrhythmias in the Aged

RAYMOND HARRIS

Introduction and Overview

Cardiac arrhythmias are not unique to the aged, but their appearance and greater frequency in the aged present special problems, because older people have greater impairment of physiological reserve and altered pharmacological response to drugs as a result of the aging process and the concurrent multiple diseases of the heart and other organs. This chapter highlights significant aspects of cardiac arrhythmias in the elderly and summarizes the newer advances in our understanding of their genesis and treatment.

Basic Considerations

Physiological Aspects

Disturbances in the rate, regularity, or origin of the heartbeat arise from an abnormality of impulse initiation—a disturbed conduction of the impulse that changes the sequence of activity of the atria or the ventricles or both (Cranefield et al. 1973). Specific pathologic lesions may cause some cardiac dysrhythmias, but many arrhythmias have not been correlated with an anatomic abnormality (Titus 1973).

RAYMOND HARRIS · Albany Medical College, Albany, New York.

Some atrial arrhythmias in the aged arise from cardiac changes attributed to the aging process, such as focal thickening of the elastic and reticular nets and infiltration of fat in and about the region of the sino-atrial (S-A) node (Harris 1970a), or a significant decrease in the amount of muscle and an increase in the percentage of fibrous tissue in the S-A node and internodal tracts of patients over 75 years of age at death, as compared with those under 50. These changes represent a slow and continuous process that starts around 60 years of age; they are unrelated to coronary artery disease, and may partially account for the ease with which atrial arrhythmias are induced in elderly hearts (Davies and Pomerance 1972).

Some common atrial dysrhythmias—atrial fibrillation, atrial flutter, and atrial tachycardia—may occur in patients with atrial pathology, such as nonspecific inflammation, degenerative and fibrotic processes, or ischemic states secondary to disease of the sinus node artery or its parent blood vessel (Titus 1973). Arteriosclerosis, acute coronary thrombosis, or shock decreasing the blood supply to the sinus node may also induce supraventricular arrhythmias in the elderly.

The activity of the autonomic nervous system and the local chemical environment of the pacemaker cells, including extracellular K^+ concentration, pH, PO_2, and the extracellular Ca^{++} concentration, also control the rate of firing of the cardiac pacemaker cells. Any physiological factor that decreases the intrinsic rate of the normal S-A nodal pacemaker or increases the automaticity of other specialized latent pacemakers can produce an arrhythmia. Increased vagal activity depressing the automaticity of the S-A node and causing the site of origin of the impulse to shift to another pacemaker proximal to the A-V node (low atrial rhythm), or to cells in the His–Purkinje system less strongly influenced by vagal activity, may contribute to some cardiac arrhythmias in this age group. Superimposed disease and the action of drugs used in therapy may cause cardiac arrhythmias by abolishing the normal physiologic overdrive suppression mechanism that ordinarily permits the sinus node to initiate the heartbeat. For example, catecholamines and digitalis may reverse the response of the automaticity cells to overdrive, so that overdrive, instead of causing depression, actually enhances automaticity and increases the possibility of escape rhythms (Cranefield et al. 1973).

Disturbances of the normal physiologic heart properties of excitability, irritability, conductivity, refractoriness, rhythmicity, and contractility must also be considered in the development of cardiac arrhythmias. Greater excitability and irritability characterize the aging myocardium; carbon dioxide retention, not uncommon in the elderly with an increased incidence of pulmonary disease, circulating catecholamines, and certain drugs, may increase excitability of heart muscle; alterations in the serum level of electrolytes, particularly potassium, influence the irritability of the heart. The serum concentration of calcium and magnesium should be checked in all patients with refractory arrhythmias. Neither conductivity nor refractoriness appears to be significantly altered in the aging heart.

Rhythmicity or automaticity enables the specialized nodal tissues of the heart to initiate rhythmic stimuli without the intervention of external agencies. Ordinarily, the S-A node tissue, building up and discharging more rapidly than the lower pacemaker centers, initiates the heartbeat. As a result, the head of the S-A node is depolarized first, then the body and tail. The activation wave passes from the sinus node through the connecting internodal pathways to the left atrium and the A-V node. These internodal pathways conduct more rapidly than the ordinary atrial myocardium, and atrial conduction is normally preferential for these particular anatomic pathways. Depolarization of the atria causes the P wave to be recorded on the ECG. After traversing the atria, the electrical impulse passes through the A-V junction, which includes the atrial approaches to the A-V node, the A-V node itself, and the penetrating portion of the bundle of His (Rosen 1973). A slightly delayed passage of the activation wave through the A-V node causes the P–R interval, which in the elderly may normally be as much as 0.21 sec. After its passage through the A–V junction, the electrical impulse traverses the remainder of the bundle of His, the bundle branches, the Purkinje fibers, and then the myocardium. The passage of the wave through the myocardium causes the QRS complex. Depolarization of the ventricular myocardium causes the T wave. The QRS time and contour in the older person are the same as in younger people, but the T waves in older people may normally be lower.

Although contractility of the heart bears little relevance to the initiation of heartbeat disorders, it is important in the hemodynamic consequences of arrhythmias in the aged patient. Certain physiological changes that characterize the aging human heart impair cardiovascular function (Table 17.1), and cardiac arrhythmias, relatively benign in younger people, may cause heart failure or death in the aged.

Cardiac arrhythmias are also more serious because they may compromise other vital organs already seriously impaired by the aging process and disease. For example, cardiac arrhythmias further decrease cerebral circulation in the presence of cerebrovascular disease.

Table 17.1. Physiological Impairment of the Cardiovascular System with Age[a]

1. Cardiac output drops 1%/yr below the normal 5 liter/min in younger persons, due to decreased stroke volume and slower heart rate.	6. Normal vasomotor tone decreases; vaginal influence increases.
2. Estimated left ventricular work at rest declines.	7. Peripheral vascular resistance rises 1%/yr.
3. Maximum blood flow through the coronary artery tree at 60 years of age is about 35% lower than in youth.	8. Heart is less sensitive to atropine and more sensitive to carotid sinus stimulation.
4. Delay in the recovery of contractility and irritability.	9. Decreased ability of heart to utilize oxygen.
	10. Increased pulse wave velocity.
5. Cardiac reserve diminishes; heart reacts poorly to sudden stress.	11. Increased cold pressor response.

[a] Adapted from Harris, R. (1970).

Cerebral blood flow in dogs decreases 7–12% during premature extrasystoles, 14% during supraventricular tachycardia, 23% during atrial fibrillation, and 40–70% during ventricular tachycardia (Samet 1973). Similar changes occur in humans. Anemia, pulmonary disorders, and other disease also aggravate the hemodynamic consequences of arrhythmias. For example, mild pulmonary congestion is more serious in an elderly patient with obstructive pulmonary emphysema than in one with normal lungs. Cardiac arrhythmias also increase anxiety in patients, leading to greater outpouring of catecholamines, with secondary adverse effects on the cardiac rhythm and peripheral vascular system (Kastor 1973). It is important, therefore, to treat promptly and properly all arrhythmias and their underlying conditions in the elderly.

Pharmacological Aspects

The pharmacological responses of the elderly differ from those of younger people. The aged are generally more sensitive to most cardiovascular drugs, and usually require smaller doses and more careful supervision. It is wise to check their medications on each visit, since they tend to continue to ingest drugs prescribed by other physicians, as well as those ordered by a new physician. In elderly patients with refractory arrhythmias, the best treatment may often be to discontinue all drugs and to start anew.

Tables 17.2 and 17.3 summarize some pertinent pharmacological aspects of antiarrhythmic drugs in the aged.

Digoxin and other shorter-acting digitalis preparations are particularly useful for the treatment of atrial fibrillation, atrial flutter, and supraventricular tachycardias. These drugs produce rapid digitalization within minutes. For most elderly patients requiring digitalis, an initial intravenous dose of 0.5 mg digoxin (Lanoxin) may be given, and additional doses (0.25–0.5 mg) at 4-h intervals, until the full digitalizing dose has been given, the arrhythmia disappears, or digitalis toxicity occurs. Reduced digitalis dosage during digitalization and maintenance is advisable in patients with potassium depletion, since the heart is more sensitive to digitalis in this situation.

Digitalis toxicity is common in elderly people. Symptoms include anorexia, vomiting, nausea, and cardiac arrhythmias, such as multifocal ventricular extrasystoles, paroxysmal supraventricular tachycardia, or atrial fibrillation with block. Although it has still not been definitely determined whether such apparent sensitivity is related to an increased sensitivity of the aged myocardium to normal concentrations of digitalis, or whether the usual dose of digitalis produces a higher myocardial concentration, it is established that such sensitivity is

TABLE 17.2. Digitalis Preparations for Geriatric Patients[a]

	Average total digitalizing dose		Average oral daily maintenance dose	Duration of effect
Preparation	Oral	i.v. or i.m.		
Shorter-Acting				
deslanoside (Cedilanid-D)	——	1.2–1.6 mg	——	24–36 h
digoxin (Lanoxin)	2–3 mg	1.2–2.0 mg	0.25–0.5 mg	24–36 h
gitalin (Gitaligin)	3–5 mg	——	0.5 mg or less	4–7 days
Longer-Acting				
digitalis leaf	1.2–2.0 g		0.1–0.2 g	17–20 days
digoxin	1.2–2 mg		0.1–0.2 mg	17–28 days

[a] Adapted from Harris, R. (1970).

TABLE 17.3. Pharmacology of Antiarrhythmic Drugs Useful in the Aged[a]

Drug	Administration	Loading dose (mg/kg)	Maintenance dose (mg/kg/day)	Therapeutic blood level (mg/liter)	Pharmacokinetic half-life (h)	Major site of inactivation
Lidocaine	i.v.	1-2	25-65	1.5-5.0	0.15-0.30	liver
	i.m.	2				
Quinidine	i.m.	2-4	12-24	3-8	4-6	kidney
	p.o.	3-6				
Procainamide	i.v.	1-2	40-80	4-10	3	kidney
	p.o.	15-20				
Atropine	i.v.	0.0086-0.015				liver
Diphenylhydantoin	i.v.	3-10		10-25	5-6	liver
	p.o.	15-30	6-12			
Propranolol	i.v.	0.05-0.15	0.5-3.0	0.015-0.08	3-4	kidney
	p.o.	0.5-1.0				
Practolol	i.v.	0.07-0.3	3.0-14.0	2.0	7-13	kidney
	p.o.	3.0-6.0				

[a] Adapted from Klein, M. D. (1975).

related in part to decreased renal excretion, digoxin being excreted mainly by the kidneys. The same dose, given to young and old subjects, produces blood level concentrations nearly twice as high and longer blood half-life in the elderly, as a consequence of their smaller body size and diminished urinary excretion. It is therefore wise to give the elderly patient slightly less than the full digitalizing dose used for younger people, and to decrease his daily maintenance dose (see Table 17.2; Harris 1970). If judicious amounts of digitalis in appropriate conditions do not effectively slow the ventricular rate to 65–95 beats/min, other forms of therapy—such as more aggressive treatment of the underlying condition, administration of antiarrhythmic agents, use of propranolol to increase A-V blockage, or cardioversion—are rational alternatives to overdigitalization.

Serum digoxin concentrations of 0.8–2 ng/ml are in the therapeutic range. Concentrations above this range are potentially toxic. For radioimmunoassay methods of measuring serum digoxin levels, blood samples should be obtained at least 5–6 h after the last dose of digoxin.

When digitalis intoxication is suspected, it is best to stop the drug. For serious digitalis-induced cardiac arrhythmias, potassium chloride may be given orally in divided doses, 4 g/day, or slowly intravenously, 40 mEq in 500 cc 5% glucose and water, and repeated as necessary. Diphenylhydantoin (Dilantin) may also be useful.

Lidocaine is effective in approximately 87% of ventricular arrhythmias, but in only 20% of supraventricular arrhythmias. It is therefore not recommended for supraventricular arrhythmias. Lidocaine exerts its antiarrhythmic effect by increasing the electrical stimulation threshold of the ventricle during diastole. It is 90% metabolized in the liver, and 10% is excreted unchanged through the kidneys.

Adverse effects in the elderly include light-headedness, drowsiness, disorientation, and convulsions, as well as hypotension, cardiovascular collapse, and bradycardia leading to cardiac arrest. Lidocaine is contraindicated in patients with Stokes–Adams syndrome, severe degrees of sino-atrial, atrioventricular, or intraventricular block, and should not be given to eliminate ventricular ectopic beats in patients with sinus bradycardia without first accelerating the heart rate by isoproterenol or electrical pacing.

For most ventricular arrhythmias, the recommended dose is a priming bolus of 50–75 mg given intravenously at a rate of 25–50 mg/min under electrocardiographic monitoring. A second dose may be repeated in 5 min if the first dose does not produce the required effect. Where indicated, a continuous infusion of lidocaine may be administered intravenously at a rate of 1–4 mg/min under constant electrocardiographic monitoring.

Procainamide hydrochloride (Pronestyl) depresses the excitability of the cardiac muscle to electrical stimulation and slows conduction in the atrium, the bundle of His, and the ventricle. It is indicated in the treatment of premature ventricular contractions, ventricular tachycardia, atrial fibrillation, and paroxysmal atrial tachycardia.

Oral or intramuscular therapy is preferable. The intravenous route should be reserved for life-threatening arrhythmias that do not respond to oral or intramuscular therapy. For premature ventricular contractions, 50 mg/kg body weight may be given orally daily in divided doses at three to four hourly intervals. For ventricular tachycardia, 1 g may be given orally and followed by a total daily dose of 50 mg/kg body weight given at three hourly intervals. For atrial fibrillation or paroxysmal atrial tachycardia, an initial oral dose of 1.25 g may be given and followed in an hour by 0.75 g if necessary. A dose of 0.5–1 g may be given every 2 h until the arrhythmia is interrupted or the limit of tolerance is reached. The suggested maintenance dose is 0.5–1 g every 4 to 6 h.

Toxic effects on the myocardium include widening of the QRS complex, prolongation of the P–R and Q–T intervals and decreased QRS and T-wave voltages. Untoward responses with normal doses may occur in elderly patients whose liver and kidney disease cause accumulation of the drug and toxic side effects, including hypotension, ventricular tachycardia, and central nervous symptoms. A syndrome resembling lupus erythematosus may occur in patients on long-term therapy. The serum antinuclear antibody titer should be determined regularly in patients receiving procainamide for a long time, or showing symptoms of a lupus-like reaction. A rising antibody titer or the appearance of clinical symptoms of lupus erythematosus demands immediate discontinuation of the drug. Although this complication is usually reversible when the drug is stopped, steroid therapy may be necessary if it continues.

Propranolol hydrochloride (Inderal), a β-adrenergic receptor blocking agent with a biologic half-life of 2 to 3 h, exerts its antiarrhythmic effects in concentrations associated with β-adrenergic blockage. It is an important drug in the management of cardiac arrhythmias due to increased levels of circulating catecholamines, or to increased sensitivity of the heart to catecholamines, as in arrhythmias associated with pheochromocytoma, thyrotoxicosis, or exercise. Propranolol is particularly useful in the management of paroxysmal atrial tachycardia, persistent symptomatic sinus tachycardia, arrhythmias due to thyro-toxicosis, atrial extrasystoles that interfere with the well-being of the patient, and atrial flutter and fibrillation when digitalis is contraindi-cated or does not adequately control the ventricular rate. It is less useful in ventricular tachycardia. Oral propranolol may reverse the tachyarrhythmia caused by digitalis intoxication that persists after digitalis is discontinued and electrolyte abnormalities have been corrected.

For the treatment of these cardiac arrhythmias, 10–30 mg may be given 3 to 4 times daily before meals and at bedtime. Intravenous administration is reserved for life-threatening arrhythmias.

This drug is contraindicated in patients with bronchial asthma, sinus bradycardia, greater than first degree A–V heart block, allergic rhinitis during the pollen season, cardiogenic shock, and right ventri-cular failure secondary to pulmonary hypertension and congestive heart failure. Sudden withdrawal of propranolol should be avoided in the elderly with coronary artery disease, since it may markedly increase the severity and frequency of angina, and cause severe arrhythmia, and even infarction (Nies and Shand 1975). It is not a drug of first choice in the elderly, whose myocardium is already compromised by age and disease and in whom propranolol may depress myocardial contractility and precipitate cardiac failure. The adverse reactions to propranolol are not related to dose, but appear with small doses early in the course of treatment (Nies and Shand 1975).

Practolol, the sole activity of which is β-adrenergic blocking, is promising for arrhythmias, although not available for clinical use in all countries.

Quinidine increases the refractory period of atrial and ventricular musculature, decreases excitability of the myocardium and conduction time in cardiac muscles, Purkinje fibers, and A–V conduction system, and suppresses automaticity. It is degraded in the liver and secreted by the kidneys.

Quinidine is effective in the treatment of paroxysmal supraventri-cular tachycardia, atrial fibrillation or flutter, ventricular tachycardia, and extrasystoles. Quinidine is the most dependable drug for the conversion of atrial fibrillation to normal sinus rhythm. The maximum effect of oral quinidine occurs within 1 to 3 h. Quinidine usually converts atrial fibrillation to normal sinus rhythm at an average plasma level of 6–8 mg/liter.

Nausea, vomiting, and diarrhea occur in some people. If these symptoms persist, the drug should be discontinued, particularly if the QRS complex widens significantly or other arrhythmic complications develop (Simon 1974).

Diphenylhydantoin sodium (Dilantin) given intravenously may control digitalis-induced arrhythmias. A dose of 5 mg/kg body weight (total dose not to exceed 300 mg) may be given intravenously in 5% dextrose and water at a rate not exceeding 50 mg/min over 1–4 min under electrocardiographic control.

This drug is contraindicated in patients with a high degree of heart block or marked bradycardia (Harris 1970), and should be used cautiously in elderly patients with hypotension and severe myocardial insufficiency. Elderly patients with impaired liver function may show early toxicity, since the liver is the site of biotransformation.

Normal Cardiac Rhythms

Extrasystoles

Minor arrhythmias that do not require treatment include extrasystoles originating in the sinus node, atria, atrioventricular junctional areas, or ventricles. Atrial premature contractions occur in 10% and ventricular premature contractions in 6% of people over the age of 65 (Mihalick and Fisch 1974). Such extrasystoles are premature in relationship to the prevailing rhythm, and may result from the increased myocardial irritability that characterizes the myocardium of elderly people, or from other functional or organic causes. Such extrasystoles usually bear a fixed or constant coupling to the preceding sinus beat and are rarely symptomatic.

Sinus Arrhythmia

This arrhythmia is common in elderly subjects. In phasic sinus arrhythmia, the sinus rate accelerates with inspiration and slows with expiration (Fig. 17.1). Nonphasic sinus arrhythmia due to shifting of the pacemaker stimulus within the sinus node is unrelated to respiration. The ECG shows P waves, variations of P–P cycles of more than 0.16 s, and a P–R interval of 0.12 s or longer.

Wandering Pacemaker

In this rhythm, the pacemaker impulse wanders to different parts of the sinus node, atria, and A–V node. The pacemaker is in the head,

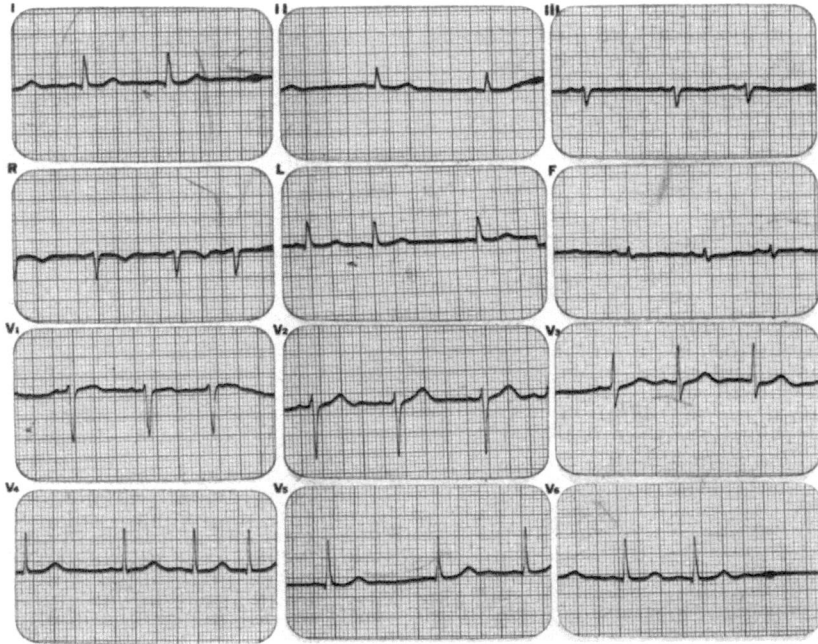

Fig. 17.1. Phasic sinus arrhythmia in an 86-year-old woman. The tracing is normal.

body, or tail of the sinus node when the ECG shows an upright P wave preceding the QRS complex in Leads I, II, and III, and a normal P–R interval of 0.12 s or longer. If antegrade and retrograde conduction are intact, a beat arising from the A–V junction produces both a retrograde P wave and a QRS of supraventricular configuration (Rosen 1973). When small P waves of variable contour precede the QRS complex in Lead I, and inverted or retrograde P waves precede the QRS complex in Leads II, III, and aVF, and the P–R interval is 0.12 sec or more in the limb leads (Fig. 17.2), the pacemaker impulse has been shown to originate in the coronary sinus area or in the inferior or low atrial region approach to the A–V junction (Rosen 1973). A–V junctional rhythm is diagnosed in the presence of retrograde P waves preceding the QRS in Leads II and III and a short P–R interval (less than 0.12 sec), or when the P wave is absent before or a retrograde P wave follows the QRS interval (see "A–V Junctional Rhythms," p. 339).

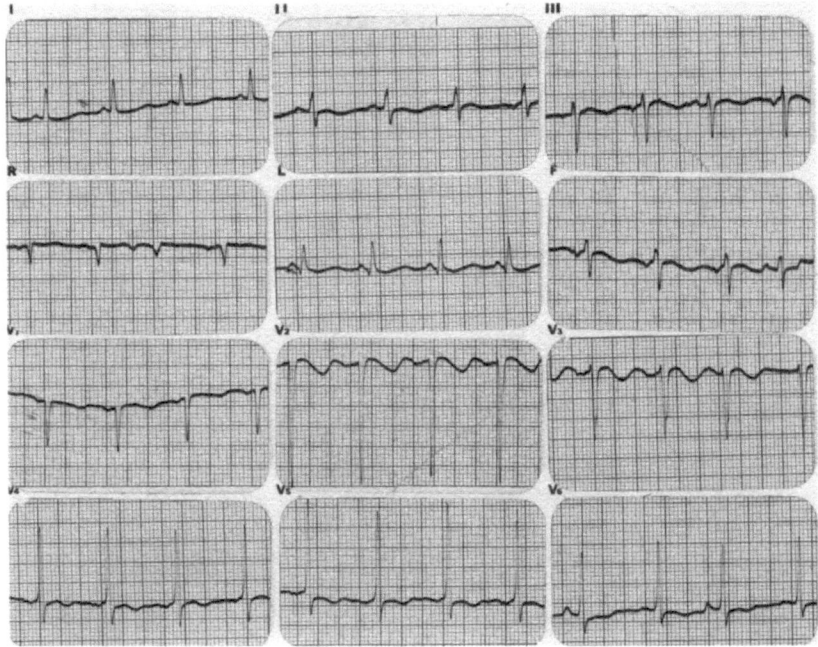

Fig. 17.2. Wandering pacemaker in a 72-year-old woman with a history of recurrent paroxysmal supraventricular tachycardia. Note the upright P waves and normal P–R interval of 0.16 sec in the first two sinus beats of Lead II. The next two beats show deformed, retrograde P waves and a slightly shorter P–R interval of 0.14 sec, indicating coronary sinus (inferior or low atrial) rhythm. Note the similar shifts of pacemaker in other leads.

Abnormal Cardiac Rhythms

Supraventricular Arrhythmias

The diagnosis of these arrhythmias is not always simple. Under unusual circumstances, the surface ECG may not readily record the P waves or atrial activity in elderly patients with atrial arrhythmias, because such recording depends on the mass of atrial depolarization and the proximity of the recording electrodes to the atrial mass (Wu et al. 1975). The surface leads that best reflect the atrial waves include Leads II, V_1, and S_5 [for which the positive electrode is over the fifth interspace to the right of the sternum and the negative electrode is over the manubrium sternum (Schamroth 1973)]. Esophageal or intracardiac recording techniques may be necessary for a more accurate diagnosis.

Supraventricular arrhythmias in which the dominant beat originates in the sinus node, atrium, or atrioventricular junction include sinus bradycardia, sinus tachycardia, sick sinus node syndrome, paroxysmal or chronic atrial tachycardia, atrial flutter, atrial fibrillation, and A–V junctional (nodal) tachycardia. The frequency of total atrial arrhythmias increases from the seventh to the tenth decade. Although multifocal atrial tachycardia has a low frequency in the geriatric population, its seriousness is probably the reason for its rarity (Mihalick and Fisch 1974).

Sinus Bradycardia. Sinus bradycardia with a heart rate below 60 beats/min may be physiologic in asymptomatic healthy old people with increased vagal tone or pathologic in those with impaired function of the S–A node due to aging changes or disease. Even rates as low as 40 beats/min may not be associated with significant hemodynamic consequences, unless the stroke volume is limited by myocardial or valvular disease, as in acute myocardial infarction or during acute stress when the heart rate cannot speed up because of a pathologic sinus node. Symptomatic sinus bradycardia with a rate of 40 or less may occur in some patients with sick sinus node syndrome, intracranial tumors, meningitis, hyperactive carotid sinus, jaundice, myxedema, beriberi, malnutrition, or mentally depressed states. Reserpine, digitalis, or β-blocking agents like propranolol or practolol may also cause a slow heart rate, and may have to be stopped in symptomatic patients. If the heart rate does not speed up or an arrhythmia occurs with exercise, disease of the S-A node should be investigated. In such patients, monitoring with a Holter-type apparatus may prove that cardiac arrhythmias are responsible for sudden falls or dizziness.

Ordinarily, no treatment is required for sinus bradycardia, except in the presence of significant hemodynamic impairment. Very slow pathologic sinus bradycardia over prolonged periods may decrease cardiac output, reduce cerebral blood flow leading to cerebral softening, and produce mental or neurologic symptoms and signs. Excessive slowing of the heart rate results in a greater disparity in the duration of action potentials and the refractory periods of cardiac tissues. This inhomogeneous electrical setting predisposes to reentrant excitation and arrhythmias. Increasing the heart rate decreases this inhomogeneity and the incidence of cardiac arrhythmias (Han et al. 1966).

Markedly slow sinus bradycardia often responds to treatment of the underlying conditions. When hypersensitive carotid sinus causes the slow heart rate, atropine, tincture of belladonna, ephedrine, or isoproterenol (Isuprel) may be given to speed up the heart rate. Some patients with symptomatic sinus bradycardia, especially those with bradytachycardia syndromes unresponsive to drug therapy, may require electrical pacing of the atrium or ventricle. Elderly patients with marked sinus bradycardia who cannot increase their ventricular rate with exercise and suffer the consequences of poor cardiac output—such as refractory congestive heart failure, azotemia due to decreased renal blood flow, lethargy, weakness, and mental confusion or other symptoms of poor blood flow—are good candidates for permanent cardiac pacing.

Sinus Tachycardia. Sinus tachycardia with a heart rate between 100 and 150 beats/min is a normal transient response to ordinary physical activity, ingestion of food, anxiety, or pain. Sinus tachycardia is rarely any faster in the elderly. When the heart rate is higher, sinus tachycardia must be differentiated from other supraventricular arrhythmias, particularly paroxysmal atrial tachycardia. Persistent sinus tachycardia suggests a chronic anxiety state, incipient heart failure, occult infection, fever, shock, hyperthyroidism, anemia, or possible digitalis toxicity.

The best treatment is directed at the underlying cause. When no cause can be found and the patient remains disturbed by the tachycardia, propranolol (10 mg q.i.d.) or reserpine (0.1–0.25 mg) orally may relieve symptoms. Diuretics, digitalis, and a low-salt diet should be prescribed for patients with sinus tachycardia due to heart failure.

Sick Sinus Node. This syndrome is common in elderly patients with impaired function of the S–A node and an abnormally unresponsive A–V junctional pacemaker due to degenerative aging changes and vascular disease of the node and the atria. Such patients may have sinus bradycardia without symptoms, or widespread abnormalities of impulse formation and conduction, in which symptomatic, often unexplained sinus bradycardia or brief or sustained sinus arrest, or both, alternate with runs of escaped beats, atrial or A–V junctional rhythm, tachybradycardia, or other disabling arrhythmias (Fig. 17.3). Patients with this syndrome may complain of fatigue, light-headedness, dizziness, sudden falls, recurrent syncope, or congestive heart failure. Prolonged sinus arrest associated with failure or a subsidiary pacemaker may cause cardiac asystole. Some patients develop chronic atrial fibrillation with slow ventricular response due to concealed conduction and concomitant disease of the A–V junction and distal pathways. In some who undergo cardioversion for atrial fibrillation or

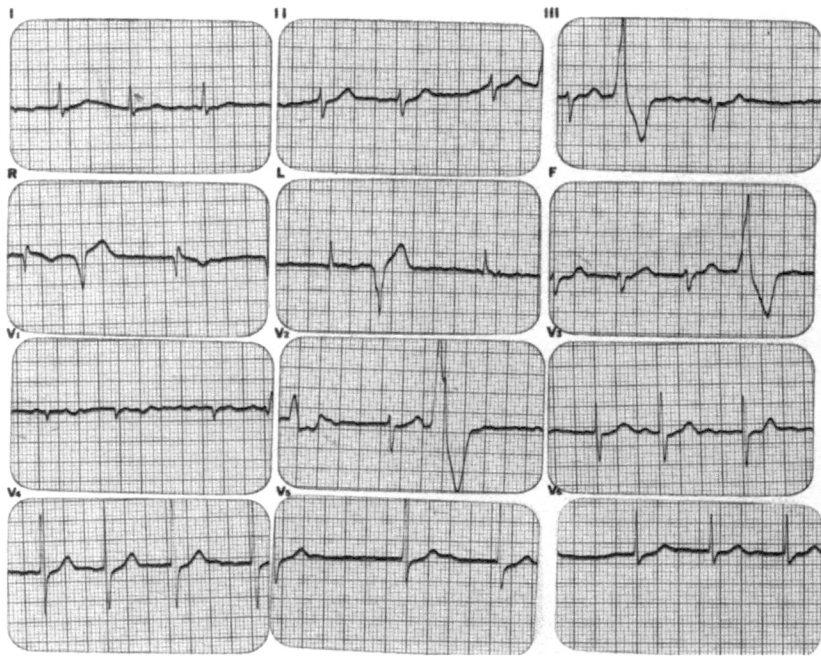

Fig. 17.3. Atrial fibrillation and ventricular extrasystoles in a 76-year-old man with sick sinus node syndrome. Atrial "F" fibrillatory waves are best seen in Lead V_1. Ventricular extrasystoles are coupled with the preceding QRS complex in Leads III, aVR, aVL, aVF, and V_2. A month previously, this patient had sinus bradycardia, a rate of 60, and frequent atrial and ventricular extrasystoles. The patient was asymptomatic and required no special treatment.

flutter, the heart may not resume sinus rhythm, and grave problems ensue (Ferrer 1968, 1973a,b).

This condition may be diagnosed when various supraventricular arrhythmias are documented on an ECG or during monitoring. This syndrome with its arrhythmias should be especially suspected in orthopedic patients hospitalized for fractures sustained during accidental falls. About one-fourth of patients with this syndrome have detectable underlying coronary artery disease.

Asymptomatic patients usually require no treatment. Artificial cardiac pacemakers may benefit those with disturbances of consciousness, syncope, or recurrent arrhythmias. Although pacing itself may not always prevent bouts of tachyarrhythmias, it permits the concur-

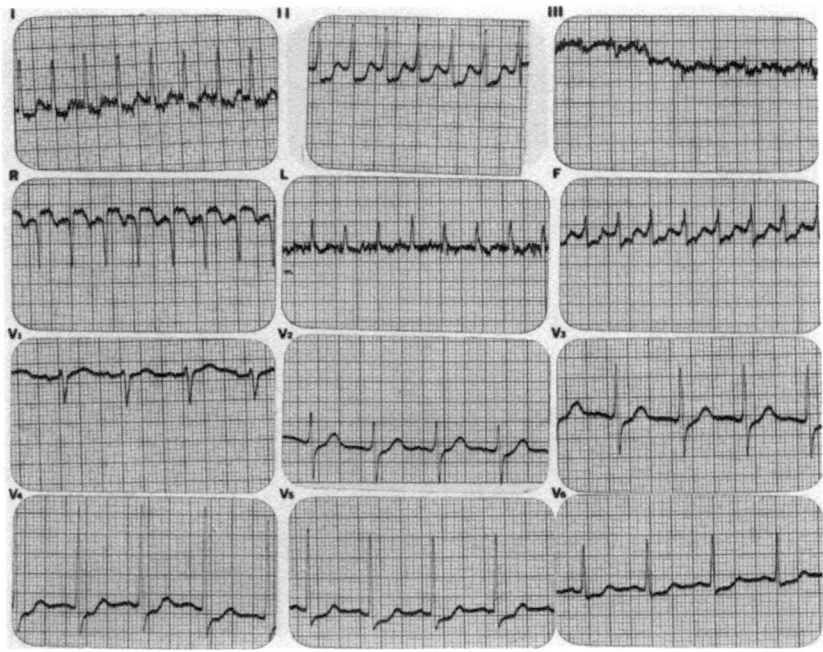

Fig. 17.4. Paroxysmal atrial tachycardia with a heart rate of 195 beats/min in limb and aV leads in a 68-year-old man. After left carotid sinus massage, sinus rhythm returned in Leads V_1–V_6.

rent addition of digitalis or antiarrhythmic agents, or both, to control the arrhythmia or heart failure without fear of aggravating the brady-cardia or sick sinus syndrome. Digitalis preparations should be used with caution in patients with sick sinus syndrome, because even small amounts may be toxic for selected patients (Margolis et al. 1975).

Supraventricular Tachycardias. Supraventricular tachycardias in-clude atrial tachycardia, atrial flutter, atrial fibrillation, and A–V junctional tachycardia. Paroxysmal supraventricular tachycardia, us-ually a reentry type of tachycardia involving the A–V node and part of the atrium, may be initiated by a properly timed atrial premature beat, junctional ectopic beat with an atrial echo, or a ventricular ectopic beat with an atrial echo and ventricular reciprocal beat (Ticzon and Whe-land 1973). Since the surface ECG does not always permit an accurate diagnosis of atrial activity, paroxysmal supraventricular tachycardia is a good term to use when it is difficult to be sure of the exact supraventricular rhythm. For example, Wu et al. (1975) reported that the surface ECG in one elderly patient suggested atrial flutter, while direct electrophysiological studies demonstrated paroxysmal left atrial tachycardia with separation of left and right atrial components of the P wave by an isoelectric period, secondary to marked interatrial conduction delay. In another patient, the surface ECG was interpreted as showing paroxysmal atrial tachycardia with block, while electrophysiological studies revealed right atrial standstill with atrial inexcitability and two dissimilar rhythms involving the left atrium.

Paroxysmal supraventricular tachycardia is characterized on the ECG by an abrupt onset and ending; a ventricular rate usually between 140 and 240 beats/min, the presence of abnormal P waves at the same rate, or absent P waves; narrow QRS complexes, except when conduction defects are present; precisely regular ventricular or atrial complexes, or both; and an absent response or abrupt ending during carotid massage (Fig. 17.4). Paroxysmal supraventricular tachycardia may be divided into paroxysmal atrial tachycardia and paroxysmal junctional tachycardia. A nonparoxysmal form of nodal tachycardia with a slow rate between 70 to 130 beats/min may occur in some elderly patients with organic disease or digitalis intoxication.

Atrial tachycardia is usually paroxysmal (see Fig. 17.4), but the chronic form with A–V heart block and a slow ventricular rate may occasionally occur (Fig. 17.5). In atrial tachycardia without atrioventricular block, the ECG shows abnormal P waves, not of a retrograde contour, that consistently precede normal-appearing QRS complexes of 0.06–0.10-sec duration, and a rate usually between 140 to 240 beats/min. At faster heart rates, A–V heart block is common in the aged because of concomitant disease of the conduction system.

Treatment of atrial tachycardia depends on the underlying cause of the arrhythmia, the patient's age and condition, and the medical history. This condition is usually associated with organic heart disease in the aged, in contrast to its appearance in young people without such disease. In the absence of serious complications such as heart failure or syncope, simple reassurance, sedation with phenobarbital, tranquilizers, or morphine and rest may permit the arrhythmia to return to sinus rhythm in a few hours. In patients with hypokalemia, correction of the low serum potassium may revert the arrhythmia spontaneously to sinus rhythm. When the serum potassium level is low, intravenous or oral potassium may be given. For intravenous therapy, 30–40 mEq potassium chloride in 500 ml of 5% dextrose in water may be given over 2–4 h, during which the ECG should be observed for prolongation of the QRS complex and increased amplitude of T waves, which would suggest toxic effects. The level of serum

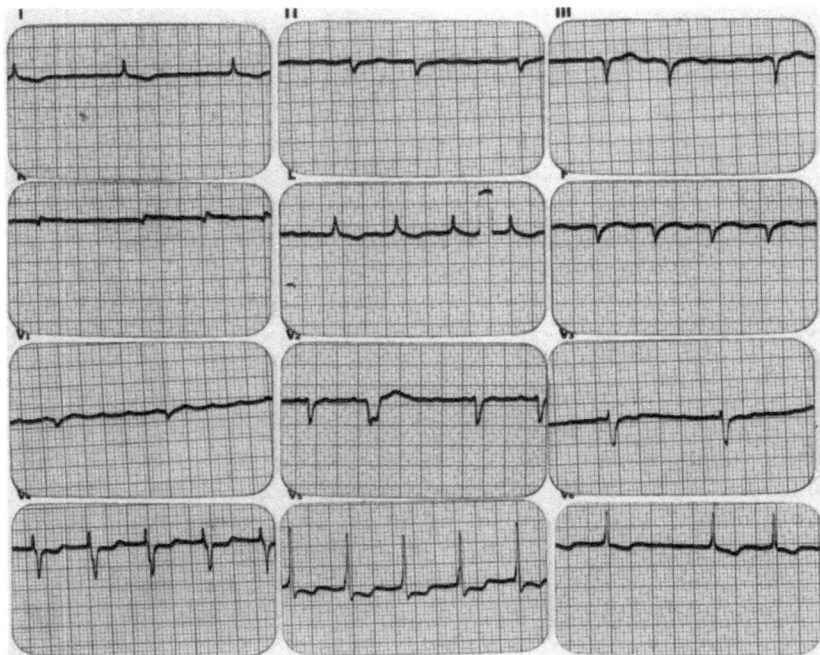

Fig. 17.5. Chronic atrial tachycardia with 4:1 conduction in a 79-year-old man. Atrial waves at a rate of 220 beats/min are best seen in V_1 and V_2. Note the 2:1 A–V conduction in V_4, V_5, and other leads. Since the patient was taking digoxin for congestive heart failure, digitalis toxicity was suspected. After digoxin was stopped, this arrhythmia persisted, indicating organic heart disease as its origin. Since a diuretic controlled the patient's heart failure and the patient tolerated this chronic atrial tachycardia with slow ventricular rate without difficulty, no other treatment was necessary. This rhythm is easily mistaken for atrial fibrillation, and emphasizes the need to look carefully at all leads before an arrhythmia is diagnosed in the elderly.

potassium should also be determined at frequent intervals to avoid hyperkalemia. Elderly patients usually suffer impaired renal function, so that special caution should be taken in giving potassium to them. Oral potassium is preferable in patients with only slightly low serum potassium levels, or in those with seriously depressed levels whose arrhythmia is not life-threatening.

Physiologic vagotonic-inducing maneuvers, such as the Valsalva maneuver, coughing, gagging, self-induced vomiting, or carotid sinus pressure, may also be effective. Carotid sinus pressure helps distinguish between sinus tachycardia and atrial tachycardia. Carotid sinus pressure slows sinus tachycardia, but either terminates paroxysmal supraventricular tachycardia (see Fig. 17.4) or produces A–V block with slowing of the ventricular but not the atrial rate. Carotid sinus pressure should be performed carefully and only under cardiographic monitoring in the aged because of their more sensitive carotid sinus and widespread atherosclerosis in the carotid or basilar arteries, which makes them more susceptible to cerebrovascular occlusion.

Digitalis is the most useful and effective therapeutic alternative in the elderly when such vagotonic maneuvers fail. Digoxin (0.5 mg) or deslanoside (Cedilanid-D, 0.4 mg) given intravenously, to depress the ectopic focus, increase vagal tone, and sensitize the carotid sinus reflex, frequently produces conversion after the initial dose. If the arrhythmia persists, subsequent doses may be given to complete digitalization (see Table 17.2). Digitalis therapy should not be continued after conversion, unless a maintenance dose is necessary to prevent the return of the arrhythmia.

Synchronized DC conversion beginning with a low dose of electrical energy such as 25–50 J and increasing the dose while the patient is monitored may be effective if the arrhythmia does not respond to the measures outlined above. It is best to do such conversion when the patient has had no digitalis, or after digitalis has been discontinued for several days. Temporary pervenous right atrial pacing or right ventricular pacing has also been useful in terminating paroxysmal supraventricular tachycardia (Ticzon and Wheland 1973).

Edrophonium bromide (Tensilon), other cholinergic drugs, and pressor agents useful in younger people may be dangerous in old people, in whom these drugs should be used cautiously, if at all. When edrophonium is used, a syringe containing 1 mg atropine sulfate should be immediately available to counteract any severe cholinergic reaction.

Quinidine may also be useful in refractory atrial tachycardias. After a test dose of 200 mg quinidine, 400 mg may be given and repeated at 2-h intervals for 5 doses; the pulse, blood pressure, and ECG should be recorded before beginning therapy and before giving the last 3 doses. The drug should be stopped immediately on return of sinus rhythm or occurrence of signs of quinidine toxicity, which include hypotension widening of the QRS to 50% of the control value, frequent ventricular premature contractions, or other abnormal arrhythmias. It is best to monitor the patient for several hours after quinidine has been stopped, since paroxysmal ventricular tachycardia or fibrillation may occur during this time.

The development of paroxysmal supraventricular tachycardia, particularly associated with A–V block, in patients on digitalis should

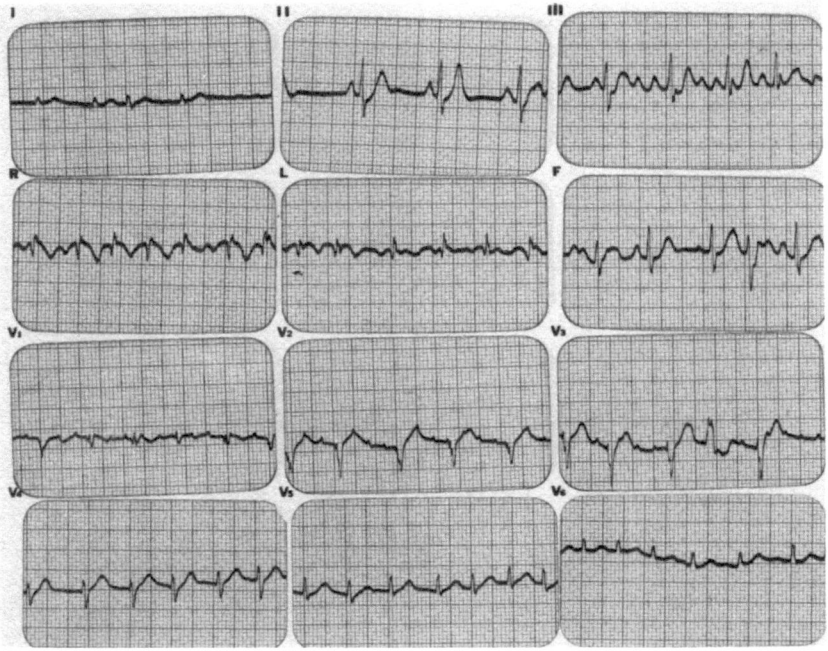

Fig. 17.6. Paroxysmal atrial flutter with an atrial flutter "F" wave rate of 370 beats/min in a 66-year-old man. These waves are best seen in the precordial leads and in Lead III. The ventricular rate is 140 beats/min. Sinus rhythm is apparently present in Lead II and sinus beats in aVF.

make the physician suspect digitalis toxicity. In this situation, it is advisable to stop digitalis and restore normal electrolyte balance. Propranolol (10–30 mg, 3 to 4 times daily), quinidine, procainamide, or diphenylhydantoin may be tried in life-threatening situations. When synchronized DC electroversion is used, it is preferable to perform this procedure after digitalis has been stopped for several days.

Patients with recurrent paroxysmal atrial tachycardia should be advised to stop smoking and not to drink coffee or other beverages with high caffeine content. Maintenance digitalis therapy or combinations of antiarrhythmic agents such as quinidine, propranolol, procainamide, and oral diphenylhydantoin may be tried prophylactically in long-term management of patients with refractory chronic supraventricular arrhythmias.

Multifocal atrial tachycardia in chronically debilitated elderly patients with chronic obstructive pulmonary disease or digitalis toxicity is characterized by multiform P waves preceding the QRS complexes, an atrial rate greater than 100 beats/min, varying P–R intervals, and irregular P–P and R–R intervals. Treatment with antiarrhythmic agents and electrocardioversion often fail, and the mortality rate is high (Donoso 1973).

Atrial flutter almost always occurs in association with organic heart disease. Pulmonary embolism should be suspected in patients with this condition.

The ECG in atrial flutter shows saw-toothed atrial flutter "F" waves, occurring regularly at a rate between 200 and 375 beats/min (Fig. 17.6), a rate much faster than that associated with atrial tachycardia, which is usually below 200 beats/min. Such "F" flutter waves are usually best seen in Leads II, III, aVF, and V₁. The average ventricular rate generally depends on the degree of A–V heart block.

Treatment of atrial flutter in the elderly depends on the underlying clinical condition. Many cardiologists believe that electroversion after diazepam (Valium, 5–15 mg) has been given intravenously for sedation and amnesia is the best immediate treatment of choice, and should be done before any initial drug therapy. Atrial flutter usually responds readily to a shock of low intensity, ranging from 10 to 25 J. In patients on digitalis, this drug should be stopped for 1 to 2 days before cardioversion is done. Digoxin is the most useful medical measure in the elderly to slow the ventricular rate and to convert atrial flutter in elderly people not already on digitalis. Many elderly patients tolerate chronic atrial flutter well when digitalis or organic A–V heart block keeps the ventricular rate between 70 and 90 beats/min. Digitalis (see the section on atrial tachycardia, p. 333, for dosage and method) may cause atrial flutter to revert directly to sinus rhythm; to change to atrial fibrillation; or to persist with a higher degree of A–V heart block and a slower, controlled ventricular rate of 60–100 beats/min that permits the patient to do well despite the arrhythmia. If atrial flutter persists after digitalization has been completed, quinidine sulfate or procainamide may be tried to restore sinus rhythm, if necessary. Very often atrial flutter will revert spontaneously to sinus rhythm once the underlying precipitating factor has been treated.

Atrial fibrillation occurs in about 8% of people over 65 years of age (Mihalick and Fisch 1974), and in 10–15% of hospitalized aged (Caird 1963). In this condition, ectopic atrial foci produce rapid, irregular depolarization of the atria. The ECG shows atrial fibrillatory waves and rapid and irregular ventricular complexes (Figs. 17.3, 17.7, and 17.8). Brief runs of paroxysmal atrial fibrillation may be noted in

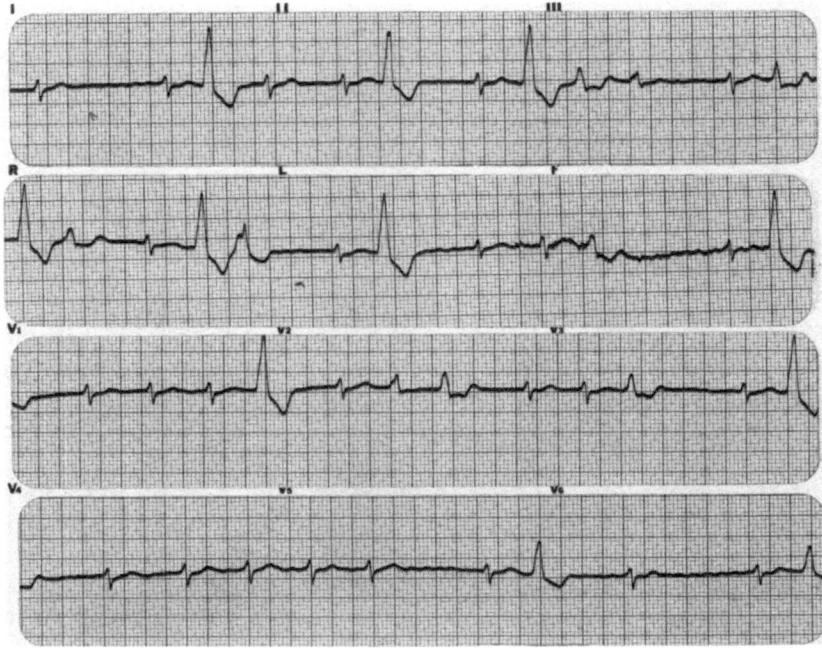

Fig. 17.7. Continuous electrocardiographic strip shows atrial fibrillation in an 88-year-old man. This rhythm is characterized by the absence of P waves, rapid undulations of the base line ("F" waves"), and irregular ventricular rhythm, with an average ventricular heart rate of 100 beats/min. The wider, taller QRS complexes, following and often coupled with the beats terminating a long diastolic interval, are ventricular extrasystoles, illustrating the "rule of bigeminy" of Langendorf et al. (1955). The fourth beat in row 3, similar to the others, occurs without a preceding long diastolic pause and tends to confirm the diagnosis of ventricular premature contractions, rather than supraventricular conducted beats with aberration.

routine ECGs in asymptomatic elderly people. Chronic atrial fibrillation is usually a manifestation of organic heart disease due to ischemic heart disease, to aging changes in and about the S-A node and the atria, and to the same causes as in younger individuals. The prognosis depends on the specific etiology. In the aged, a rheumatic etiology is less likely, and atrial fibrillation may be the only evidence of masked hyperthyroidism, which occurs more frequently in this group. Although atrial fibrillation is more common in the geriatric population, no definite age-related trend is noted in patients over the age of 70 (Mihalick and Fisch 1974).

Lone auricular fibrillation (benign idiopathic arteriosclerotic or senile fibrillation without heart disease), an interesting variant found in middle-aged and older people without evidence of structural heart disease (Evans and Swan 1954), is more common in men and does not appear to affect longevity. Most patients are asymptomatic and require no treatment. Digitalis may be useful in those complaining of palpitations or whose heart rate becomes much faster after exertion.

The primary objective in treating atrial fibrillation is to maintain an acceptable heart rate between 60 and 80 beats/min at rest and rising to no more than 110 beats/min with exercise or after the administration of atropine. Treatment depends on the clinical condition. Correction of the underlying condition often spontaneously restores sinus rhythm. When atrial fibrillation is present with a ventricular rate less than 100 beats/min and no heart failure, rest, reassurance, and a salt-restricted

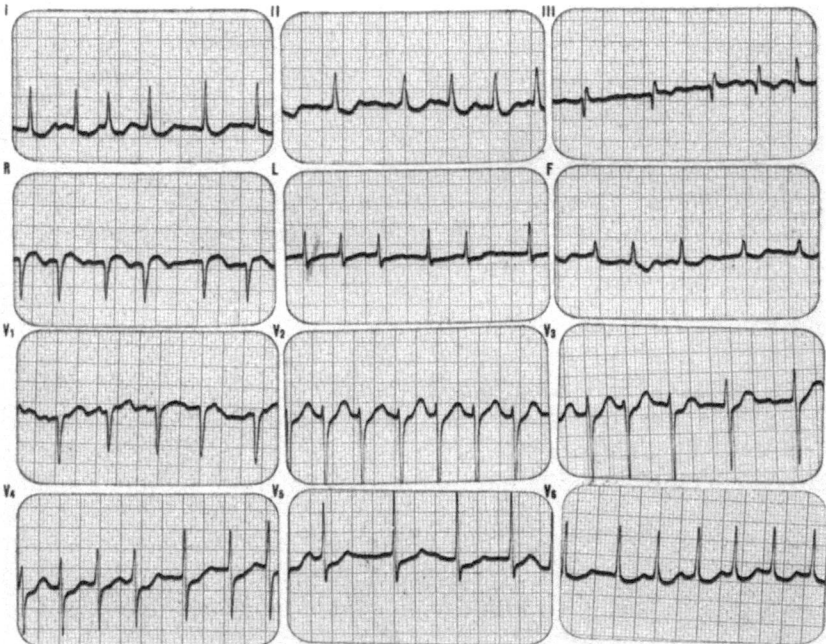

Fig. 17.8. Atrial fibrillation with an average ventricular rate of 130 beats/min and nonspecific S-T–T wave changes in a 96-year-old woman with congestive heart failure, requiring digitalization.

diet may be enough. When a rapid ventricular rate with or without heart failure is present, digitalis is needed to slow the ventricular rate and improve diastolic ventricular filling, coronary artery blood flow, and myocardial function. Enough digitalis should be given to maintain the heart rate between 70 and 80 beats/min. Propranolol may be added to slow the heart rate when fast atrial fibrillation does not respond sufficiently to digitalis.

Most elderly patients tolerate chronic atrial fibrillation well when the ventricular rate is between 60 and 80 beats/min, and conversion to sinus rhythm is unnecessary, except in the presence of refractory heart failure or recurrent emboli. Pharmacological conversion is usually simpler and safer in elderly patients with symptomatic atrial fibrillation. Digitalis or quinidine therapy converts atrial fibrillation to sinus rhythm in about 80% of patients with arteriosclerotic heart disease, and in about 40% of those with rheumatic heart disease. If the atrial fibrillation persists after the patient has been digitalized, an oral test dose of quinidine sulfate (200 mg) may be given. If no untoward effects occur, 200 mg may be given orally every 6 h for the first day. If the arrhythmia persists, the dose may be increased to 400 mg every 8 h on the second day and to every 6 h on the third day. Rarely is it justified in the elderly to use doses of quinidine of 500 mg or more. During this procedure, the patient should be monitored. Quinidine should be discontinued if any signs of toxicity occur (see the section on atrial tachycardia, p. 333). Once sinus rhythm has returned, quinidine sulfate (200–400 mg) may be given 3 to 4 times daily to prevent the return of the arrhythmia.

Synchronized DC cardioversion may be necessary in some patients with atrial fibrillation and rapid ventricular rate that fail to respond to drug therapy, and in whom hyperthyroidism and electrolyte imbalance have been excluded. This procedure is successful in about 92% of patients with atrial fibrillation. Ordinary indications include congestive heart failure uncontrolled by ordinary therapy, refractory angina pectoris, peripheral or pulmonary emboli originating from the atria, a rapid ventricular rate uncontrolled by digitalis, and persistent atrial fibrillation after hyperthyroidism has been controlled. Relative contraindications include asymptomatic patients whose ventricular rate is easily controlled with or without digitalis therapy or propranolol, or both; digitalis toxicity; quinidine intolerance; recurrence of atrial fibrillation after conversion, despite adequate prophylactic therapy; complete heart block; and a giant left atrium (Hurst et al. 1964). Any decision to use this method must consider that the elderly patient ordinarily tolerates slow atrial fibrillation well, and following conversion, normal sinus rhythm may last from only a few seconds to as long as several years. Furthermore, many elderly people with atrial fibrillation also have sinus node pathology, and electrocardioversion may be hazardous. The sick sinus node may fail to take over atrial fibrillation, or a more dangerous arrhythmia may follow the attempted conversion.

Electrocardioversion is best performed after diuretics, rest, digoxin, and oxygen have improved the cardiac status. When time and the patient's condition permit, the patient should first be digitalized with digoxin and given anticoagulation therapy for 7–10 days to lessen the risk of systemic emboli. Then, digitalis should be stopped for 2 days and quinidine sulfate (400 mg) tried 4 times daily for 3 days. If the arrhythmia persists, electrocountershock may be administered after diazepam (5–15 mg) has been given intravenously for sedation and amnesia. Following successful electroversion, a maintenance dose of quinidine sulfate (400 mg) should be prescribed every 6 h to prevent return of the arrhythmia. Procainamide may also be useful for long-term suppression.

A–V junctional rhythms: The A–V junction consists of the atrial approaches to the A–V node, the A–V node itself, and the penetrating portion of the bundle of His (Rosen 1973). In some arrhythmias, the A–V junction serves as an ectopic pacemaker or a site of reentry. A beat arising in the proximal A–V junction is more likely to show a retrograde P wave preceding the QRS complex; one arising distally is more likely to have a retrograde P wave following the QRS complex or buried within the QRS or S–T segments and not seen.

A–V junctional rhythm should be diagnosed when the ECG shows retrograde P waves in Leads II, III, and aVF, and a P–R interval shorter than normal (less than 0.12 sec); or an absent P wave preceding regular QRS complexes; or a retrograde P wave following the QRS interval. Retrograde P waves visible in the S–T segments or absent because they are buried in the QRS complex suggest A–V junctional rhythm. In A–V junctional tachycardia, the QRS complex suggest A–V junctional rhythm. In A–V junctional tachycardia, the QRS complex is of normal width unless bundle branch block is present, and occurs regularly at a rate of 140–240 beats/min. A–V junctional rhythm should be distinguished from coronary sinus, inferior, or low atrial rhythms in which inverted or deformed P waves precede the QRS complex in Leads II, III, and aVF, and the P–R interval is 0.12 sec or more in the limb leads (see Fig. 17.2). There is still considerable controversy concerning the origin of such rhythms, but there is a growing tendency to call this type of rhythm inferior or low atrial rhythm, rather than the more specific coronary sinus rhythm (Rosen 1973). A–V junctional rhythm and inferior or low atrial rhythms require no treatment when the heart rate is between 60 and 100 beats/min and the patient is asymptomatic. When digitalis toxicity or other drugs produce these arrhythmias, the offending medications should be reduced or eliminated. When the ventricular heart rate is rapid and there is danger of impending heart failure or other complications, treatment similar to that described under paroxysmal atrial tachycardia (p. 331) should be undertaken.

Ventricular Arrhythmias

Ventricular Extrasystoles. Occasional ventricular extrasystoles are usually asymptomatic and rarely require treatment. When they occur more frequently than 5 beats/min or close to the preceding T wave, or when multifocal ventricular extrasystoles are present, treatment with oral procainamide (250 mg or more) or quinidine (200 mg) q.i.d. is indicated. Multifocal ventricular extrasystoles, especially common in elderly patients on digitalis whose myocardium is particularly sensitive to this drug, are more serious. When such extrasystoles increase after digitalis, it is wise to decrease or stop the drug, rule out hypokalemia, and give procainamide or quinidine. In the absence of impending or actual heart failure, propranolol (10 mg q.i.d. alone or combined with procainamide to obtain a synergistic effect) may help as a last resort to control ventricular extrasystoles, which by their frequency or proximity to the preceding T wave may relapse into paroxysmal ventricular tachycardia. Parenteral lidocaine or procainamide may be necessary as a temporary expedient when oral therapy fails.

Paroxysmal Ventricular Tachycardia. Paroxysmal ventricular tachycardia is commonly associated with coronary artery disease, and may result from partial depolarization and depression of excitability in focal or extensive areas of the ventricular conducting system secondary to hypoxia or poor perfusion. It indicates a serious heart condition and carries a poor prognosis, which is determined by the severity of the underlying heart disease and the promptness of reversion. The myocardium of the average elderly patient, weakened by the pathology of aging and disease, cannot tolerate this arrhythmia too long without developing myocardial failure or ventricular fibrillation and death. In more than 50% of cases, ventricular tachycardia follows a recent myocardial infarction in elderly subjects and may be the first evidence of such infarction. Sustained ventricular tachycardia unrelated to acute myocardial infarction occurs generally beyond the fifth decade and is more common in males. Straining at stool or digital stimulation of the rectum can precipitate it. Intermittent paroxysmal ventricular tachycardia may be noted in routine ECGs of elderly patients who may be asymptomatic, or complain of dizziness, "blackout," or falling.

The ECG in this condition shows wide QRS complexes of 0.12 sec or more, a heart rate of 150 or more beats/min, and slight irregularity of the ventricular rhythm (Fig. 17.9a). Retrograde P waves may be detected after the ventricular complexes. Since the incidence of bundle branch block pattern is higher in the elderly, it may be difficult to differentiate supraventricular arrhythmias with bundle branch block pattern from paroxysmal ventricular tachycardia. A helpful diagnostic rule of thumb is that supraventricular tachycardia is the more likely diagnosis in the presence of right bundle branch block pattern;

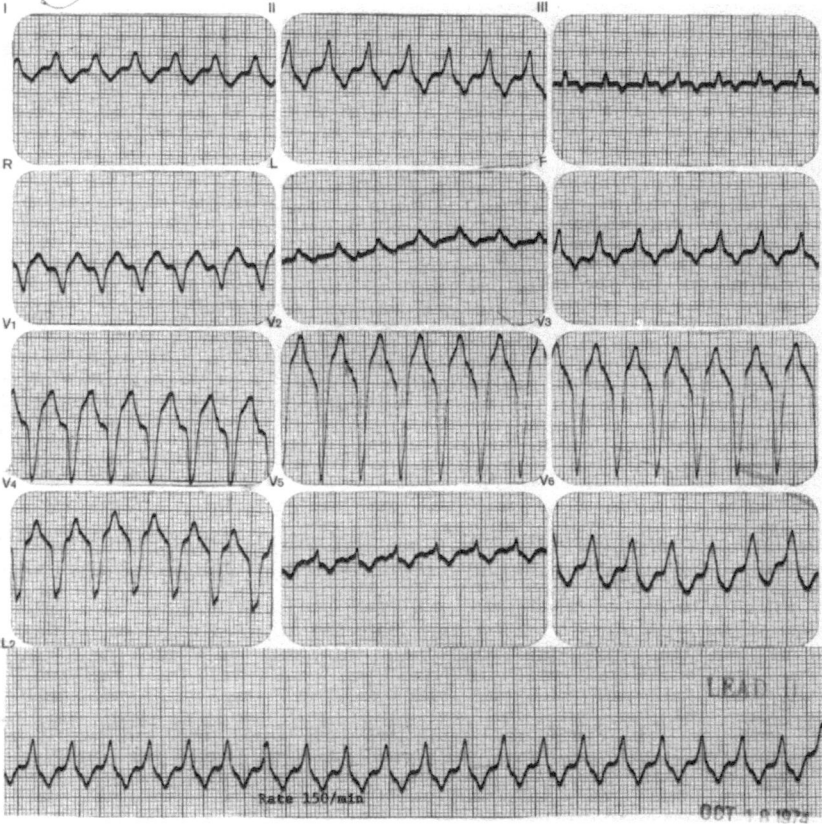

Figure 17.9a. Paroxysmal ventricular tachycardia with a heart rate of 150 beats/min in a 74-year-old man. Note the wide QRS complexes of 0.12-sec duration and the slight irregularity of rhythm.

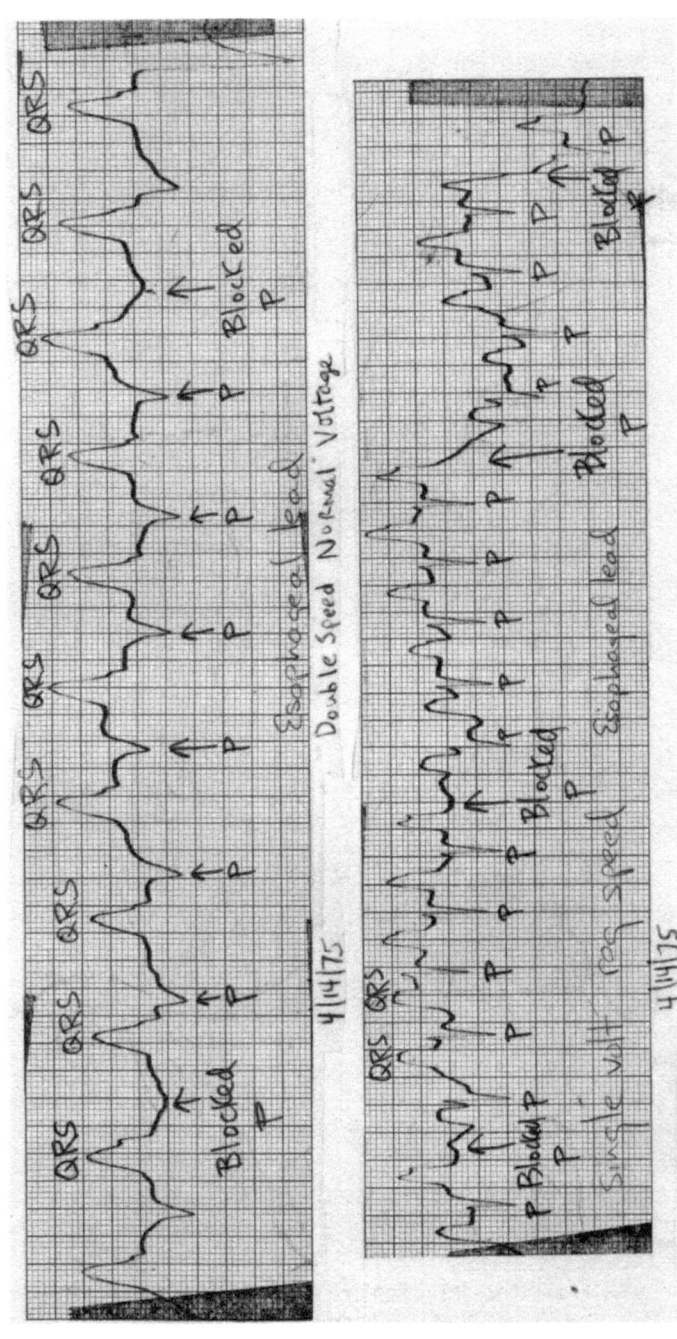

Fig. 17.9b. Esophageal leads confirm paroxysmal ventricular tachycardia with retrograde P waves and Wenckebach block. Top tracing recorded at 50 mm/sec; lower strip, at 25 mm/sec.

Following myocardial infarction in 1956 at the age of 55, this man subsequently averaged one or two bouts of tachycardia yearly. These bouts were usually interpreted as paroxysmal ventricular tachycardia, but some electrocardiographers suspected supraventricular tachycardia with left bundle branch block. At first, these attacks responded readily to the oral administration of procainamide and intravenous lidocaine, but recent years required progressively larger amounts of such medications. The tracing on 10/18/74 (Fig. 17.9a) shows paroxysmal ventricular tachycardia, which proved refractory to usual drug therapy. When the patient went into heart failure, DC synchronized cardioversion with 10 J easily reverted this arrhythmia. He was maintained on 500 mg procainamide every 4 h with no recurrence of his ventricular tachycardia until 4/12/75, when it returned while he was climbing the stairs in a New York City opera house. It persisted for two days, and he was hospitalized for treatment on 4/14/75. His ECG on this date was similar to that on 10/18/74 (Fig. 17.9a). Administration of intravenous lidocaine and procainamide failed to convert the arrhythmia. Since the exact nature of the arrhythmia was always questioned, an esophageal lead was recorded on 4/14/75 (this figure). This tracing established the diagnosis of paroxysmal ventricular tachycardia with retrograde P waves and Wenckebach block. An attempt at synchronized DC cardioversion, first with 10 J and then with larger doses, failed to convert the arrhythmia until 400 J were used. After a few minutes of sinus bradycardia, paroxysmal ventricular tachycardia returned, despite the prophylactic administration of procainamide (750 mg) prior to cardioversion. It was decided to try a combination of procainamide (750 mg) every 4 h and propranolol (10 mg q.i.d.) for several days while the patient was investigated further for possible causes of his recurrent and refractory ventricular tachycardia. When a small left ventricular aneurysm was detected on fluoroscopy, coronary arteriography, pacemaker therapy, and ventricular aneurysmectomy were considered, but it was decided to try cardioversion again before submitting the patient to these procedures, especially since it was felt that such surgical procedures at his age might be dangerous. This time, synchronized DC cardioversion with only 10 J easily converted the ventricular tachycardia to sinus rhythm. Sinus rhythm was maintained for several weeks by the combination of procainamide (750 mg every 4 h) and propranolol (10 mg q.i.d.), and thereafter by procainamide (750 mg every 4 h) alone. When the paroxysmal ventricular tachycardia recurred several months later, a permanent transvenous cardiac pacemaker was inserted and the patient was given procainamide, digoxin, and propranolol with good results.

ventricular tachycardia, in the presence of left bundle branch block pattern. At times, esophageal or right atrial intracavitary leads may be necessary to identify this arrhythmia precisely (Fig. 17.9b).

The best treatment for uncomplicated ventricular tachycardia is synchronized DC electrical countershock, beginning with a low electrical energy of 10 J, and repeating with an additional stronger countershock if necessary. This method is effective in 98% of episodes. Before conversion, quinidine or procainamide should be given to prevent the recurrence of the tachycardia, and diazepam (5–15 mg) injected intravenously for sedation and amnesia.

When electrical countershock cannot be given or fails, a lidocaine drip infusion of 1–4 mg/min (1 g lidocaine in 500 ml 5% dextrose and water) may be tried. If this fails, procainamide may be given orally (0.5 g every 2 or 3 h) or intramuscularly (0.5–1 g every 1 or 2 h) until the arrhythmia responds or toxic effects occur. In critical conditions, a drip of procainamide (1 g in 500 cc 5% glucose and water) may be given intravenously at a rate of 100 mg/min under continuous electrocardiographic control. Widening of the QRS interval, additional arrhythmias, profound shock, or other toxic effects may necessitate stopping the drug. In patients not already on digitalis, a short-acting digitalis preparation may succeed when lidocaine or procainamide fails. After the paroxysmal ventricular tachycardia has reverted to sinus rhythm, procainamide (250 mg or more) or quinidine sulfate (200–400 mg or more) may be given orally at 3- to 4-h intervals to maintain a therapeutic blood level (see Table 17.3) and to prevent the return of the arrhythmia. Combinations of quinidine and procainamide or propranolol, or all three, may prevent the arrhythmia when individual drugs fail. When drug therapy or cardioversion fails to control paroxysmal ventricular tachycardia, electrical pacing to override the arrhythmia or ventricular aneurysmectomy, or both, may be necessary.

Intermittent ventricular tachycardia is best managed pharmacologically, trying a bolus of lidocaine (1–2 mg/kg body weight) given intravenously and repeated in 10–20 minutes if a satisfactory response is not achieved. This dose may be followed by a lidocaine infusion of 1–4 mg/min, the total amount not to exceed 400–500 mg/h. Mental agitation is a common side effect of lidocaine in the elderly, and can best be avoided by smaller doses. If the arrhythmia persists, procainamide may be tried, making sure a therapeutic blood level of 4–10 mg/liter is obtained. Quinidine sulfate may also be useful if a therapeutic level of 3–8 mg/liter (see Table 17.3) is obtained.

Atropine, 0.5–1.0 mg, may be given intravenously in patients with slow ventricular rates resulting from sinus bradycardia or atrioventricular block between bouts of ventricular tachycardia. Permanent cardiac pacing may be necessary for long-term control of bradyarrhythmias in such patients.

Ventricular fibrillation requires immediate defibrillation by electrical countershock and other measures (see the next section). For refractory digitalis-induced ventricular tachycardia or fibrillation, intravenous injections of diphenylhydantoin or potassium chloride may be tried if lidocaine and procainamide fail to control the arrhythmia.

Acute Stokes–Adams Syndrome. This syndrome, which is characterized by transient episodes of syncope, may be caused by slow heart rates due to complete A–V heart block, sino-atrial block, marked sinus bradycardia, or by very fast rates due to ventricular fibrillation or other supraventricular or ventricular tachycardias producing cerebral ischemia. Ventricular tachycardia causes Stokes–Adams syndrome and circulatory failure in 10–25% of patients with heart block (Harris 1970).

Treatment requires immediate cardiac resuscitation, including striking the anterior chest wall to restore cardiac action, external cardiac massage, and artificial ventilation, on the assumption that cardiac arrest is responsible. An ECG should be taken as soon as possible to identify the cardiac rhythm. In cardiac arrest due to ventricular standstill, an external pacemaker, preferably battery-operated, can be used for emergency external pacing during ventricular asystole, one electrode being placed over the manubrium of the sternum and the other over the apex of the heart. An infusion of 2 mg isoproterenol in 500 cc of 5% glucose in water should be started immediately, at a rate that restores a ventricular rate of 40–50 beats/min without causing ventricular extrasystoles or other arrhythmias. This drip should be continued until a temporary pacemaker can be inserted (Dack 1967). In an emergency, a needle electrode can be inserted percutaneously through the chest wall into the ventricular muscle and attached to the internal terminals of a cardiac pacemaker. Assisted ventilation and closed-chest massage should be maintained until adequate heart contractions and a palpable pulse are observed. Epinephrine, isoproterenol, phenylephrine, or other vasopressor agents should be given to maintain the blood pressure, and sodium bicarbonate for acidosis. During ventricular fibrillation, injection of epinephrine may be harmful. Steroids may also be useful to manage complete heart block (Aber and Jones 1965). Molar sodium lactate (5–7 cc/kg) may be given under constant electrocardiographic monitoring for Stokes–Adams seizures associated with hyperpotassemia, acidosis, and cardiac arrest. Ventricular fibrillation is best treated by electroshock, followed by cardiac pacing, if necessary.

A permanent artificial cardiac pacemaker is recommended for

patients with recurrent Stokes–Adams attacks related to ventricular standstill or ventricular tachycardia, severe heart block, or sinus bradycardia who cannot increase their ventricular rate with exercise. Such artificial pacemaking has restored many bedridden elderly patients to more active and happier lives (Harris 1970b).

References

Aber, C., and Jones, E. (1965) *Br. Heart J.* **27**, 56.

Caird, F. (1963) *Postgrad. Med. J.* **39**, 408.

Cranefield, P. F., Wit, A. L., and Hoffman, B. F. (1973) *In* Donoso, E. (ed.), *Symposium Cardiac Arrhythmias*, American Heart Association Monograph No. 40, The American Heart Association, New York, p. 24.

Dack, S. (1967) *J. Am. Med. Assoc.* **201**, 868.

Davies, M., and Pomerance, A. (1972) *Br. Heart J.* **34**, 150.

Donoso, E. (1973) *In* Donoso, E. (ed.), *Symposium Cardiac Arrhythmias*, American Heart Association Monograph No. 40, The American Heart Association, New York, p. 1.

Evans, W., and Swann, P. (1954) *Br. Heart J.* **16**, 189.

Ferrer, M. I. (1968) *J. Am. Med. Assoc.* **206**, 645.

Ferrer, M. I. (1973a) *Circulation* **47**, 635.

Ferrer, M. I. (1973b) *In* Donoso, E. (ed.), *Symposium Cardiac Arrhythmias*, American Heart Association Monograph No. 40, The American Heart Association, New York, p. 67.

Han, J., Millet, D., Chizzonitti, B., and Moe, G. K. (1966) *Am. Heart J.* **71**, 481.

Harris, R. (1970a) *The Management of Geriatric Cardiovascular Disease*, J. B. Lippincott Co., Philadelphia, p. 10.

Harris, R. (1970b) *idem*, p. 265.

Hurst, J., Paulk, E., Proctor, D., and Schlant, C. (1964) *Am. J. Med.* **37**, 728.

Kastor, J. A. (1973) *In* Donoso, E. (ed.), *Symposium Cardiac Arrhythmias*, American Heart Association Monograph No. 40, The American Heart Association, New York, p. 113.

Klein, M. D. (1975) *In* Lown, B. (ed.), *Clinical Sudden Death*, Medcom, Inc., New York, p. 42.

Langendorf, R., Pick, A., and Winternitz, M. (1955) *Circulation* **11**, 422.

Mihalick, M. J., and Fisch, C. (1974) *Am. Heart J.* **87**, 117.

Margolis, J. R., Strauss, H. C., Miller, H. C., Gilbert, M., and Wallace, A. G. (1975) *Circulation* **52**, 162.

Nies, A. S., and Shand, D. (1975) *Circulation* **52**, 6.

Rosen, K. M. (1973) *In* Donoso, E. (ed.), *Symposium Cardiac Arrhythmias*, American Heart Association Monograph No. 40, The American Heart Association, New York, p. 86.

Samet, P. (1973) *idem*, p. 39.

Schamroth, L. (1973) *idem*, p. 60.

Simon, A. P. (1974) *Am. Fam. Physician* **9**, 127.

Ticzon, A. R., and Whalen, R. W. (1973) *In* Donoso, E. (ed.), *Symposium Cardiac Arrhythmias*, American Heart Association Monograph No. 40, The American Heart Association, New York, p. 74.

Titus, J. L. (1973) *idem*, p. 4.

Wu, D., Denes, P., Leon, F., Chhablani, R., and Rosen, K. (1975) *Am. J. Cardiol.* **36**, 91.

18

Management of Heart Block

HAROLD SIDDONS

Syncope and the ECG

Syncope or dizzy spells with near syncope are common in the elderly. Whether or not there is gross bradycardia, such symptoms require, among other investigations, an ECG. If the ECG taken between attacks shows complete block, the likelihood is that the syncope (Stokes–Adams attack) is due to a temporary cessation of the cardiac rhythm. Asystole, ventricular tachycardia, or ventricular fibrillation may each occur. Such attacks can be reliably prevented only by artificial pacing. Although long-acting isoprenaline has often been used, there is little or no evidence that any drug therapy is effective. If the ECG taken between syncopal attacks shows lesser degrees of block or bundle branch block, it is highly probable that the syncope is cardiogenic, although many of these rhythms without syncope are relatively benign. Syncope from cessation of the heartbeat is exceptional when the ECG between attacks shows no conduction defect. Syncopal attacks associated with block are usually both infrequent and unpredictable; thus, continuous monitoring to determine the rhythm during an attack is usually impractical.

Because electrocardiographic proof of the diagnosis of the cause of syncope is usually lacking, and because artificial pacing can transform the outlook both for the length of survival and for the quality of life, the diagnosis based on clinical features is critically important.

HAROLD SIDDONS · St. George's Hospital, Hyde Park Corner, London, SW1X 7EZ, England.

Clinical Diagnosis of Syncope

Circumstances of the Attack

Syncope or near syncope must first be distinguished from muscular weakness causing falls, which can result in injuries that produce unconsciousness. Postural hypotension without arrhythmia may produce gross dizziness, particularly on changing posture, such as on rising to stand. Head movement immediately preceding an attack favors cerebral ischemia from vertebrobasilar disease. In contrast, Stokes–Adams attacks can occur at any time, and are not infrequent in bed. Attacks have often been observed with an ECG monitor during sleep, and may wake the patient. There is no preceding aura, as in some epileptics, although patients with syncope associated with block may have enough warning of an attack to sink to the floor without injuring themselves.

During the Attack

The critical feature for diagnosis is the absence of a pulse during the attack, but it is rare for the pulse to have been reliably taken, even in the hospital. The length of unconsciousness is quite variable; incontinence may occur.

Recovery from an Attack

Unlike recovery from vasovagal attacks and some other causes of cerebral ischemia, recovery is abrupt (although attacks may be repeated); it is often associated with flushing, which the patient may be aware of. This feature is diagnostic. The pulse returns abruptly, and at this stage a marked bradycardia strongly favors an arrhythmic basis. Several attacks may occur inexplicably over a period of days or weeks, and be followed by years without symptoms. Repeated attacks can occur every few minutes, and may not allow full recovery of consciousness. There is strong evidence that attacks during operations, whether under general or local anesthesia, are common.

Associated Valve Disease

Attacks of dizziness on exertion, with or without syncope, are common in aortic stenosis. Because an aortic systolic murmur is common in sclerosis without stenosis, a murmur alone must not be taken to indicate stenosis. The slow pulse in block accentuates the murmur. Before syncope is attributed to aortic valve disease, other features of stenosis must be elicited; the slow-rising carotid pulse associated with enlargement of the left ventricle is helpful. It must be remembered that in long-standing bradycardia from complete block, the heart will increase in size, with a normal aortic valve.

Complete Block Without Syncope

Perhaps a third of all patients with complete block never have syncopal attacks, but they are liable to sudden death. It might be stated, alternatively, that the first syncopal attack may be fatal.

A bradycardia below 40 beats/min, the most common cause of which is complete block, may result in various manifestations of inadequate cardiac output, such as poor cerebration, fatigue on slight exertion, cardiac failure, or renal failure. These are collectively termed "the low-output syndrome."

Many patients with complete block are symptom-free, and it is not exceptional to find an elderly patient leading a reasonably active life with a pulse below 40.

Prognosis in Acquired Complete Block Without Pacing

It is usually stated that the mortality is 50% within a year of diagnosis. Johansson's (1966) prospective study and some others put the outlook as slightly better than this. A rather better outlook can be anticipated if the A–V dissociation is associated with a long history of block; the absence of syncope, or freedom from syncope for many months; a heart rate above 40, particularly if the rate increases by 5 beats/min on exercise; and a QRS complex of normal width. Even with these features, mean life expectancy is not likely to be over 2 years, and there is a risk of sudden death.

The return of conducted rhythm at times does not carry with it any improvement in outlook. There is a minority who live long with complete block. Unfortunately, it is not yet possible to select these patients, and the decision whether or not to pace must therefore be based on the overall picture.

It might be hoped that the cause of the block could be determined and a prognosis based on this. The wide variety of underlying pathology is discussed in Chapter 3. Unfortunately, it is possible to establish etiology in only very few living patients. Of many possible causes, there are only three that are likely to be diagnosed in the elderly, and it is important to identify them, because management differs for the three types. They are digitalis overdosage, acute myocardial infarction, and calcification extending from the aortic or mitral valve rings.

With poor renal function, digitalis blood levels may reach the toxic range with relatively small dosage. Digitalis overdosage is reversible, but it may take more than a week after stopping the drug for the excess to be cleared. Digitalis serum levels are valuable in excluding or establishing this cause.

Block in the acute phase of myocardial infarction is discussed in Chapter 16. The persistence of complete dissociation even intermittently for more than 10 days is an indication for pacing for at least several years, because such patients are liable to sudden arrhythmic death, which it is reasonable to suppose might be avoided by pacing. Lesser degrees of block persisting after the acute phase may also indicate long-term pacing, but the need in this condition is not yet certain.

It is often difficult to decide in retrospect whether an incident that occurred in the past at the onset of block was in fact an acute myocardial infarction or simply the result of the onset of a slow heart rate. If cardiac pain was a feature of the incident, acute infarction is likely. The diagnostic electrocardiographic features of infarction may be completely obscured if there is bundle branch block. To be fully confident that block is due to an ischemic incident, it is necessary to have recorded the changing ECG and enzyme levels at the time.

The third specific cause of heart block that is diagnosable in life is calcific disease extending from the aortic and mitral ring into the conducting tissue. X-ray screening or tomography should reveal the calcification. The prognosis in these patients without pacing is better than average, and might be considered as a relative contraindication to pacing.

Drug Treatment of Complete Block

With so unpredictable a course, it is very difficult to assess the value of drugs. Isoprenaline (Isuprel) given by intravenous drip is undoubtedly beneficial in the acute situation when cardiac asystole is occurring frequently, and to cover danger periods such as the insertion of pacing electrodes. Its effect must be monitored by ECG, and multiple ventricular ectopics or ventricular tachycardia are danger signals that suggest overdosage. The effect can be counterbalanced by intravenous lignocaine, which is used in syncopal attacks seen to be due to ventricular tachycardia or fibrillation.

Isoprenaline linguets dissolved under the tongue provide a fairly rapid means of administering the drug, but the effect is not controllable. The slow-release form of isoprenaline (Saventrine) raises the blood catecholamine level, but does not achieve stable levels. Large dosage is undoubtedly dangerous, and dosage small enough to avoid risk may have no demonstrable effect or speed the pulse only a few beats a minute. Because syncopal attacks are so unpredictable in frequency, their control would have to be demonstrated in a very large number of unpaced patients before lessening of the attacks could be attributed to the drug; that there are occasional patients who have no attacks while taking the drug cannot be used as evidence of its efficacy. The danger of overdosage must be accepted as contraindicating a drug without proven use in the chronic situation.

Steroids have been recommended at the onset of complete block, and in individual cases have been reported to reverse complete block. There is no good evidence that they have a long-term therapeutic value. There are no drugs known to prevent the occasional progress from partial to complete block (except in hypothyroid block).

Because toxic blood levels of digitalis cause heart block, the drug is contraindicated in partial block. In the presence of complete block from other causes, there is no contraindication to its use, and it may prove most valuable in the management of failure.

For some patients with arrhythmias, suppressive drugs, in particular β-blockers, are therapeutically desirable. When they are required in considerable dosage, however, they may cause a serious bradycardia. The risk of such bradycardia can be eliminated by pacing, and pacemakers are being used increasingly often on this basis. The need to use digitalis in a patient with bradycardia from partial heart block is also regarded as an indication for pacing.

Indications for Pacing

The indications for permanent pacing are summarized in Table 18.1. On the basis of expectation of life discussed above, there is a strong reason for pacing in complete block. It is necessary, however, always to take into consideration another less tangible factor, the quality of life. If there are symptoms that will be relieved by pacing,

TABLE 18.1. Indications for Permanent Pacing

Complete block:	Whether intermittent or not (except transient in the acute phase of myocardial infarction, or from digitalis overdose).
Second degree block:	If associated with cardiogenic syncope or bradycardia with low-output symptoms.
Bundle branch block:	If associated with cardiogenic syncope or near syncope, particularly if trifascicular or bifascicular block.
Sino-atrial disease:	With transient symptoms from sinus arrest or sino-atrial block, or with symptoms from slow rates.
Bradycardias:	Of various types, if resistant to other treatment and producing low-output symptoms, including slow atrial fibrillation to cover the risk of bradycardia, etc., from high dosage of β-blockers and other drugs.

the choice is clear. In those with few or no symptoms, the decision to pace will be taken only after the risks and discomforts of the technique have been weighed against the desirability of prolonging life.

Partial Block and Bundle Branch Block

There is a great variety of forms of partial block, and it is commonplace for one form to change to another from time to time. Although the transition from partial block to complete block is known to occur, there is little firm evidence to indicate which patients are likely to develop complete block. Most partial blocks are benign and do not need treatment. A problem arises in partial block with dizzy spells and such transient symptoms suggesting an arrhythmic basis.

The significance of the various combinations of bundle branch block (RBBB and LBBB) and axis deviation (RAD and LAD) has been clarified by Rosenbaum's (Rosenbaum et al. 1970) concept of three fascicles of conducting tissue below the bifurcation of the bundle of His. The conducting tissue to the left ventricle arises as a number of branches, but his concept considers them as two main fascicles, one going anteriorly and one posteriorly; the right bundle branch forms a third fascicle. The following bundle branch ECG patterns can then be explained as block in two of the three fascicles (i.e., bifascicular block):

1) LBBB
2) RBBB with LAD ($-60°$ or more)
3) RBBB with RAD ($+110°$ or more)

All three fascicles are compromised (trifascicular block) when there is second degree block, alternating LBBB and RBBB, or RBBB with alternating LAD and RAD.

It has been postulated that with bifascicular or trifascicular block, associated syncope is likely to be arrhythmic, and that even asymptomatic patients are at risk of an arrhythmic death, which could be prevented by pacing. Prospective studies of patients with these forms of block are as yet limited, and we do not always accept these forms of block in the absence of symptoms as indications for pacing.

A new method of locating the site of block in partial block is by His-bundle ECGs (Narula et al. 1968; Narula 1973, Scherlag et al. 1969). These tracings indicate whether the delay in conduction lies above or below the site in the His bundle that gives rise to the detectable His deflection. It has been postulated that disease below this site is more likely to progress to complete block. If complete dissociation does occur, the rhythm center taking over control is likely to be less reliable, possibly allowing syncope or sudden death. If this hypothesis is true, an increased His-to-ventricle (H–V) time would be a relative indication for pacing. Studies so far have not substantiated this hypothesis. An increase in H–V time does not correlate closely with syncope. As more experience accumulates, however, its significance may become clearer.

Another technique that may prove of value in selecting patients for pacing is the sinus node recovery time. This time is particularly applicable to sino-atrial disease, a condition in which A–V conduction may remain intact, but the sinus node becomes erratic. To test its reliability, the atrium is temporarily paced at various rates; when pacing is stopped, the time before the node takes over and produces a natural impulse is measured. A long recovery period suggests a liability to Stokes–Adams attacks and indicates pacing.

Sino-Atrial Disease and Other Indications

Various manifestations of sino-atrial disease may require permanent pacing. Sinus bradycardia is occasionally slow enough to give rise to low-output symptoms, but it is the incidence of sinus arrest and paroxysmal bradycardias, as in the "brady-tachy syndrome," that offers a serious risk, preventable by pacing (Schoenfeld and Bhardwaj 1975). Atrial fibrillation with a very slow ventricular rate is another form of bradycardia that may require pacing, particularly if it is desirable to give digitalis for failure. These various forms of bradycardia other than block represent an increasing proportion of patients coming to pacing.

Heart Failure

Heart failure that is resistant to diuretics, and is due to a persistent bradycardia of less than 45 beats/min, is a clear indication for pacing. Pacing in itself, however, rarely improves the pump action sufficiently to do without diuretics. Renal failure and symptoms from peripheral atherosclerosis may be marginally improved if the prepacing rate is very slow.

Temporary Pacing to Cover Operations

In complete block, and to a lesser degree with 2° block, there is a real risk of cardiac arrest during surgical procedures, particularly during anesthetic induction. This risk can be eliminated by temporary pacing, which should be continued for 3 days after a major procedure.

Methods of Pacing

The endocardial (transvenous) electrode is the most suitable for elderly patients. Attaching epicardial electrodes to the heart requires an operation of greater magnitude, even though this attachment may be done through an epigastric or similar approach that does not involve a thoracotomy. In the elderly, the epicardial technique should be reserved for those who run into difficulties with the endocardial method.

A unipolar electrode is preferred to a bipolar for various reasons, including its smaller size. The most suitable vein is the cephalic in the deltopectoral fold. If this vein proves too small, a skilled operator will be able to dissect deeper and use the axillary or subclavian veins, into which it drains. Alternatively, the external jugular, or, if none of these is available, the internal jugular can be used.

The greatest drawback of the endocardial methods is the possibility of *displacement* from a position of good electrical contact in the right ventricle. It usually occurs within the first week, and displacement rates of 1–20% have been recorded. Reports giving low displacement rates all come from experienced operators, and many reports emphasize that high displacement rates occur with inexperienced operators. Electrode contact can be tested by using the electrode as an intracardiac ECG lead; marked elevation of the S–T is a reliable sign of good physical contact, and the potential of the QRS complex should not be less than 3 mV, peak to peak. The threshold required to pace varies with the surface area and other features of the electrode, but a site with the threshold above 0.5 V at 2 msec should not be accepted. The stability of the electrode can be tested if the patient is conscious by getting him to cough, or take deep breaths while observing on an X-ray screen, using an image amplifier.

If an electrode does displace, or if it penetrates the wall of the ventricle, pacing is likely to stop and a syncopal attack may occur. *Penetration into the pericardium* during or soon after placement of the electrode is a comparatively common event and is surprisingly harmless. It may result in an audible pericardial rub, but clinical evidence of tamponade is extremely rare. Perforation can sometimes be seen on X-ray, and the ECG may show that the left ventricle is being stimulated before the right. If the electrode is used as an intracardiac ECG lead, the change in the pattern on withdrawing the electrode is almost diagnostic of perforation.

It might be thought that the risk of displacement carries with it an unacceptable risk to life. In 649 patients paced endocardially at St. George's, there were no deaths attributable to this cause, and there was only 1 unexplained death within 4 weeks of electrode placement. Other relevant reports also indicate that death from this cause is rare (Siddons 1974). Electrode displacement after 2 weeks is rare, although it may occur if the wire is pulled on when the pacemaker is changed.

Pacemaker implantation, like electrode placement, can be done satisfactorily under local anesthesia, which is preferable in elderly patients, because they are particularly prone to thrombotic and chest complications after a general anesthetic.

Provided the patient is not very thin with inelastic skin, and the pacemaker to be implanted is not too thick, the axilla is a satisfactory site. The usual alternative is the anterior chest wall. If this site is used, the pacemaker should be placed deep to the fascial sheath of the pectoralis major; otherwise, it is likely to be mobile and come through the skin, even in women when there appears to be ample space behind the breast.

The early surgical complications most likely to mar the result are *infection* or *hematoma* formation. Comparatively minor wound contamination may give rise to lasting sepsis in the presence of an implanted foreign body, and sepsis rates of up to 5 or 6% have been recorded. With due care, this rate can be reduced to 1%, a rate that has been achieved without the use of prophylactic antibiotics (Siddons and

Nowak 1975). Signs of low-grade sepsis may be long delayed. Hematomata can be avoided by meticulous *hemostasis*. Some surgeons feel that brief drainage reduces wound infection by avoiding hematoma formation, but drainage is not recommended, because the drain track inevitably provides a path for skin bacteria to enter the foreign-body pocket.

With an electrode providing a low-resistance pathway to the heart, there is some risk in the use of *diathermy* during operation. Although this risk is probably remote with reasonable care, it is recommended that diathermy not be used when implanting pacemakers. The 1% infection rate quoted above was achieved without using diathermy, without drainage, and without routine antibiotic prophylaxis.

Necrosis of skin over the most prominent part of the pacemaker remains an important problem. It occurs late, and may develop years after an otherwise satisfactory implantation. It depends on the thinness of the overlying tissue and the lack of skin elasticity, together with the size and smoothness of the pacemaker. The incidence can be reduced by care in selecting the implant site and adequate soft tissue cover when implanting the pacemaker. The incision should be designed so that it does not lie over the pacemaker. The *incidence of infection and skin necrosis* totals about 5–7% (Siddons and Nowak 1975) in most reports, although some claim a rate below 1% and several give a higher incidence.

There is, fortunately, very little risk of *thromboembolic complications* from transvenous pacing. The incidence of pulmonary embolism is certainly lower than following operation to place epicardial electrodes. Rarely, thrombosis of the axillary vein occurs when a cephalic vein has been used for the electrode wire. Although some clot may be seen at autopsy along the vascular course of the wire, significant embolism from this site has been recorded only very rarely. A few cases of *septicemia* have been reported; it has usually been explained by contamination at the time of electrode placement (Siddons and Nowak 1975).

Fixed-Rate vs. Demand Pacing

In many patients requiring pacing, complete block is only intermittent, and when the conducted rate exceeds that of the fixed-rate pacemaker, there is competition. There are several reasons for supposing that such competition is undesirable, and it is regarded by some as dangerous.

The artificially stimulated beats occur without the physiologic aid of filling from atrial systole, and those that occur shortly after a natural beat allow inadequate time for ventricular filling. They thus produce a small stroke volume and are wasteful of energy.

The artificial stimulus may fall in the vulnerable phase of the cardiac cycle of a conducted beat, and it is well recognized that in the experimental animal and in various abnormal states in the human subject, a stimulus in this phase can cause ventricular fibrillation. Acute myocardial infarction, gross electrolyte disturbance (particularly of potassium), and hypoxia are all states in which there is a real danger that the mistimed stimulus will produce dangerous arrhythmia. Fixed-rate pacing should therefore not be used in these situations. In treating patients with long-standing block, and when using endocardial electrodes and implantable pacemakers, the theoretical risk of producing dangerous arrhythmias has not been borne out. Perhaps the reason is that operative exposure of the pericardium with its inevitable pericardial reaction is avoided, and the modern implantable pacemaker has a limited stimulus output. It is difficult to obtain conclusive evidence on this point, but our analysis of the published evidence and our own experience of pacing 168 patients with competition does not suggest a significant risk of sudden death with competition from conducted beats (Siddons 1974).

The *demand pacemaker* is designed to avoid competition. The cardiac electrode senses the natural QRS, and as a result the artificial pacemaker does not fire until after an appropriate interval. The demand mode has certain inherent disadvantages. Its more complex mechanism carries an expected higher failure rate. In practice, most demand pacemakers use more current and therefore do not last as long as fixed-rate units. Because these pacemakers must be designed to sense very small impulses, they may be affected by extraneous electrical fields from such sources as radar or microwave ovens, and occasionally by the electropotential of the patient's own muscular activity. The possibility that such interference or any inherent fault could suppress pacing when it is required cannot be totally ignored, but has been largely eliminated by design features.

The economics of the two types of pacemakers are an important consideration. At present, the British fixed-rate pacemaker costs 40% less than its demand counterpart, and can be relied on to last about 50% longer.

For a new patient, we usually select a demand pacemaker, unless the block is complete and has been observed over a long period not to be intermittent. In patients who have been observed for only a month or so, conduction may recover intermittently after pacing is started, and it is not possible to foretell which patients will experience this recovery of conduction. If a patient comes from a change of pacemaker and competition has never been observed, a fixed-rate model is used.

Pacing Failure

Failure of the pacing system from whatever cause may result in a syncopal attack, even if the patient has never suffered syncope before. In most patients, however, a slow bradycardia takes over, and the patient notices no change or has a recurrence of symptoms of low output. If the pulse is found to be slow and regular, failure of pacing is immediately apparent. The diagnosis is more difficult when the output of the pacemaker falls to the level of the threshold required to pace and only occasional beats are dropped. The size of the stimulus artifact on the ECG does not alter sufficiently to show a significant drop in power, although its total absence is, of course, important. Prolonged observation of the ECG may be required before a stimulus is seen to fall in an appropriate phase of the cardiac cycle that is not followed by a QRS complex. A single proven failure to follow an appropriately timed stimulus requires action.

When a demand pacemaker that is inhibited by a competing rhythm is to be tested, it must be changed to its fixed-rate mode. To meet this requirement, demand pacemakers have a built-in reed switch controllable by a magnet held on the skin over the implant.

If appropriate stimuli are not being followed by contractions of the heart, an intravenous drip is set up so that isoprenaline and lignocaine can be given as required, and the pacemaker is then explored under local anesthesia. If syncopal attacks occur, a temporary electrode is passed by an arm vein to gain pacing control. The electrode is first detached from the implanted pacemaker and the threshold required for pacing measured. The acceptable minimum depends on both the make of the electrode and the output of the pacemaker. A threshold rise within a month or so of pacing is likely to be due to displacement of the tip, and the electrode should be repositioned until a stable low-threshold position is achieved.

A relatively small or intermittent rise in threshold may be due to an insulation leak in the electrode wire; this cause can sometimes be established by showing that manipulation of the wire affects the threshold. Fracture of the conduction filament is very uncommon; it is one of the causes of complete absence of the stimulus artifact on the ECG.

Determining When to Change a Pacemaker

It has been generally assumed that the failure of a pacemaker to provide adequate stimulus for pacing will almost always be due to battery depletion, not to failure of other components. It will be seen below that this assumption is not fully justified, and as power sources become longer-lasting and more reliable, it will become even less true. Nevertheless, pacemaker management is at present largely based on the detection of battery depletion, and the methods used may continue to be of importance.

Current drain differs from patient to patient (particularly with demand pacemakers, which stimulate only when required), so that even if the total life output of the power source could be exactly forecast, it would not be possible to predict accurately when the power source would run out. As experience accumulates with a particular model, it becomes possible to state that depletion is extremely unlikely up to a given number of months of implantation; the time for changing the unit can be based on this experience, but in order to be safe, many pacemakers will have to be removed unnecessarily early. Any change made by the manufacturers in the nature of the batteries or the circuitry invalidates such a method until experience with the modified pacemaker has been acquired. It is clear, therefore, that a scheme is required that can test the battery state from time to time in the life of each implant.

Most manufacturers have designed their pacemaker circuitry so that a fixed-rate pacemaker (or a demand pacemaker when switched for testing to the fixed-rate mode) slows as the battery becomes depleted. The degree of significant slowing may be several beats a minute, which can be detected by careful counting over one or two minutes, or may require an electronic counter to detect the change. This dependence on accurate rate measurement has led to the development for clinics of a system by which a patient telephones the clinic at appropriate intervals and places over his implanted pacemaker a portable instrument that converts the impulse into an audible signal. This system can be supplemented, if required, by transmitting ECGs over the telephone.

The method of telephone transmission has not been much used in Britain, for various reasons; it is expensive, a high proportion of pacemaker patients do not have ready access to a telephone, and some geriatric patients find the method too complex. British clinics tend to rely on hospital visits, which need be very few in the early life of the pacemaker, but more frequent later. At such hospital visits, it is possible, with the aid of ECG limb leads and a standard measuring oscilloscope, to measure other parameters as well as rate—for instance, pulse width, which with some makes of pacemaker is more significant and reliable in detecting battery change. The oscilloscope trace may also enable determination of impending failure of the electrode wire or its insulation before pacing fails. Various instruments have been specifically designed to show the rate and pulse width of implanted pacemakers; some are readily portable and can be carried and used by the more intelligent patients, or used by their doctors. The success of these various methods depends on many factors: some are more suitable for certain makes of pacemaker than for others; some are suitable for clinics caring for large numbers of pacemaker patients, some for smaller clinics.

A different approach has been used by some pacemaker manufacturers, who have designed models with built-in features that enable the application of external magnets to reduce output to a controllable degree. It is then possible to show how great is the margin between output and the threshold required for pacing. In particular, the Elema Vario and the GEC pacemaker have these features.

However close the surveillance of patients may have been, reports show that a proportion of pacemakers stop functioning without the stoppage having been predicted by these various tests. An analysis at St. George's Hospital (J. G. Davies, personal communication) suggests that the gradual drop of voltage from the mercury cells as they become depleted is not the usual reason for these unpredicted failures. The majority fail because some electrolyte has leaked from the battery and affected other components. The next most common cause of failure is the formation of a bridge of mercury within one or more cells. Primary failure of other components is rare. Whether this explanation of the mode of failure is accepted as the common cause or not, it has been widely reported that voltage drop is usually much more rapid than was anticipated from cell exhaustion.

Pacemaker Longevity

Comparison of the longevity of different models of pacemaker is not straightforward. Even if a standard method of presentation using clearly defined terms as suggested by Green (1974) were to be universally adopted, the apparent longevity of pacemakers would still be dependent on how often the rate or pulse width was measured and on whether small changes in these parameters were taken to indicate explanation. Pacemakers left unobserved until they failed would obviously appear to have a longer life than those removed prophylactically.

By the time sufficient numbers of any pacemaker model have been observed in use for their longevity to be proved, the manufacturer has usually made significant changes in the design of the current model. Even without a planned alteration in design, there have been several instances in which batches of batteries or other components have proved less reliable than the standard, resulting in early failure of a batch of pacemakers. No model is immune from such a defect.

An example of the variation of reliability between different models made by a single manufacturer was reported by Green (1974), who used 98 Model 5870C Medtronic pacemakers, testing the rate "periodically." A significant rate change or failure to pace had

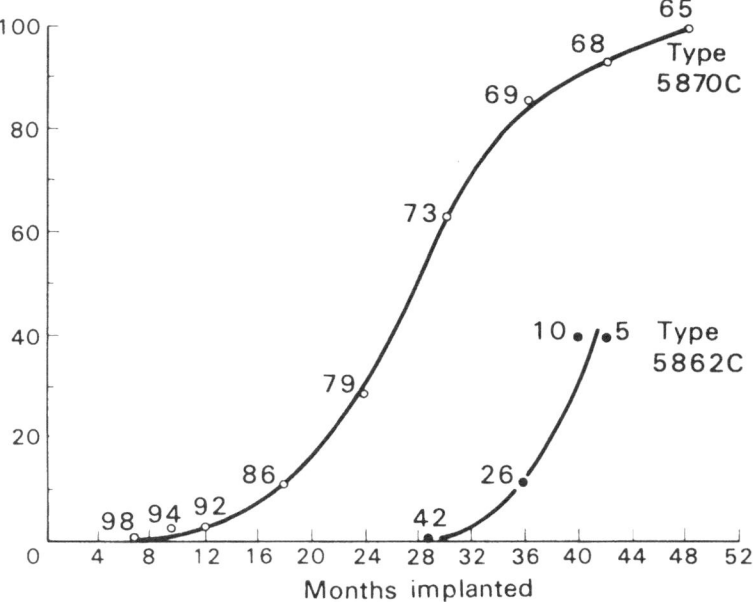

Fig. 18.1. Percentage failures of Medtronic asynchronous generators (7/66–12/73). Reproduced from Green (1974). Green defines "failed implant lifetime" as the time between implantation and the occurrence of a technical fault in the generator.

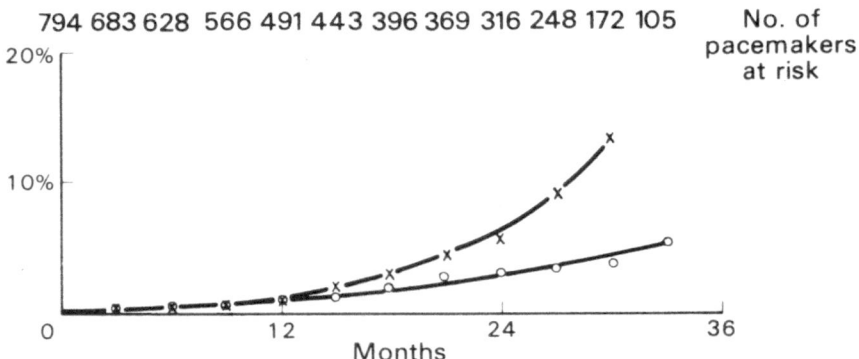

Fig. 18.2. All Devices fixed-rate (Model 2970) implants at St. George's Hospital from 1970 to 1974, inclusive, followed to 12/31/74 (×, stopped pacing or prophylactic change; ○, stopped pacing).

necessitated explantation in 10% by 18–21 months, and in 50% by 30 months, as shown in Fig. 18.1. By the time this information had been obtained, Medtronic had withdrawn this model from the market. The report shows that Model 5862C was subsequently used, and it was found that none of 42 implants had required changing for these reasons after 30 months' implantation. This is an exceptionally good record.

At St. George's Hospital, the policy has been to test for rate or pulse width changes only occasionally for the first 2 years, and thereafter at about 4-month intervals. With this regime, the life of 794 Devices "fixed-rate" pacemakers (Model 2970) was observed. Figure 18.2 shows the percentage of pacemakers that had been removed after various periods either because they had failed to pace the patient or because the pulse width had altered sufficiently to indicate a prophylactic change. Fewer than 10% of the pacemakers had been removed after 27 months' implantation. The policy adopted when this series was collected was to remove these pacemakers after 30–36 months' implantation, with the result that further significant figures could not be obtained (e.g., Furman et al. 1973).

Longer-Lasting Power Sources

Nearly all pacemaker failures are attributable to the mercury cells that power them. In most models, the battery is encased in epoxy resin, which may or may not be covered with silicone rubber. A very small amount of moisture penetrates this coating, and it may be that this moisture is the cause of some of the battery failures. There are now on the market one or two models in which a case of titanium is used (Telectronics of Australia and some models of Medtronic U.S.A.). With such an impervious case, special provision must be made for the absorption of the small quantity of gas that the mercury cell gives off. It is anticipated that these metal-coated models may last 50% longer than their counterparts in epoxy resin. The real hope for the future, however, probably lies in a different power source.

The use of a power source outside the body transmitting to a relatively simple implanted apparatus was developed in Birmingham by Abrams 14 years ago. It depends on *simple induction* to a secondary coil implanted beneath the skin. Power is derived from household flashlight batteries, which the patient can change himself at 3-week intervals, and no further operation is required after the initial electrode and receiving coil are placed. The simplicity of the method makes it very reliable, but a transmitting coil must be kept adhering to the skin exactly overlying the implant. Some patients find this a practical method, but the psychological disadvantage of seeing and handling apparatus that controls life is not acceptable to many, and the method has never achieved widespread use despite its cheapness and the avoidance of repeated hospitalization. The method's most serious disadvantage is that it is not suitable for demand pacing.

Several pacemakers dependent on an *implanted battery* unit that is *charged* at intervals *from outside* have been used. Pacesetters of Baltimore markets such a product containing nickel–cadmium cells. Recharging is required every 1 to 4 weeks and can be done in the home. As yet, these pacemakers have not been in use long enough to know how long the batteries will last. A life of 5–10 years is anticipated.

The *isotope* pacemaker powered by plutonium-238 has been in use for several years. The temperature difference between the center and the surface of the unit is converted by thermopiles to provide electrical energy. It is necessary to protect the radioactive material in an exceptionally strong case, both to absorb radiation and to withstand trauma from, for example, a road or air traffic accident. The radioactive material must not be released even after the patient's death, and must therefore withstand cremation. These precautions result in a pacemaker rather larger than conventional units with mercury cells. The power source can be expected to last 10–15 years, and so far the pacemaker has proved reliable. Its greatest disadvantage for widespread use is its cost, which is about 10 times that of the cheaper mercury cell models with a 3-year life.

TABLE 18.2. Age of 948 Adults When
First Paced

Age	No. of Patients
15–19	2
20–29	4
30–39	10
40–49	32
50–59	103
60–69	289
70–79	369
80–89	132
90–99	7

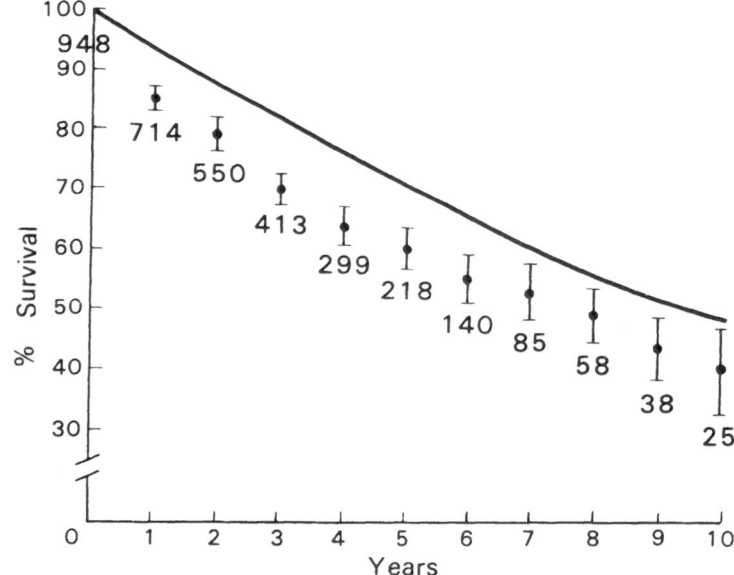

Fig. 18.3. Survival of 948 paced adults with complete heart block matched for age and sex with population of England and Wales. The *brackets* above and below the plotted points indicate twice the standard deviation; the *figures* indicate the number at risk. The *solid line* indicates the population survival figures, which are derived from the last available unabridged Life Tables of the Registrar General (England and Wales 1961). More up-to-date survival figures are not available, as detailed tables have not yet been published, but the Registrar General's abridged Life Table 1971–1973 shows that there has been an appreciable improvement in life expectancy since 1961.

Two years ago, Greatbatch introduced the *lithium-iodide* cell, which he had designed specifically for pacemakers, and which has an anticipated life of over 10 years. It has been reliable over the first 2 years of life. The cell is less bulky than either mercury cells or the isotope power source. Pacemakers with lithium-iodide cells are already marketed by various manufacturers in the U.S., Australia, France, and Holland. All are smaller than previous products. They are much less costly than the isotope-powered pacemaker and, if their initial promise is maintained, are likely to be widely used.

Results of Pacing

It has already been observed that the *expectation of life* with complete heart block *without pacing* is poor, 50% surviving 1 or 2 years. There are now plenty of reports of paced patients with 50% survival to 5 years. Table 18.2 shows the age distribution of 948 adults paced at St. George's Hospital for complete block. Their survival curve is shown and compared with the general population matched for age and sex in Fig. 18.3. The mortality in the paced patients is greater in the first year, but thereafter the two curves run almost parallel.

Figure 18.4 shows that the expectation of life in the 139 of these patients who were over 80 is almost exactly that of the general population. In this age group, there has been no greater mortality in the first year of pacing.

The quality of life cannot be quantified, but almost all patients are thankful and able to lead a more active life. The prime benefit for those who have had Stokes–Adams attacks is the release from fear of an attack. The relief of other symptoms is dependent on their relationship to the slow heart. Dizziness and near syncope are often partially, if not completely, relieved; increased physical energy and mental alertness can be expected, if the pulse before pacing was below 40. Relief of cardiac failure has been less dramatic; only a few of those previously dependent on diuretics have been able to do without them, although some improvement can be expected.

Size of the Pacing Problem

If the incidence of complete block and the other arrhythmias requiring pacing is similar in Britain to that in the rest of Europe and in North America, it must be anticipated that there will be a great

Harold Siddons

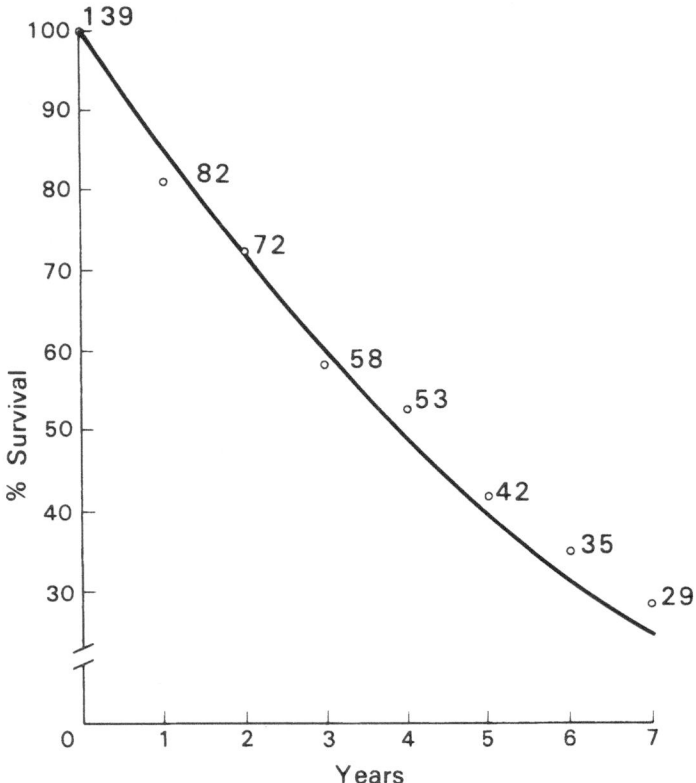

Fig. 18.4. Survival of 139 patients over 80, paced for complete heart block. The *solid line* shows the survival curve for the general population of England and Wales matched for age and sex with the 139 patients. The *circles* indicate the survival of the patients; the *figures* indicate the number at risk.

increase in the number of patients in Britain treated by pacing in future years. The number first paced in 1973 was estimated to be 22 per million of population. This is about a quarter of the number per million in Canada, France, Sweden, the U.S., and West Germany, where it has been estimated that about one person in 1,500 has a pacemaker (various authors; see Thalen 1974).

References

Furman, S., Escher, D. J. W., and Parker, B. (1973) *In* Dreifus, L. S., and Likoff, W. (eds.), *Cardiac Arrhythmias,* Grune and Stratton, New York, p. 183.

Green, G. D. (1974) *J. Electrocardiol. (San Diego)* **7**, 375.

Johansson, B. W. (1966) *Acta Med. Scand.* **180,** Suppl. 451.

Narula, O. S. (1973) *In* Samet, P. (ed.), *Cardiac Pacing,* Grune and Stratton, New York, p. 331.

Narula, O. S., Lister, J. W., Cohen, L. S., and Samet, P. (1968) *Circulation* **38,** Suppl. VI, 146.

Rosenbaum, M. B., Elizari, M. V., and Lazzari, J. O. (1970) *In: The Hemiblocks,* Tampa Tracings, Oldsmar, Florida, p. 8.

Scherlag, B. J., Laus, H., Helfant, R. H., Berkowitz, W. D., Stein, E., and Damato, A. N. (1969) *Circulation* **39,** 13.

Schoenfeld, C. D., and Bhardwaj, P. (1975) *In* Samet, P. (ed.), *Cardiac Pacing,* Grune and Stratton, New York, p. 143.

Siddons, H. (1974) *Br. Heart J.* **36,** 1201.

Siddons, H., and Nowak, K. (1975) *Br. J. Surg.* **62,** 929.

Thalen, H. M. Th. (1974) Editor, *Fourth International Symposium on Cardiac Pacing,* Van Gorcum, Netherlands, p. 143.

19

Cardiac Surgery in the Elderly

ALBERT STARR and ROBERT LAWSON

Introduction

Reports in 1948 and 1949 of series of young patients undergoing closed transatrial mitral commissurotomy (Harken et al. 1948, Bailey 1949), later modified to a transventricular approach (Logan and Turner 1959), were in time followed by documentation of successful open-heart procedures on older patients (Spencer et al. 1964, Bowles et al. 1966, Ahmad and Starr 1969). The intervening 20 years saw the development of cardiopulmonary bypass in 1954 (Gibbon 1954), the replacement of diseased aortic and mitral valves by ball-valve prostheses in 1960 (Harken et al. 1960, Starr and Edwards 1961), the use of homografts in 1962 (Ross 1962), and the beginnings of direct surgical treatment for coronary artery disease in 1964 (Effler et al. 1964). The latter has now been extended to include surgical treatment for the complications of myocardial infarction.

The performance of open-heart surgical procedures on elderly patients has been the natural sequel to earlier success with this treatment in younger patients, and requires special consideration.

ALTERT STARR and ROBERT LAWSON · Division of Cardiopulmonary Surgery, University of Oregon Medical School, 3181 S.W. Sam Jackson Park Road, Portland, Oregon 97201.

General Assessment

Evaluation of the elderly patient for cardiac surgery requires an accurate knowledge of the natural history of the patient's cardiac pathological condition, assessment of the stage of the patient's cardiac disease, a knowledge of the operative mortality and the late survival characteristics for the operation envisaged, and a thorough knowledge of any concomitant pathology present in the patient. Particular attention in this age group must be directed to cerebral, renal, peripheral vascular and pulmonary status, both preoperatively and intraoperatively. Historical or clinical evidence of cerebrovascular or peripheral vascular insufficiency may necessitate angiography. Positive results may affect arterial cannulation sites or change operation sequences; e.g., carotid stenoses may require relief prior to cardiac surgery, or combined procedures may be advisable (Bernhard et al. 1972). High intraoperative perfusion pressures may similarly be necessary in such patients to avoid cerebral or peripheral vascular damage. Patients with

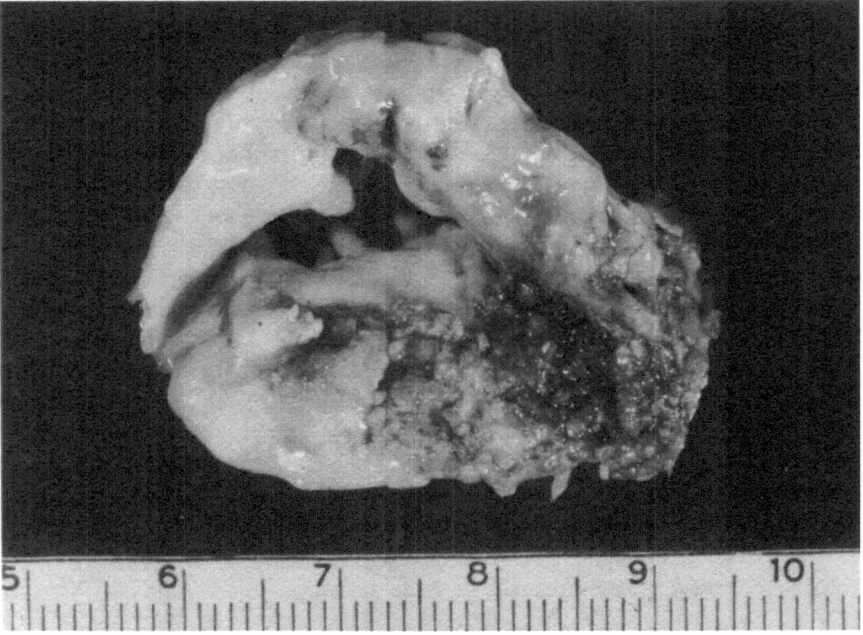

Fig. 19.1. Mitral stenosis (left atrial view). Note the thickened leaflets and chordae, restricted orifice, and exuberant calcification of anterior leaflet.

impaired renal function (serum creatinine greater than 2 mg/100 ml) will require vigorous intraoperative and postoperative diuresis and possible dialysis. Prostatic obstruction may necessitate careful preoperative bouginage and catheterization and further definitive management postoperatively. Patients with pulmonary insufficiency require preoperative assessment of remaining lung function, and may benefit from preoperative chest physiotherapy and intermittent positive-pressure breathing.

Postoperative management may include breathing exercises, intermittent positive-pressure breathing, mucolytic agents and bronchial relaxants, blood-gas monitoring, and, if necessary, tracheal or bronchoscopic suction. Avoidance of confusional and paranoid states necessitates that these patients should be returned from the impersonal and exhausting atmosphere of the intensive care unit to a friendly ward atmosphere and then to a stable home environment as soon as possible.

If a prosthesis is to be used, its durability, hemodynamic characteristics, complication rates, and functional capacity should be known (Rahimtoola 1975). Data obtained with a particular prosthetic model cannot be extrapolated to another model, and results obtained in one center where, say, obstructive and restrictive airway disease is rare will not necessarily apply where both are commonplace.

Mitral Valve Disease

Mitral Stenosis

Etiology and Pathology. A possible history of rheumatic fever is noted in about 65% of patients (Wood 1954). Rheumatic involvement of the free leaflet edges results in cusp thickening and rigidity. Commissural fusion reduces the valve orifice (Brock 1952); subsequent subvalvular chordal thickening and shortening and further commissural fusion may critically reduce the valve orifice size and cause hemodynamically significant stenosis (Fig. 19.1).

Natural History. The gradual onset of shortness of breath and effort intolerance due to elevated pulmonary venous pressures reflects the slow fibrosis occurring in the mitral valve. Significant stenosis occurs during exercise when the valve orifice is reduced to 1.5–2.5 cm^2 (normal 4.0–6.0 cm^2). This stenosis commonly occurs in the fourth decade of life (Bland and Jones 1951). Further reduction in valve orifice size to 1.0–1.5 cm^2 results in obstruction to flow at rest, with symptoms of orthopnea and paroxysmal nocturnal dyspnea. Pulmonary vascular resistance frequently increases, followed by right ventricular failure, tricuspid incompetence, congestive failure, and death. Survival depends on the stage of disease at diagnosis (Rapaport 1975). Thus, 40% of Functional Class III patients were dead at 5 years and 60% at 10 years after diagnosis (Olesen and Baden 1969), whereas only 7% had died at 10 years in a series of mainly Functional Class I patients (Wilson and Lim 1957). In a series of medically treated patients diagnosed initially at different stages of disease, 80% were alive at 5 years and 60% at 10 years (Rapaport 1975).

Mitral Regurgitation

Etiology and Pathology. Rheumatic heart disease is the most common cause of mitral incompetence, usually with associated stenosis of varying degrees. Other relatively common causes of mitral incompetence in older patients, however, are degenerative valve diseases with chordal rupture or floppy valve, papillary muscle rupture secondary to myocardial infarction, and dilatation of the mitral ring secondary to left ventricular failure. Indeed, degenerative valve disease is the most common cause of pure mitral regurgitation in the elderly.

Natural History. With acute mitral regurgitation, such as from ruptured chordae, left ventricular hypertrophy does not have time to develop; acute left ventricular distention and failure may rapidly result in pulmonary edema or circulatory failure, or both. In chronic mitral incompetence, the gradually increasing ventricular preload and the diminution in afterload produces an increase in end-diastolic volume and, through the Frank–Starling mechanism, an increase in stroke volume. The left ventricle hypertrophies, but left ventricular end-diastolic pressure does not rise because of an increase in left ventricular compliance, and thus increased pulmonary capillary hypertension and congestion do not readily occur in the early stages of the disease. Survival of medically treated patients with mitral incompetence was 80% at 5 years and 60% at 10 years (Rapaport 1975). Survival of similarly treated patients with mixed mitral stenosis and mitral incompetence was considerably poorer, with 66% surviving 5 years and 33% surviving 10 years (Rapaport 1975).

Surgical Implications

The natural history and progression of disease in patients with seriously symptomatic mitral valve disease (Functional Classes III and

IV) confirms the necessity for surgical intervention. Recent evidence indicating significant correlations between postoperative functional class and preoperative duration of symptoms and response to medical therapy (Bonchek et al. 1974) suggests that surgery should be offered earlier to moderately disabled patients responding to medical therapy. Findings at the Mayo Clinic that a large left atrium and advanced functional impairment were associated with a greater operative risk, and that increased atrial size was also associated with a higher late mortality (Barnhorst et al. 1975), add further weight to the case for earlier surgery. Because of the poor prognosis with medical therapy, urgent mitral valve replacement is usually indicated in patients sustaining acute mitral incompetence.

Operation

Mitral Stenosis. Although closed mitral valvotomy is still practiced in many centers (Hurst et al. 1974), we prefer to take advantage of the increased precision of an open technique for all mitral valve surgery. Following a median sternotomy, the patient is placed on cardiopulmonary bypass, utilizing caval cannulation for venous drainage and ascending aortic intubation for arterial return. High flow (2.4 liters/min/m^2), moderate hypothermia (32°C), and fluid prime are used. Ventricular pacing wires are stitched to the heart and used for operative fibrillation and postoperative pacing. Following aortic cross-clamping, the interatrial groove is dissected, the heart is fibrillated, and the left atrium is entered. Two or more traction sutures are then inserted into the mitral valve leaflets, and a thorough assessment of the valve is performed. If the valve is adequate for valvotomy, following suture traction, each commissure is incised to the valve ring, taking care to maintain chordae to each separated valve cusp. The chordae are then separated down to and into the papillary muscles. When commissurotomy is not feasible, the valve is excised to the tips of the papillary muscles. A prosthetic valve of suitable size is then inserted, using simple interrupted sutures of 2.0 Tevdek. Aortic cross-clamping is released at 15-min intervals to allow a 3- to 4-min period of coronary perfusion in the fibrillating heart. The valve is rendered incompetent by a Foley catheter during atrial closure. Following open mitral commissurotomy, the left ventricle is allowed to fill to check mitral valve competence. The left atrium is then partially closed with the valve tripped, all air evacuated from the left atrium and pulmonary veins, the heart defibrillated, and the left atrial closure completed on the beating heart.

Mitral Incompetence. In the presence of annular dilatation with intact chordae and pliable leaflets, we now prefer valvuloplasty techniques utilizing a ring prosthesis (Carpentier et al. 1971) to annuloplasty procedures used previously (Merendino et al. 1959). Localized rupture of posterior chordae may be treated in a manner suggested by McGoon (1960). Most incompetent and mixed mitral valve lesions, however, will require mitral valve replacement, especially in elderly patients with poor tissues for repair.

Postoperative Care

Atrial pacing for 48–72 h is employed when necessary to control heart rate, diminish atrial arrhythmias, and improve cardiac output (Friesen et al. 1968). In the presence of atrial fibrillation, ventricular pacing may be similarly used. Preoperative digitalis is continued, and anticoagulation is started on the second postoperative day for all valve cases, except postvalvotomy patients in sinus rhythm. A β-stimulator (isoprenaline, Isuprel) is commonly used in the early postoperative period, especially in the presence of pulmonary hypertension, to enhance cardiac output.

Results

Of 100 patients undergoing open mitral commissurotomy between 1960 and 1974, 9 were at least 60 years of age. No hospital deaths occurred in these older patients, and only 1 early death occurred in this series (Bonchek 1975). No deaths were noted in 7 patients over 60 undergoing closed mitral valvotomy (Oh et al. 1973). Hospital mortality rates of 18% and 20% have been noted for mitral valve replacement (prostheses and homografts) in patients over 60 and 65 years, respectively (Oh et al. 1973, Barnhorst et al. 1974). Our own experience with patients over 60 years of age undergoing prosthetic mitral valve replacement from 1961 to 1974 reveals a 16% hospital mortality, a 59% actuarially assessed 5-year survival, and a 39% 10-year survival (see Fig. 19.2). Early deaths were commonly due to myocardial infarction and low-output states, and late deaths to cardiac failure and endocarditis.

Improvements in valve prostheses have resulted in a gratifying decrease in the incidence of postoperative thromboembolism. A recent review of 363 patients (mean age 50 years, range 15–74 years) undergo-

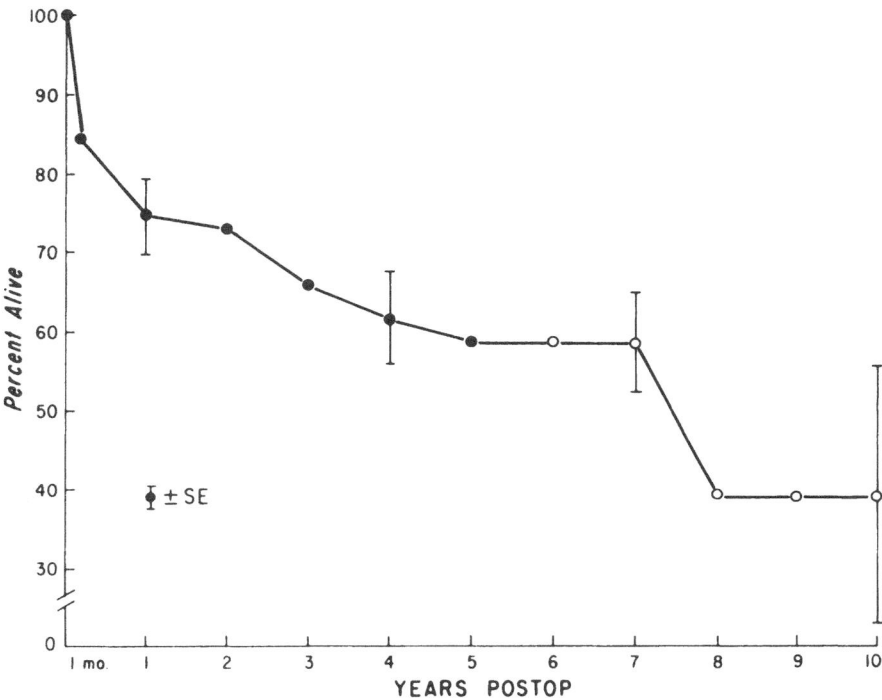

Fig. 19.2. Survival curve for 89 isolated mitral valve replacements in patients over 60 years of age at the University of Oregon Medical School. Open circles indicate fewer than 20 patients at risk.

ing mitral valve replacement at this center revealed 1.9 emboli/100 years of patient follow-up in cloth-covered prostheses (Starr-Edwards Model 6310/6320), with a mean follow-up of 2.5 years, and 6 emboli/ 100 patient-years in non–cloth-covered prostheses (Starr-Edwards Model 6120), with a mean follow-up of 6 years (Bonchek and Starr 1975). Emboli with cloth-covered valves occurred mostly in the first year, and all occurred within 3 years of insertion, whereas the threat of embolism is of greater duration with non–cloth-covered prostheses. Although no reoperation was needed at 5 years for the Model 6120 prosthesis, 4% of those with the Model 6310/6320 required it, mainly for thrombosis. Although satisfactory early results have been noted after homograft replacement of the mitral valve (Yacoub et al. 1972), comparable long-term survival and thromboembolic data for alternative ball, disc, or homograft prostheses are not yet available.

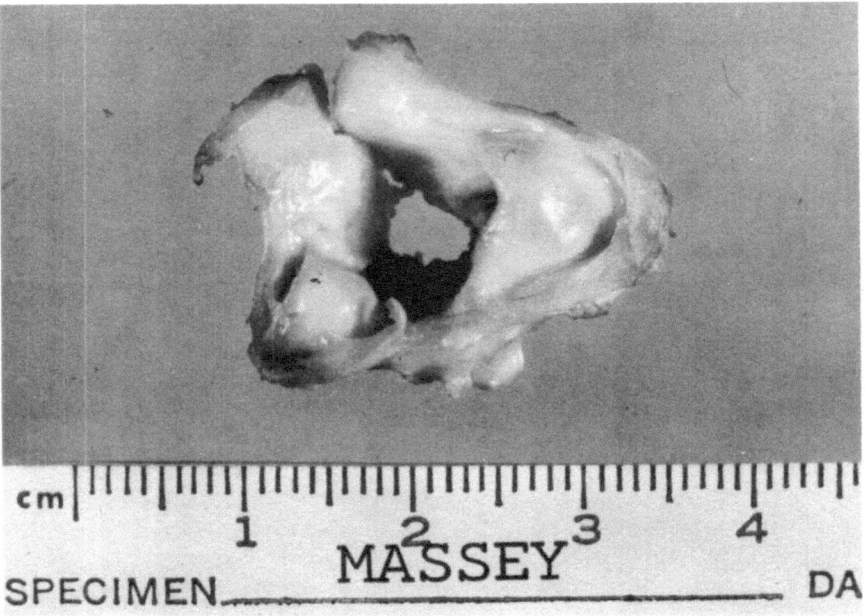

cm ‖‖‖‖|‖‖‖|‖‖‖|‖‖‖|‖‖‖|‖‖‖|‖‖‖|‖‖‖|‖‖‖|

                    1   2   3   4

SPECIMEN_____ MASSEY _____ DA

Fig. 19.3. Aortic stenosis (aortic view). Note the commissural fusion, calcification and fibrosis of cusps, and markedly reduced orifice.

Aortic Valve Disease

Aortic Stenosis

Etiology and Pathology. Stenosis of a congenital bicuspid valve is a more common obstructive cause than rheumatic disease in the elderly (Pomerance 1972). Degenerative disease is less common in patients in their early 60's, but it becomes the most common obstructive cause in extreme old age (Pomerance 1972, Roberts et al. 1971, Fig. 19.3). In a recent review of 63 patients more than 60 years of age under our care, stenosis was from a congenitally bicuspid valve in 44%, from rheumatic fever in 21%, from degenerative disease in 10%, and from an uncertain origin in 22%. Significant coronary artery disease (greater than 50% lumen reduction) was noted in 50% of patients more than 60 years and in 7 of 8 patients over 70 years of age (Lawson et al. 1976). A high incidence of coronary artery disease has also been noted in these old patients with aortic stenosis by other workers (Oh et al. 1973, Austen et al. 1970).

Natural History. Progressive aortic valve stenosis results in left ventricular hypertrophy with little increase in heart size. Increased left atrial contraction results in an adequate left ventricular end-diastolic stretch, despite a fall in left ventricular diastolic compliance. Mean left atrial and pulmonary capillary pressures eventually rise as left ventricular failure occurs. These increased pressures are transmitted back to the right heart, giving rise to right ventricular failure, the end stage of aortic stenosis. The appearance of more and older patients with aortic stenosis suggests either that the heart is better able to tolerate a pressure load for longer than previously appreciated (Campbell 1968) or that some of these valves do not become critically obstructed until later in life.

Although aortic stenosis may be tolerated for long periods without symptoms (Campbell 1968, Ross and Braunwald 1968), 80% of patients dying of aortic stenosis had symptoms for less than 4 years (Ross and Braunwald 1968). The average survival from the onset of angina, syncope, dyspnea, or congestive heart failure ranged from 3 to $1\frac{1}{2}$ years. Of 15 patients with severe aortic stenosis (aortic valve index less than 0.7 cm/m²), 36% were dead at 3 years, 52% at 5 years, and 90% at 10 years (actuarial determinations; Frank, Johnson, and Ross 1973). There was no correlation between symptomatology and survival and hemodynamic parameters in these patients. Sudden death due to probable dysrhythmia secondary to myocardial hypoxia has been noted in 7% of children with congenital aortic stenosis (Reynolds et al. 1960), and in 20% of older patients (Hurst et al. 1974).

Analysis of hemodynamic data in 63 patients more than 60 years of age with aortic stenosis confirmed that most patients were able to generate high left ventricular systolic pressures even in the face of the added afterload of systemic hypertension. Mean left ventricular systolic pressure in the 14 patients with systolic blood pressure greater than 130 mm Hg was 230 mm Hg, whereas the overall mean left ventricular systolic pressure in the whole series was 213 mm Hg. Mean pulse pressure in the same 14 patients was 83 mm Hg, whereas mean pulse pressure in the remainder was 40.4 mm Hg. There was no evidence of age-related changes in parameters of left ventricular function, i.e., left ventricular systolic pressure, left ventricular end-diastolic pressure and volume, cardiac index, and ejection fraction. Mean ejection fraction in 20 patients was within normal limits despite significant coronary artery disease in 8 of these, and mean left ventricular end diastolic volume was higher, but not significantly so, in those with coronary artery disease (122 ml/m²) than those without (96 ml/m²) (Lawson et al., 1975, 1976).

Aortic Incompetence

Etiology and Pathology. Aortic incompetence may result from aortic cusp deformity or loss of substance, secondary to rheumatic valvulitis, subacute bacterial endocarditis, trauma, or other conditions, or from dilatation of the aortic annulus secondary to cystic medial necrosis, syphilis, bacterial endocarditis, arteriosclerotic aneurysm formation, or rheumatoid disease. Dissection of the ascending aorta into the sinuses of Valsalva may also produce aortic incompetence by loosening the aortic valve cusp attachments. In 17 patients over the age of 60 years of age undergoing aortic valve replacement for aortic incompetence in our service, incompetence was caused by syphilis in 6 patients, by rheumatic fever in 4, by cystic medial necrosis in 3, by arteriosclerosis in 2, by rheumatoid disease in 1, and by dissection in 1.

Natural History. The sudden increase in volume load thrown on the left ventricle in acute aortic incompetence results in acute ventricular dilation. Compensatory left ventricular hypertrophy may not have time to develop, and increasing pulmonary capillary pressure rapidly results in pulmonary edema. A prohibitive medical mortality may necessitate emergency valve replacement. Chronic aortic incompetence may be tolerated well for many years. Gradual left ventricular hypertrophy accompanies increasing left ventricular end-diastolic volume, while increasing left ventricular compliance prevents large increases in left ventricular end-diastolic pressure. A 75% 5-year and 50% 10-year survival have been noted in patients with significant aortic incompetence treated medically (Rapaport 1975). Death frequently follows within 2 years of signs of decompensation (Massell et al. 1966). Angina, frequently occurring in the presence of cardiac failure and poor ventricular function, is a late and sinister symptom (Basta et al. 1975).

Surgical Implications

The danger of sudden death and the poor prognosis that follows development of symptoms indicate that aortic valve replacement should be advised in patients with a critical aortic orifice valve and gradients in excess of 50 mm Hg, whether symptomatic or not.

Although mild aortic incompetence may be well tolerated for years, improvements in valve design, reductions in operative mortality, evidence that depressed left ventricular function persists despite postoperative functional and hemodynamic improvement (Gault et al. 1970), and findings that operative mortality is related to preoperative functional class and late mortality to left ventricular size (Barnhorst et al. 1975) suggest the logic of earlier surgery. All symptomatic patients with aortic insufficiency should be offered surgery in the absence of a strong contraindication such as major degenerative diseases of other organ systems. While we recommend operation to selected young individuals with asymptomatic aortic insufficiency (Spagnuolo et al. 1971), this type of prophylactic surgery may not be wise in the elderly.

Operation

The operative approach, cannulation method, and perfusion technique are similar to those used for mitral valve replacement. The left ventricular apex is vented, the aorta cross-clamped, and the aortic valve inspected through a transverse aortotomy. In a few instances, incompetence is due to thickening and irregularity of the free cusp margins, which may be successfully rendered competent by shaving the cusp edge to allow cusp opposition. Commonly, calcific rigid cusps, dilated aortic roots, or fenestrated cusps will necessitate valve removal and prosthetic replacement. Adequate myocardial perfusion during aortic cross-clamping will enable the heart to take over circulation following cessation of cardiopulmonary bypass. We now utilize continuous coronary perfusion at 32°C in the beating heart, since spontaneous fibrillation in hypertrophied ventricles during bypass results in increased coronary vascular resistance, increased coronary sinus lactate production, lowered coronary sinus pH, loss of intracellular potassium ions, and depressed postbypass function (Hottenrott et al. 1973). Thorough debridement, allowing satisfactory seating and lessening the risk of perivalvular leak, precedes valve insertion. The valve itself is inserted using interrupted 3-0 Tevdek sutures. The aortic root is then closed, and, following removal of all air, cardiopulmonary bypass is terminated and the heart allowed to take over the circulation. In addition to temporary ventricular and atrial pacing wires, a permanent ventricular lead is placed in any patient who shows persistent or impending evidence of heart block at operation. This lead is buried in the subcutaneous tissues of the upper abdominal wall, and may be connected to a permanent pacemaker unit at a later date. In the rare case of aortic incompetence due to dissection, the ascending aorta is transected above the valve, the two cut ends are oversewn, thus resuspending the cusps, and the aorta is reconstituted (Hufnagel and Conrad 1962).

Postoperative Care

Attention is directed toward maintaining adequate cardiac and urinary output and blood-gas levels. Cardiac output may be improved by increasing ventricular preload, as monitored by mean left atrial pressure, to 15 mm Hg (Kouchoukos et al. 1971). Persistent low cardiac output with adequate left atrial mean filling pressures may require the inotropic effects of digitalis, or dopamine. The reduction in ventricular afterload and improved coronary diastolic filling pressure generated by the balloon pump (Kantrowitz et al. 1969) may be required in the recalcitrant case. Cardiac tamponade, which impairs diastolic filling and thus cardiac output (Isaacs et al. 1954), and which has been shown experimentally to promote subendocardial ischemia (Wechsler et al. 1974), must always be excluded both in the early postoperative phase and also in later convalescence. Therapeutic modification of classic signs of tamponade must be noted. We have recently seen that a fall in urinary output, previously considered a constant and reliable early sign of tamponade, may not occur in the presence of dopamine therapy, despite the presence of considerable tamponade. Intermittent positive-pressure breathing is needed to reduce the work of breathing and allow adequate rest and sedation in the early postoperative period. Confusion, paranoia, and dysrhythmias may signify hypoxia in older patients and necessitate a return to mechanical ventilation. Following 48 h of complete rest on the respirator, many elderly patients will go on to an uneventful recovery. Postoperative telemetry is especially valuable in older patients, as it permits a continuous central ECG display without interfering with the patient's freedom of movement in his hospital room.

Results

Hospital mortality rates varying from 3 to 33% have been recorded for aortic valve replacement with prostheses and homografts in older patients (Oh et al. 1973, Barnhorst et al. 1974, Austen et al. 1970, Ross and Braunwald 1968, Henze 1974, Guthrie et al. 1972, Angell et al. 1972). In a series of 221 patients over age 60 operated on between 1962 and 1974, a hospital mortality of 16% was recorded. Actuarially assessed 5-year survival was 58%, and 10-year survival was 41% (see

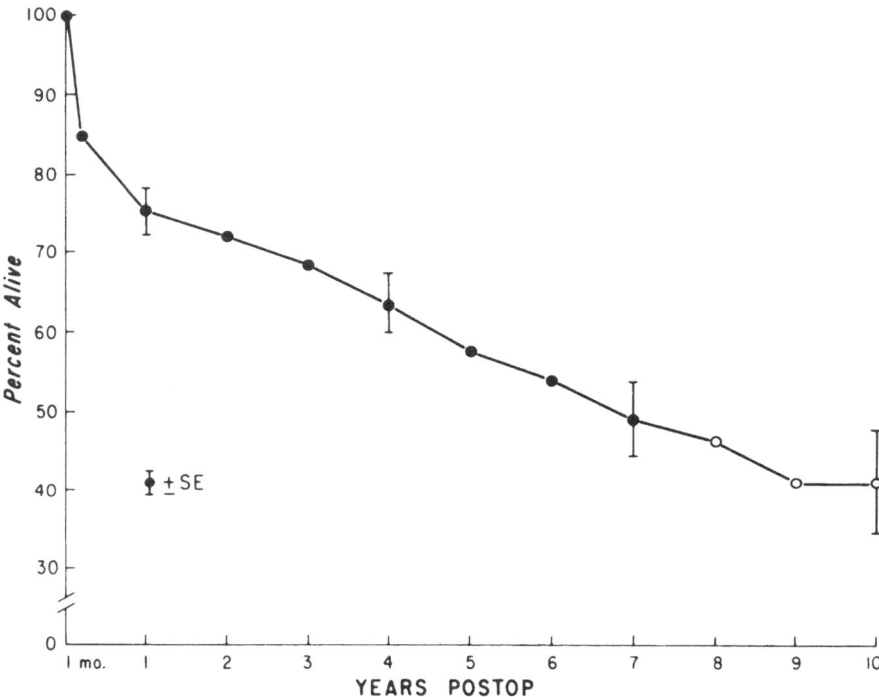

Fig. 19.4. Survival curve for 221 isolated aortic valve replacements in patients over 60 years of age at the University of Oregon Medical School. Open circles indicate fewer than 20 patients at risk.

Fig. 19.4). Some of the early deaths were due to technical problems related mainly to arteriosclerosis; many of the late deaths were due to cerebral vascular accidents or congestive heart failure.

A recent review of 549 patients (mean age 55 years, range 17–79 years) undergoing aortic valve replacement revealed a 4.2 emboli/100 patient-years of follow-up in anticoagulated non-cloth-covered valves (Starr-Edwards Model 1200/1260), with a mean follow-up of 4.3 years; 8.8 emboli/100 patient-years of follow-up on nonanticoagulated cloth-covered valves (Starr-Edwards Model 2310/2320), with a mean follow-up of 1.7 years; and no emboli in the anticoagulated cloth-covered valves, with a mean follow-up of 3.1 years. Patients whose anticoagulation was stopped, however, had 29.4 emboli/100 patient years, with a mean follow-up of 2 years. The reoperation rate at 5 years was 1% for Model 1200/1260 (infection) and 8% for Model 2310/2320 (leaks and anemia mainly secondary to cloth tears). Similar detailed long-term analyses for disc and homograft replacements are not yet available.

Multiple-Valve Disease

Rheumatic fever may damage several valves and necessitate multiple-valve surgery. Aortic or mitral disease or both may be accompanied by intrinsic tricuspid disease in 10–15% of patients (Cooke and White 1941). More commonly, tricuspid incompetence follows the right ventricular hypertension or right ventricular dilatation of long-standing mitral stenosis. Mixed valvular lesions will usually necessitate valve replacement, but pure regurgitation with normal cusps may respond to annuloplasty or insertion of a prosthetic ring (Carpentier et

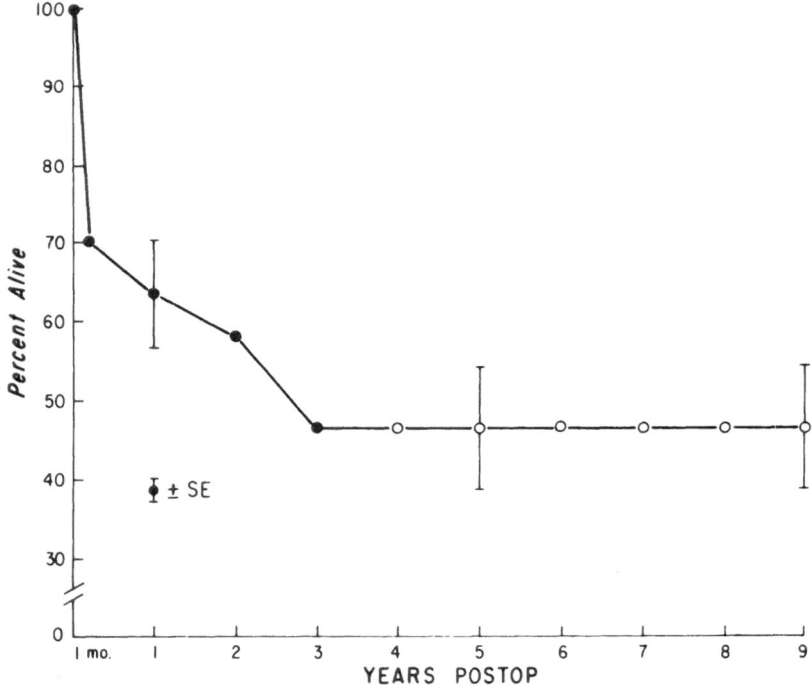

Fig. 19.5. Survival curve for 50 multiple valve replacements in patients over 60 years of age at the University of Oregon Medical School. Open circles indicate fewer than 20 patients at risk.

al. 1971). Downstream lesions will usually be made worse following relief of proximal stenosis, whereas proximal lesions may be lessened following relief of a distal stenosis.

Operation

Following institution of cardiopulmonary bypass and aortic cross-clamping, the aortic root is opened. The aortic valve is assessed, excised if necessary, and continuous coronary perfusion is commenced. The left atrium is then opened, and the mitral valve is either repaired or replaced. The left atrium is then closed, the aortic valve replaced, the aortic root closed, the left heart vented of air, and bypass discontinued. Tricuspid valve surgery, if needed, follows aortic and mitral valve surgery.

Results

We noted a 30% hospital mortality in patients over 60 years of age undergoing multiple valve surgery between 1962 and 1974. Actuarially assessed 5-year survival was 47% (see Fig. 19.5). Early deaths were due to myocardial infarction and left ventricular failure and late deaths mainly to congestive heart failure. Hospital mortalities of 42.4% (Barnhorst et al. 1975) and 60% (Oh et al. 1973) have recently been documented in patients of similar age.

Ischemic Heart Disease

Although surgery for ischemic heart disease is still in its early stages, and future follow-up data may modify current indications for surgery, certain facts are already clear. Preoperative evaluation should include graded stress-testing for patients with angina; estimation of SGOT, LDH, and CPK for baseline levels; and high-resolution three-plane coronary arteriography. Since operative risk and prognosis are closely related to left ventricular function, left ventricular cineangiography, left ventricular end-diastolic pressure, left ventricular end-diastolic volume, and ejection fraction should all be accurately ascertained prior to operation. When assessing coronary arteriograms, it must be remembered that appraisal accuracy is highest in poststenotic vessels with antegrade filling, is lower beyond occlusions with generous retrograde collateral flow, and is least in postocclusion vessels filled by insufficient collaterals (Roesch et al. 1973). Congestive cardiac failure is the single most severe risk factor, but generalized or localized hypokinesis, high left ventricular end-diastolic pressure, and cardiomegaly all increase operative risks; increasing age did not do so (Loop et al. 1975, Brown and Harrison 1974).

In discussing the role of cardiac surgery for ischemic heart disease in the elderly, we shall initially deal with angina pectoris (stable and unstable) and uncomplicated myocardial infarction, and then discuss surgery for the complications of infarction—namely, cardiogenic shock, ventricular septal defect, mitral incompetence, ventricular aneurysm, and congestive cardiac failure.

Natural History

Stable Angina Pectoris. An 80–85% 4-year survival from the onset of angina pectoris has been documented (Frank, Weinblatt, and Shapiro 1973; Kannel and Feinlieb 1972). Since angina may occur in the presence of normal coronary arteries in up to 10% of patients (Scanlon et al. 1973), a group with a normal life expectancy (Kemp et al. 1973), a more accurate survival assessment must be performed on patients with demonstrated coronary artery disease. Survival of patients with coronary artery disease has been shown to be related to the number of vessels involved (Oberman et al. 1972, Friesinger et al. 1970, Bruschke et al. 1973). In a study of 590 patients with greater than 50% diameter stenosis, a 5-year cardiac mortality of 34.4% was noted. This total was made up of 14.6% for one-vessel disease, 37.8% for two-vessel disease, 53.8% for three-vessel disease, and 56.8% for left main coronary disease. A further lesion of 30–50% stenosis in patients with single-vessel disease significantly increased the 5-year mortality rate, from 14.6% to 23.2% (Bruschke et al. 1973).

Unstable Angina Pectoris. Variations in the definition of unstable angina pectoris complicate assessment of survival data. Wood, in 1961, recorded a 22% infarction rate, of which 70% died within 3 months of their first symptoms (Wood 1961). Survival at 5 years in this series was 50%. A prospective study 10 years later documented an 82% 1-year survival, a 69% 3-year survival, and a 61% 5-year survival (Gazes et al. 1973). A high-risk subgroup with continued pain following 48 h of bedrest in a hospital had a 57% 1-year survival, a 37% 3-year survival, and a 27% 5-year survival. Infarction mortalities of 2% (Fulton et al. 1972) and 22% (Krauss et al. 1972) have also been noted at follow-up at 14 and 21 months, respectively. Coronary arteriograms, however, had not been performed in any of these series.

Myocardial Infarction. Mortality rates of 20% have been reported in patients being treated in coronary care units for myocardial infarction (Miller et al. 1972). The current consideration for early revascularization of patients with myocardial infarction is based on experimental evidence of reversal of ischemic damage around infarcts in animals (Maroko et al. 1972, McNamara et al. 1974, Cox et al. 1968). These studies suggest that revascularization should be done within 3 to 6 h of the onset of ischemia, but such findings cannot necessarily be extrapolated to human hearts with collateral development.

Operation

Cardiopulmonary bypass is instituted in the same way as for valvular surgery. Particular attention is directed, however, to maintaining mean perfusion pressures in excess of 80 mm Hg by using α-stimulators (e.g., metaraminol, Aramine) if necessary and to avoiding increased cardiac oxygen uptake caused by β-stimulators (e.g., isoprenaline). Lesions of the left main coronary artery frequently require rapid establishment of cardiopulmonary bypass, and preliminary pump priming is therefore advised for these cases (Zeft et al. 1974). After cooling to 32°C, the aorta is cross-clamped, and the heart is fibrillated and further cooled with ice-cold Ringer's solution on the pericardium. A vein graft is inserted into the significantly narrowed coronary artery (greater than 50% reduction in lumen diameter, which is equivalent to 75% reduction in a cross-sectional area of the lumen). The anastomosis is made with running 7-0 Proline sutures commencing at the heel of the anastomosis and continuing around in a counterclockwise direction. The proximal anastomosis to the ascending aorta is made over a side-biting clamp with the heart beating. Further grafts are performed as necessary, the heart being resuscitated during the construction of proximal anastomoses. Occluded or severely narrowed vessels may be manually endarterectomized. Anastomoses must be meticulous and graft length appropriate. We have used the saphenous vein as first choice, the cephalic vein when the leg vein is diseased or absent, and, rarely, the internal thoracic artery. In the presence of acute myocardial infarction, grafts are initially inserted into ischemic areas, as assessed visually or suggested by ECG (Starr 1975). Left ventricular venting is not employed unless there is associated aortic incompetence.

Postoperative Care

Postoperative care is similar to that given to other open-heart patients. Mechanical ventilation is usually maintained until the first

postoperative morning. Patients with preoperative angina are digitalized prior to surgery, and usually maintained for 2 months postoperatively. Unless contraindicated, anticoagulants are given for about 4
weeks to diminish the risk of leg vein thromboses and pulmonary
emboli. Atrial arrhythmias occur in about 20% of our patients, but
invariably respond to increased digitalis or antiarrhythmic therapy, or
both. Ventricular arrhythmias have rarely proved fatal unless associated with myocardial infarction. In a recent series of 220 patients
(mean age 55 years) undergoing coronary artery bypass surgery, we
noted a perioperative myocardial infarction rate of 5.5%; infarction
was fatal in one patient.

Results

Relief of angina is noted in approximately 90% of the patients
(Anderson, Rahimtoola, Bonchek, and Starr 1974), and symptomatic
relief and objective evidence of increased exercise capacity is significantly related to graft patency (Kassebaum et al. 1969, Lapin et al.
1973). Reports on cardiac function after coronary artery bypass surgery
are controversial; improvement (Chatterjee et al. 1972, Rees et al. 1971,
Bolooki et al. 1971), no change (Bolooki et al. 1971, Arbogast et al.
1973), and deterioration (Shepherd et al. 1974) have all been recorded.
These discrepancies probably reflect variation in degrees of coronary
artery disease and associated cardiac function, differences in restudy
intervals, and variations in surgical technique. Early postoperative
myocardial infarction has been noted in from 7 to 20% of patients
(Morris et al. 1972, Alderman et al. 1971, Brewer et al. 1973); evidence
of myocardial injury following coronary artery bypass as assessed by
enzyme studies has been noted in 80% of patients (Oldham et al.
1973). The effects on long-term cardiac function of this type of injury
are as yet uncertain. The long-term function of bypass grafts is also
still uncertain. Vein patency rates of 70–80% are generally noted at 6
months to 1 year after surgery (Anderson, Rahimtoola, Bonchek, and
Starr 1974; Effler et al. 1971; Grondin et al. 1971), and current evidence
suggests little further attrition in the first 3 postoperative years
(Lesperance et al. 1973). Patency depends on adequate run-off, with
grafts carrying less than 40 ml/min unlikely to remain patent for 2
years (Walker et al. 1972). Marked discrepancy between vein and
artery size may also result in high occlusion rates (Furuse et al. 1972).
The palliative nature of the surgery is further reflected in reports of
accelerated closure of coronary stenoses in some bypassed vessels
(Aldrich and Trimble 1971) and pathological changes in veins.

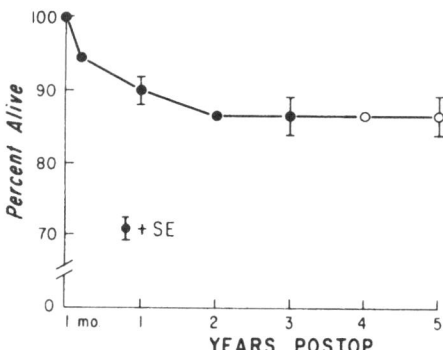

Fig. 19.6. Survival curve for 290 aorta–coronary artery–saphenous vein bypass graft procedures in patients over 60 years of age at the University of Oregon Medical School. Open circles indicate fewer than 20 patients at risk.

The effect of coronary artery bypass on the longevity of patients with chronic angina is not yet known, although there is some evidence that surgery may improve long-term survival (Anderson, Rahimtoola, Bonchek, and Starr 1974; Spencer et al. 1974).

Preliminary results of prospective studies of randomized medical vs. surgical therapy for patients with coronary insufficiency indicate no difference in mortality or incidence of myocardial infarction, but surgically treated patients had significantly higher exercise tolerance and less myocardial hypoxia (Selden et al. 1974, Conti et al. 1975). Our own experience (Bonchek et al. 1974; Lawson, Chapman, Wood, and Starr 1975) suggests that surgery is particularly safe and effective in patients with coronary insufficiency.

Further clinical trials will be necessary to determine whether early myocardial revascularization will reduce the extent of necrosis in patients with myocardial infarction. Results will have to be correlated with the elapsed time between infarction and surgery. Surgery for infarction occurring at cardiac catheterization proved highly lethal in our experience, whereas an operative mortality of 16% was recorded in 21 patients operated on within 2 h to 21 days of infarction (Starr 1975).

The results in all patients 60 years of age or over undergoing coronary artery bypass surgery for chronic angina, coronary insufficiency, and postmyocardial infarction for 1968–1974 are illustrated in Fig. 19.6. Overall operative mortality was 5%, and actuarially assessed 4-year survival was 87%. Early deaths were due mainly to myocardial infarction and late deaths to congestive heart failure.

Complications of Myocardial Infarction

Over 80% of the patients sustaining a defect following myocardial infarction died within 2 months of the infarct (Oyamada and Quenn 1961, Sanders et al. 1956) from left and right heart overload. Many of these patients had multiple perforations, coronary artery disease, and associated left ventricular aneurysms or akinetic segments, or both. Acute papillary muscle rupture has proved equally lethal, 70% of patients dying within 24 h and less than 20% living a few weeks (Sanders et al. 1957). The prognosis for congestive cardiac failure due to previous myocardial infarction or to ischemia (ischemic cardiomyopathy; Burch et al. 1970) is also extremely poor. Survival with left ventricular aneurysm is slightly better, 73% dying at 3 years and 88% at 5 years (Schlichter et al. 1954) from congestive failure, further myocardial infarction, and arterial embolization. Cardiogenic shock following myocardial infarction was almost invariably fatal prior to the use of intra-aortic balloon pump assistance, as it commonly represents a loss of at least 40% of left ventricular muscle mass (Page et al. 1971).

Surgical Implications. The poor survival recorded with conservative modes of therapy has prompted surgical treatment for the various complications of myocardial infarction. If the patient's condition permits, ventricular septal defect repair should be delayed for at least 6 weeks to allow fibrous septal healing and consequently better repair material. The high incidence of coronary artery disease and left ventricular wall motion abnormalities in these patients demands preoperative coronary arteriography and left ventricular cineangiography and concomitant surgical correction of these lesions when present. Although congestive cardiac failure is the most severe risk factor in the surgery of ischemic heart disease, the presence of concurrent angina indicating ischemic but viable myocardium has a more favorable prognosis (Mundth et al. 1971). Patients with cardiogenic shock or severe left ventricular failure after myocardial infarction can often be hemodynamically improved by intra-aortic balloon pump assistance. Acute revascularization of these patients is based on the premise that at least part of the myocardial damage may be reversed if adequate circulation can be established at an early enough stage. Additional resection of large akinetic or dyskinetic segments of infarcted myocardium may further acutely improve myocardial function (Buckley et al. 1971).

Operation. The patient is placed on cardiopulmonary bypass as previously described. A left ventriculotomy allows easy visualization and repair of the postinfarction ventricular septal defect and removal of a left ventricular aneurysm when present. Small ventricular septal defects may be sutured over Teflon felt; larger defects require a Dacron patch. Left ventricular aneurysms are excised to leave a rim of scar tissue, which is then closed over a Teflon bolster. Elective fibrillation and aortic cross-clamping may be used to prevent dislodgement of mural thrombi during manipulation of the aneurysm. In the rare case with concomitant mitral regurgitation, the mitral valve may be repaired or replaced through the same left ventriculotomy. Coronary artery bypass grafts, when necessary, are usually inserted more easily after removal of an aneurysm. Obtuse marginal grafts are placed prior to mitral valve replacement. Solitary mitral valve replacement is done in the manner noted earlier. Intra-aortic balloon pump assistance may be used pre-, intra-, or postoperatively in these ill patients to improve cardiac performance and survival.

Results. The results of surgery for complications of myocardial infarction are better when limited amounts of ventricular muscle damage has occurred. Thus, patients with extensive left ventricular damage will usually present early in the postinfarction stage and have a very high operative risk. A survival rate of 80% has been recorded following early (4–10 days) closure of a ventricular septal defect and resection of an infarct, whereas all patients undergoing closure of a ventricular septal defect after 3–6 months survived (Buckley et al. 1971). A 58% 2-month and 32% 12-month postoperative survival were noted in a series of 65 patients undergoing postinfarction ventricular septal defect repair (Kitamura et al. 1971).

Operative mortalities of 50% after early replacement and 17% after later replacement were noted following mitral valve replacement for mitral valve dysfunction or papillary muscle rupture (Buckley et al. 1971) in a group of 22 patients. We also recorded a 46% operative mortality in 13 patients undergoing mitral valve replacement for mitral dysfunction and coronary artery disease (Anderson, Bonchek, Wood, Chapman, and Starr 1974).

A 9.8% overall operative mortality was noted in 400 patients undergoing left ventricular aneurysm excision with or without coronary artery bypass (Loop et al. 1973). These workers emphasize the fall in their operative mortality that has occurred with the introduction of concomitant vein graft bypasses, which are now performed in 70% of their operations for left ventricular aneurysms. An 8.4% operative mortality was noted in 226 of the patients undergoing excision of a left ventricular aneurysm only. Long-term follow-up revealed a 76% 4-year survival. Follow-up at 29 months revealed that 91% of patients with congestive failure secondary to aneurysms due to left anterior descending artery occlusion, and a similar number of patients with angina only, were improved.

Of patients with a previous aneurysm and multiple coronary artery disease, 74% were also improved, and of patients operated on for pure arrhythmia, 77% had no further symptoms. No late emboli occurred in patients whose aneurysms were excised because of previous embolization.

Results of revascularization with or without infarctectomy for congestive cardiac failure are related to the severity of the failure. A 25% operative mortality with a further 12% mortality at 1 year and little or no improvement in left ventricular function was noted in patients with intractable failure (Spencer et al. 1971). An operative mortality of 15%, however, was noted in patients with lesser degrees of failure, and 62% of them had improvement in left ventricular function (Mundth et al. 1971). In another series, only one operative death occurred in 17 patients with ejection fractions of less than 40% following resection and vein graft insertion. Improvement in left ventricular function occurred postoperatively, but did not return to normal in any case (Lefemine et al. 1974). Survival from cardiogenic shock has been improved by the early use of intra-aortic balloon pumping (Buckley et al. 1971), early angiography, and revascularization with or without infarctectomy in specialized centers (Buckley et al. 1971, O'Rourke et al. 1975).

Congenital Lesions

Primary operations for correction of congenital heart defects in patients over 60 years of age are quite rare. In a review of cases for the first 10 years of congenital heart surgery (1954–1964), there were 2,353 cases under 35 years of age and only 167 over 35 (Cooley et al. 1966). Of those over 35, only a very few (but unspecified number) were over 60. More recently, of 303 such congenital procedures in adults (over 21 years of age), only 24 were over 50 years old (Gerbode et al. 1969). Thus, few congenital heart lesions are compatible with old-age survival without surgical treatment.

The most common congenital heart defect that permits long-term survival is ostium secondum atrial septal defect (Cooley et al. 1966, Cohn and Kelly 1969, Ellis et al. 1960). Uncomplicated, this lesion permits survival to even the ninth or tenth decade; however, practically all who survive to age 60 are symptomatic (Perloff and Lindgren 1974). Of more than 300 patients treated for this defect, only 5 were

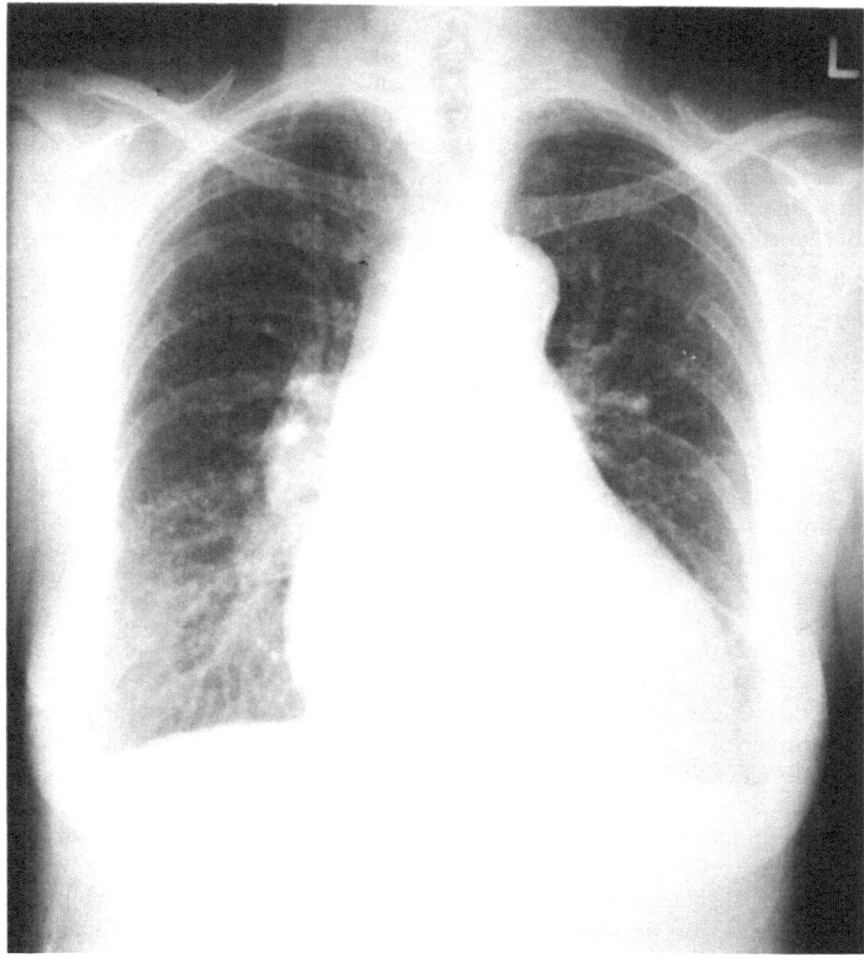

Fig. 19.7. Preoperative chest X ray of 64-year-old female with patent ductus arteriosus. Note the enlarged heart with left ventricular hypertrophy, prominent main pulmonary artery with enlarged right and left pulmonary artery branches, and pulmonary overcirculation.

more than 65 years old; all were performed successfully, and all 5 were improved symptomatically (Ellis et al. 1960).

The other types of congenital defects for which survival to age 60 is possible are, roughly in order of decreasing frequency, bicuspid aortic valve, coarctation of the aorta, valvular pulmonary stenosis, patent ductus arteriosus (Fig. 19.7), and ventricular septal defect (Perloff and Lindgren 1974). These defects are quite rare in the aged population, however, and should become even more infrequent in the future, with the trend toward earlier total correction. We have corrected all of these lesions in the elderly in the presence of significant functional impairment. With ductus, we prefer ligation to division in this age group. With coarctation, a bypass graft from ascending to descending aorta may be safer than resection and end-to-end anastomosis.

Conclusion

The severe and progressive functional deterioration that marks the later stages of valvular heart disease should be avoided in older patients, as in younger, by timely surgical intervention. There is increasing evidence that earlier intervention will improve operative and late prognosis. Coronary artery bypass surgery has thus far frequently proved symptomatically successful, and appears to significantly improve exercise tolerance in surgically treated patients. Improvement in longevity after coronary artery bypass has yet to be proved. The indications for surgery for acute myocardial infarction are still uncertain, although there is considerable experimental and accruing clinical evidence of the value of early revascularization in selected cases. The generally poor prognosis with nonsurgical management of the complications of infarction has stimulated an aggressive surgical approach to these problems. Severe ventricular damage usually results in the rapid onset of symptoms; accordingly, operative mortality is high. Operative mortality for surgery carried out later in the postinfarction stage continues to improve, however, with an increasing awareness of the importance of attempting full correction of all lesions. The use of intra-aortic balloon pumping appears to have salvaged a few patients who would otherwise certainly have died.

The preservation of good ventricular function that we and others have noted in many old patients, the overall cardiac surgical mortality and survival characteristics, and the frequently poor natural history of the particular disease process—all indicate that age alone should not be considered a contraindication to surgical treatment. However, common sense and sound surgical judgment are essential ingredients in the management of heart disease in the elderly.

References

Ahmad, A., and Starr, A. (1969) *N. Engl. J. Med.* **239,** 801.

Alderman, E. L., Enright, L. P., Cohn, L. H., Isaeff, D. M., Shumway, N. E., and Harrison, D. C. (1971) *Circulation* **44,** Suppl. 11, 134.

Aldrich, H. E., and Trimble, A. S. (1971) *J. Thorac. Cardiovasc. Surg.* **62,** 7.

Anderson, R. P., Bonchek, L. I., Wood, J., Chapman, R., and Starr, A. (1974) *Am. J. Surg.* **128,** 282.

Anderson, R. P., Rahimtoola, S. H., Bonchek, L. I., and Starr, A. (1974) *Circulation* **50,** 274.

Angell, W. W., Shumway, N. E., and Kosek, J. C. (1972) *J. Thorac. Cardiovasc. Surg.* **64,** 329.

Arbogast, R., Solignac, A., and Bourassa, M. G. (1973) *Am. J. Med.* **54,** 290.

Austen, W. G., de Sanctis, R. W., Buckley, M. J., Mundth, E. D., and Scannel, J. G. (1970) *J. Am. Med. Assoc.* **211,** 624.

Bailey, C. P. (1949) *Dis. Chest* **15,** 377.

Barnhorst, D. A., Giuliani, E. R., Pluth, J. R., Danielson, G. K., Wallace, R. B., and McGoon, D. C. (1974) *Ann. Thorac. Surg.* **18,** 81.

Barnhorst, D. A., Oxman, H. A., Connolly, D. C., Pluth, J. R., Danielson, G. K., Wallace, R. B., and McGoon, D. C. (1975) *Am. J. Cardiol.* **35,** 228.

Basta, L. L., Raines, D., Najjar, S., and Kioschos, J. M. (1975) *Br. Heart J.* **37,** 150.

Bernhard, V. M., Johnson, W. D., and Peterson, J. J. (1972) *Arch. Surg.* **105,** 837.

Bland, E. F., and Jones, T. P. (1951) *Circulation* **4,** 836.

Bolooki, H., Rubinson, R. M., Michie, D. D., and Jude, J. R. (1971) *J. Thorac. Cardiovasc. Surg.* **62,** 543.

Bonchek, L. I. (1975) *In: Results of Valvular Commissurotomy,* presented at ACC Symposium, Progress in Coronary Artery and Valvular Heart Diseases, Portland, Oregon.

Bonchek, L. I., Anderson, R. P., and Starr, A. (1974) *J. Thorac. Cardiovasc. Surg.* **67,** 93.

Bonchek, L. I., Rahimtoola, S. H., Anderson, R. P., McAnulty, J. A., Rösch, J., Bristow, J. B., and Starr, A. (1974) *Circulation* **50,** 972.

Bonchek, L. I., and Starr, A. (1975) *Am. J. Cardiol.* **35,** 843.

Bowles, L. T., Hallman, G. L., and Cooley, D. A. (1966) *Circulation* **33,** 540.

Brewer, D. L., Bilbro, R. H., and Bartel, A. G. (1973) *Circulation* **47,** 58.

Brock, R. (1952) *Br. Heart J.* **14,** 489.

Brown, B., and Harrison, D. C. (1974) *Circulation* **49,** 77.

Bruschke, A. V. G., Proudfit, W. L., and Sones, F. M. (1973) *Circulation* **47,** 1147.

Buckley, M. J., Mundth, E. D., Daggett, W. M., de Sanctis, R. W., Sanders, C. A., and Austen, W. G. (1971) *Surgery* **70,** 814.

Burch, G. E., Giles, T. D., and Colcolough, H. L. (1970) *Am. Heart J.* **79,** 291.

Campbell, M. (1968) *Br. Heart J.* **30,** 514.

Carpentier, A., Deloche, A., Dauptain, J., Soyer, R., Blondeau, P., Piwnica, A., and Dubost, C. (1971) *J. Thorac. Cardiovasc. Surg.* **61,** 1.

Chatterjee, K., Swan, H. J. C., Parmley, W. W., Sustaita, H., Marcus, H., and Matolott, J. (1972) *N. Engl. J. Med.* **286,** 1117.

Cohn, K. E., and Kelly, J. J. (1969) *Postgrad. Med.* **46,** 103.

Conti, C. R., Gilbert, J. B., Hodges, M., Hutter, A. M., Jr., Kaplan, E. M., Newell, J. B., Resnekou, L., Rosati, R. A., Ross, R. S., Russell, R. O., Jr., Schroeder, J. S., and Wolk, M. (1975) *Am. J. Cardiol.* **35,** 129.

Cooke, W. T., and White, P. D. (1941) *Br. Heart J.* **3,** 147.

Cooley, D. A., Hallman, G. L., and Hammam, A. S. (1966) *Am. J. Cardiol.* **17,** 303.

Cox, J. L., McLoughlin, V. W., Flowers, N. C., and Horan, G. (1968) *Am. Heart J.* **76,** 650.

Effler, D. B., Favaloro, R. G., Groves, L. K., and Loop, F. D. (1971) *J. Thorac. Cardiovasc. Surg.* **62,** 503.

Effler, D. B., Groves, L. K., Sones, F. M., Jr., and Shirey, E. K. (1964) *J. Thorac. Cardiovasc. Surg.* **47,** 98.

Ellis, F. H., Brandenburg, R. O., and Swan, H. J. C. (1960) *N. Engl. J. Med.* **262,** 219.

Frank, C. W., Weinblatt, E., and Shapiro, S. (1973) *Circulation* **47,** 509.

Frank, S., Johnson, A., and Ross, Jr. (1973) *Br. Heart J.* **35,** 41.

Friesen, W. G., Woodson, R. D., Ames, A. W., Herr, R. H., Starr, A., and Kassebaum, D. G. (1968) *J. Thorac. Cardiovasc. Surg.* **55,** 271.

Friesinger, G. C., Page, E. E., and Ross, R. S. (1970) *Trans. Assoc. Am. Physicians* **83,** 78.

Fulton, M., Lutz, W., Donald, K. W., Kirby, B. J., Duncan, B., Morrison, S. L., Kerr, F., Julian, D. B., and Oliver, M. F. (1972) *Lancet* **1,** 860.

Furuse, A., Klopp, E. H., Brawley, R. K., and Gott, V. L. (1972) *Ann. Thorac. Surg.* **14,** 282.

Gault, J. H., Covell, J. W., Braunwald, E., and Ross, J., Jr. (1970) *Circulation* **42,** 773.

Gazes, P. C., Mobley, E. M., Jr., Faris, H. M., Jr., Duncan, R. C., and Humphries, G. B. (1973) *Circulation* **48,** 331.

Gerbode, F., Sanchez, P. A., and Jessen, C. (1969) *J. Thorac. Cardiovasc. Surg.* **3,** 81.

Gibbon, J. H., Jr. (1954) *Minn. Med.* **37,** 171.

Grondin, C. M., Meere, C., Castonguay, Y. R., Lepage, G., and Grondin, P. (1971) *Ann. Thorac. Surg.* **12,** 574.

Guthrie, R. B., Spellberg, R. D., Benedict, J. S., and Buhl, T. L. (1972) *Arch. Surg.* **105,** 42.

Harken, D. E., Ellis, L. B., Ware, P., and Norman, L. R. (1948) *N. Engl. J. Med.* **239,** 801.

Harken, D. E., Soroff, H. S., Taylor, W. J., Lefemine, A. A., Gupta, S. K., and Lunzer, S. (1960) *J. Thorac. Cardiovasc. Surg.* **40,** 744.

Henze, A. (1974) *Scand. J. Thorac. Cardiovasc. Surg.* **8,** 1.

Hottenrott, C. E., Towers, B., Krukji, H. J., Maloney, J. V., and Buckberg, G., (1973) *J. Thorac. Cardiovasc. Surg.* **66,** 742.

Hufnagel, C. A., and Conrad, P. W. (1962) *Surgery* **51,** 84.

Hurst, J. W., Logue, R. B., Schlant, R. C., and Wenger, N. K. (1974) *In: The Heart, Arteries and Veins,* 3rd edition, McGraw Hill Book Company, New York, Ch. 46.

Isaacs, J. P., Berglund, E., and Sarnoff, S. J. (1954) *Am. Heart J.* **48,** 66.

Kannel, W. B., and Feinlieb, M. (1972) *Am. J. Cardiol.* **29,** 154.

Kantrowitz, A., Krakauer, J. S., Rosenbaum, A., Butner, A. N., Freed, P. S., and Jaron, D. (1969) *Arch. Surg.* **99,** 739.

Kassebaum, D. G., Judkins, M. P., and Griswold, H. E. (1969) *Circulation* **40,** 297.

Kemp, H. G., Jr., Vokonas, P. S., Cohn, P. F., and Gorlin, R. (1973) *Am. J. Med.* **54,** 735.

Kitamura, S., Mendez, A., and Kay, J. H. (1971) *J. Thorac. Cardiovasc. Surg.* **61,** 186.

Kouchoukos, N. T., Kirklin, J. W., Shepherd, L. C., and Roe, P. A. (1971) *Surg. Forum* **22,** 126.

Krauss, K. R., Hutter, A. M., Jr., and de Sanctis, R. W. (1972) *Circulation* **45,** Suppl. 1, 66.

Lapin, E. S., Murray, J. A., Bruce, R. A., and Winterscheid, L. (1973) *Circulation* **47,** 1164.

Lawson, R. M., Chapman, R., Wood, J., and Starr, A. (1975) *Br. Heart J.* **37**, 1053.

Lawson, R. M., Murphy, E., Griswold, H. E., Starr, A., and Rahimtoola, S. H. (1976) *In: Associated Coronary Disease State of Left Ventricular Function and Long Term Results of Surgery* (in preparation).

Lefemine, A. A., Moon, H. S., Flessas, A., Ryan, T. J., and Ramaswamy, K. (1974) *Ann. Thorac. Surg.* **17**, 1.

Lesperance, J., Bourassa, M. G., Saltiel, J., Campeau, L., and Grondin, C. M. (1973) *Circulation* **48**, 633.

Logan, A., and Turner, R. (1959) *Lancet* **2**, 874.

Loop, F. D., Berrettoni, J. N., Pichard, A., Segel, W., Razavi, M., and Effler, D. B. (1975) *J. Thorac. Cardiovasc. Surg.* **69**, 40.

Loop, F. D., Effler, D. B., Navia, J. A., Sheldon, W. C., and Groves, L. K. (1973) *Ann. Surg.* **178**, 399.

Maroko, P. R., Ginks, W. R., Libby, P., Sobel, B. E., Shell, W. E., and Ross, J., Jr. (1972) *Am. J. Cardiol.* **29**, 278.

Massell, B. F., Amezcua, F. J., and Czoniczer, G. (1966) *Circulation* **34**, Suppl. III, 164.

McGoon, D. C. (1960) *J. Thorac. Cardiovasc. Surg.* **39**, 357.

McNamara, J. J., Smith, G. T., Suehiro, G. T., Soeter, J. R., Anema, R. J., Morgan, A. L., Jr., and Liao, S. K. (1974) *J. Thorac. Cardiovasc. Surg.* **68**, 248.

Merendino, K. A., Thomas, G. I., Jesseph, J. E., Herron, P. W., Winterscheid, L. C., and Vetto, R. R. (1959) *Ann. Surg.* **150**, 5.

Miller, D. C., Cannom, D. S., Fogarty, T. J., and Schroeder, J. S. (1972) *Circulation* **47**, 234.

Morris, G. C., Jr., Reul, G. J., Howell, J. F., Crawford, E. S., Chapman, D. W., Beazley, H. L., Winters, W. L., Peterson, P. K., and Lewis, J. M. (1972) *Am. J. Cardiol.* **29**, 180.

Mundth, E. D., Harthorne, J. W., Buckley, M. J., Dinsmore, R., and Austen, W. G. (1971) *Arch. Surg.* **103**, 529.

Oberman, A., Jones, W. B., Riley, C. P., Reeves, T. J., Sheffield, L. T., and Turner, M. E. (1972) *Bull. N.Y. Acad. Med.* **48**, 1109.

Oh, W., Hickman, R., Emmanuel, R., McDonald, L., Sommerville, J., Ross, D., Ross, K., and Gonzalez-Lavin, L. (1973) *Br. Heart J.* **35**, 174.

Oldham, H. N., Jr., Roe, C. R., Young, W. G., Jr., and Dixon, S. H., Jr. (1973) *Surgery* **74**, 917.

Olesen, K. H., and Baden, H. (1969) *Scand. J. Thorac. Cardiovasc. Surg.* **3**, 119.

O'Rourke, M. F., Chang, Y. P., Windsor, H. M., Shanahan, M. X., Hickie, J. B., Morgan, J. J., Gunning, J. F., Seldon, A. W., Hall, G. V., Michell, G., Goldfarb, D., and Harrison, D. G. (1975) *Br. Heart J.* **37**, 169.

Oyamada, A., and Quenn, F. B. (1961) Presented at the Panpacific Pathology Congress.

Page, D. L., Caulfield, J. B., Kastor, J. A., de Sanctis, R. W., and Sanders, C. A. (1971) *N.. Engl. J. Med.* **285**, 133.

Perloff, J. K., and Lindgren, K. M. (1974) *Geriatrics* **29**, 94.

Pomerance, A. (1972) *Br. Heart J.* **34**, 569.

Rahimtoola, S. H. (1975) *Am. J. Cardiol.* **35**, 711.

Rapaport, E. (1975) *Am. J. Cardiol.* **35**, 221.

Rees, G., Bristow, J. D., Kremkau, E. L., Green, G. S., Herr, R. H., Griswold, H. E., and Starr, A. (1971) *N. Engl. J. Med.* **284**, 1116.

Reynolds, J. L., Nadas, A. S., Rudolph, A. M., and Gross, R. E. (1960) *N. Engl. J. Med.* **262**, 276.

Roberts, W. C., Perloff, J. K., and Costantino, T. (1971) *Am. J. Cardiol.* **27,** 497.

Roesch, J., Dotter, C. T., Antonovic, R., Bonchek, L. I., and Starr, A. (1973) *Circulation* **48,** 202.

Ross, D. N. (1962) *Lancet* **2,** 487.

Ross, J., Jr., and Braunwald, E. (1968) *Circulation* **38,** Suppl. V, 61.

Sanders, R. J., Kern, W. H., and Blount, S. G., Jr. (1956) *Am. Heart J.* **51,** 736.

Sanders, R. J., Neuberger, K. T., and Ravin, A. (1957) *Dis. Chest* **31,** 316.

Scanlon, P. J., Nemickas, R., Moran, J. F., Talano, J. V., Amirparviz, F., and Pifarre, R. (1973) *Circulation* **47,** 19.

Schlichter, J., Hellerstein, H. K., and Katz, L. N. (1954) *Medicine* **33,** 43.

Selden, R., Anderson, R. P., Titzmann, L. W., and Neill, W. A. (1974) *Circulation* **50,** Suppl. III, 34.

Shepherd, R. L., Itscoitz, S. B., Glancy, D. L., Stinson, E. B., Reis, R. L., Olinger, G. N., Clark, C. E., and Epstein, S. E. (1974) *Circulation* **49,** 467.

Spagnuolo, M., Kloth, H., Taranta, A., Doyle, E., and Pasternack, B. (1971) *Circulation* **44,** 368.

Spencer, F. C., Green, G. E., Tice, D. A., Wallsh, E., Mills, N. L., and Glassman, E. (1971) *J. Thorac. Cardiovasc. Surg.* **62,** 529.

Spencer, F. C., Isom, O. W., Glassman, E., Boyd, A. D., Engelman, R. M., Reed, G. E., Pasternack, B. S., and Dembrow, J. M. (1974) *Ann. Surg.* **180,** 439.

Spencer, F. C., Trinkle, J. K., Eiseman, B., Reeves, J. T., and Surawicz, B. (1964) *J. Am. Med. Assoc.* **189,** 103.

Starr, A. (1975) *Early Experience with Surgery for Acute Myocardial Infarction* (submitted for publication).

Starr, A., and Edwards, M. L. (1961) *Ann. Surg.* **154,** 726.

Walker, J. A., Friedberg, H. D., Flemma, R. J., and Johnson, W. D. (1972) *Circulation* **45,** Suppl. 1, 86.

Wechsler, A. S., Auerbach, B. J., Graham, T. C., and Sabiston, D. C. (1974) *J. Thorac. Cardiovasc. Surg.* **68,** 847.

Wilson, M. G., and Lim, W. N. (1957) *Circulation* **16,** 700.

Wood, P. (1954) *Br. Med. J.* **1,** 1051.

Wood, P. (1961) *Br. Med. J.* **1,** 1779.

Yacoub, M., Towers, M., and Somerville, W. (1972) *Circulation* **45,** Suppl. I, 44.

Zeft, B. J., Manley, J. C., Huston, J. H., Tector, A. J., Auer, J. E., and Johnson, W. D. (1974) *Circulation* **49,** 68.

Glossary of Drug Names

British Approved Name	U.S. Adopted Name	British Trade Name	U.S. Trade Name
adrenaline	epinephrine	———	Adrenalin
amiloride	amiloride	Midamor	Colectril
aminophylline	aminophylline	Theodrox, Aminodur	Lixaminol
amiphenazole		Daptazole	
amoxycillin	amoxicillin	Amoxil	Amoxil, Larocin
ampicillin	ampicillin	Penbritin	Penbritin, etc.
bendrofluazide	bendroflumethiazide	Aprinox, Neonaclex, etc.	Benuron, Naturetin
bumetanide	bumetanide	Burinex	
carbimazole	carbimazole	Neomercazole	Methimazole
chlormethiazole	clomethiazole edisylate	Heminevrin	
chlorthalidone	chlorthalidone	Hygroton	Hygroton
chlorothiazide	chlorothiazide	Saluric	Diuril
choline theophyllinate	oxtriphylline	Choledyl	Choledyl
clofibrate	clofibrate	Atromid-S	Atromid-S
clonidine	clonidine	Catapres	Catapres, Combipres
clopamide	clopamide	Brinaldix	
cloxacillin	cloxacillin	Orbenin	Tegopen
cyclopenthiazide	cyclopenthiazide	Navidrex	
debrisoquine	debrisoquine	Declinax	
	deslanoside	———	Cedilanid-D
diazepam	diazepam	Valium	Valium
diazoxide	diazoxide	Eudemine	Hyperstat
digitoxin	digitoxin	Digitaline	Crystodigin, Digitaline
		Nativelle	Nativelle, Purodigin
digoxin	digoxin	Lanoxin	Lanoxin
edrophonium	edrophonium	Tensilon	Tensilon
ethacrynic acid	ethacrynic acid	Edecrin	Edecrin
frusemide	furosemide	Lasix	Lasix
———	gitalin		Gitaligin

glyceryl trinitrate	nitroglycerin	Trinitrin	Nitrol
guanethidine	guanethidine	Ismelin	Ismelin
hydrallazine	hydralazine	Apresoline	Apresoline
hydrochlorothiazide	hydrochlorothiazide	Esidrex	Hydrodiuril, Oretin
hydroflumethiazide	hydroflumethiazide	Naclex	Diucardin, Saluron
isoprenaline	isoproterenol	Saventrine	Isuprel
lanatoside-C	lanatoside-C	Cedilanid	Cedilanid
levodopa	L-dopa	Larodopa, Brocadopa,	Levodopa, Bendopa,
		Sinemet, Madopar	Dopar, Larodopa
lignocaine	lidocaine	Xylocaine	Xylocaine
mefruside	mefruside	Baycaron	
metaraminol	metaraminol	Aramine	Aramine
methyldopa	methyldopa	Aldomet	Aldomet
minoxidil	minoxidil		
nikethamide	nikethamide	Coramine	Coramine
ouabain	ouabain	Ouabaine	Ouabain
oxprenolol	oxprenolol	Trasicor	
phenylbutazone	phenylbutazone	Butazolidin	Butazolidin
phenylephrine	phenylephrine	Neosynephrine	Neosynephrine
phenytoin	phenytoin	Epanutin	Dilantin
pindolol		Visken	
practolol	practolol	Eraldin	
procainamide	procainamide	Pronestyl	Pronestyl
propanolol	propanolol	Inderal	Inderal
proxyphylline		Thean	
quinidine	quinidine		Quinidine Sulfate
reserpine	reserpine	Serpasil	Serpasil, etc.
salbutamol	salbutamol	Ventolin	Ventolin
spironolactone	spironolactone	Aldactone	Aldactone
thioridazine	thioridazine	Melleril	Mellaril
triamterene	triamterene	Dytac	Dyrenium
warfarin	warfarin	Marevan	Coumadin, etc.

Index